CORE CURRICULUM FOR
PROFESSIONAL EDUCATION IN PAIN

Mission Statement of IASP Press®

The International Association for the Study of Pain (IASP) is a nonprofit, interdisciplinary organization devoted to understanding the mechanisms of pain and improving the care of patients with pain through research, education, and communication. The organization includes scientists and health care professionals dedicated to these goals. The IASP sponsors scientific meetings and publishes newsletters, technical bulletins, the journal *Pain,* and books.

The goal of IASP Press is to provide the IASP membership with timely, high-quality, attractive, low-cost publications relevant to the problem of pain. These publications are also intended to appeal to a wider audience of scientists and clinicians interested in the problem of pain.

CORE CURRICULUM FOR PROFESSIONAL EDUCATION IN PAIN

Editor

J. Edmond Charlton, MBBS, FRCA

**Committee on Education
of the International Association for the Study of Pain**

J. Edmond Charlton, MBBS, FRCA, United Kingdom, *Chair*
Pedro F. Bejarano, MD, Spain
Michael J. Bond, MD, PhD, DSc, DUniv, FRCS, FRCPsych,
FRCP, FRCA, FRSE, FRSA, United Kingdom, *ex officio*
Stephen H. Butler, MD, Sweden
Geoffrey Gourlay, PhD, BPharm, Australia
Dilip Kapur, MB ChB, United Kingdom
Patricia A. McGrath, PhD, Canada
Barry J. Sessle, MDS, PhD, Canada
Olaitan A. Soyannwo, MMed, DA, FWACS, Nigeria
Masaya Tohyama, MD, PhD, Japan
Dennis C. Turk, PhD, USA
Paul J. Watson, MSc, MCSP, United Kingdom
C. Peter N. Watson, MD, FRCP, Canada
Harriet M. Wittink, PhD, PT, USA

IASP PRESS • SEATTLE

Library of Congress Cataloging-in-Publication Data

Available from the publisher.

Published by:

IASP Press
International Association for the Study of Pain
909 NE 43rd St., Suite 306
Seattle, WA 98105-6020, USA
Fax: 206-547-1703
www.iasp-pain.org
www.painbooks.org

Contents

Part IV. Clinical States

Contributing Authors

Anna Maria Aloisi, MD
Instituto di Fisiologia Umana
Universito degli Studi di Siena
Via Aldo Moro
53100 Siena
Italy

Ralf Baron, MD
Klinik für Neurologie
CAU-Kiel
Niemannsweg 147
24105 Kiel
Germany

Rae F. Bell, BA, MD
Department of Anaesthesia and
  Intensive Care
Haukeland University Hospital
5021 Bergen
Norway

Richard E. Berger, MD
Department of Urology
Health Sciences Building
University of Washington
Box 356510
1959 NE Pacific
Seattle, WA 98195
USA

Nikolai Bogduk, MD, PhD
Newcastle Bone and Joint Institute
David Madison Building
Royal Newcastle Hospital
Newcastle, NSW 2300
Australia

Lynn M. Breau, PhD
Pediatric Pain Management Program
University of Dalhousie and IWK
  Health Centre
Halifax, NS B3H 4H7
Canada

Brenda Bursch, PhD
Neuropsychiatric Pain Service
UCLA Westwood Plaza
Los Angeles, CA 90024
USA

M. Catherine Bushnell, PhD
Center for Research on Pain
Room M-19 Strathcona A&D Building
McGill University
3640 University Street
Montreal, PQ H3A 2B2
Canada

Michael J. Butler, MB ChB, DOb(NZ),
  FRCP, FRACP, FFPMANZCA
Rheumatology Department Building 7
Private Bag 92024
1 Auckland
New Zealand

Stephen H. Butler, MD
Department of Anesthesia and
  Intensive Care
University Hospital
75185 Uppsala
Sweden

J. Edmond Charlton, MBBS,
  DObstRCOG, FRCA
1 The Wynding
Bamburgh
Northumberland NE69 7DB
United Kingdom

Fernando Cervero, MD, PhD, DSc
Anesthesia Research Unit Room 1207
McGill University McIntyre Medical
  Building
3655 Promenade Sir William Osler
Montreal, PQ H3G 1Y6
Canada

C. Richard Chapman, PhD
Pain Research and Management Center
University of Utah
615 Arapeen Drive #200
Salt Lake City, UT 84108
USA

David A Cherry, MBBS, FFARACS
Pain Management Unit
Flinders Medical Centre
Bedford Park, SA 5042
Australia

Jose Closs, PhD, MPhil, RGN
Department of Nursing Research
School of Healthcare Studies
Baines Wing
University of Leeds
Woodhouse Lane
Leeds LS2 9UT
United Kingdom

Beverly J. Collett, MBBS, FRCA
Pain Management Centre
Leicester Royal Infirmary
Infirmary Square
Leicester LE1 5WW
United Kingdom

Peggy Compton, RN, PhD
Acute Care Section
UCLA School of Nursing
4-246 Factor Building
Los Angeles, CA 90095
USA

Sandra J. Counts, MD, FASAM
4131 42nd NE
Seattle, WA 98105
USA

Edward C. Covington, MD
Section on Pain Medicine
Cleveland Clinic Foundation
9500 Euclid Avenue
Cleveland, OH 44106
USA

Michael J Cousins, AM, MB, MS,
  MD, FANZCA, FFPMANZCA
Department of Anaesthesia and Pain
  Management
University of Sydney
Royal North Shore Hospital
St Leonards, NSW 2065
Australia

Kenneth D. Craig, PhD
Department of Psychology
University of British Columbia
2136 West Mall
Vancouver, BC V6T 1Z4
Canada

Anthony H. Dickenson, PhD
Department of Pharmacology
University College London
Gower Street
London WC1E 6BT
United Kingdom

Robert H. Dworkin, PhD
Department of Anesthesiology
University of Rochester Medical
  Center
601 Elmwood Drive, Box 604
Rochester, NY 14642
USA

W. Thomas Edwards, MD, PhD
Harborview Medical Center
Anesthesiology Box 359724
Seattle, WA 98104
USA

John T. Farrar, MD, PhD
Center for Clinical Epidemiology and
  Biostatistics
University of Pennsylvania
423 Guardian Dr., Blockley Hall,
  Room 816
Philadelphia, PA 19104
USA

Roger B. Fillingim, PhD
University of Florida
Public Health Service and Research
PO Box 100404
1600 SW Archer Road, Room D8-44A
Gainesville, FL 32610
USA

Maria Fitzgerald, PhD
Department of Anatomy and
  Developmental Biology
University College London
Gower Street
London WC1E 6BT
United Kingdom

Roeland Gaymans, MD, PhD
Lignestraat 15
4921 ET Made
The Netherlands

Stephen J. Gibson, PhD
National Ageing Research Institute
PO Box 31
Parkville, VIC 3052
Australia

Gerald F. Gebhart, PhD
Department of Pharmacology
Bowen Science Building
University of Iowa
Iowa City, IA 52242
USA

Douglas Gourlay, MD, MSc, FRCPC,
  FASAM
Centre for Addiction and Mental
  Health
Wasser Pain Management Centre
Mount Sinai Hospital
University of Toronto
600 University Avenue
Toronto, ON M5G 1X5
Canada

Geoffrey Gourlay, PhD,
  FFPMANZCA
Pain Management Unit
Flinders Medical Centre
Bedford Park, SA 5042
Australia

Ruth E. Grunau, PhD
Centre for Community Child Health
  Research
University of British Columbia
F605B 4480 Oak Street
Vancouver, BC V6H 3V4
Canada

Thomas Hadjistavropoulos, PhD
Department of Psychology
University of Regina
3737 Waskana Parkway
Regina, SK S4S 0A2
Canada

Ji-Sheng Han, MD
Neuroscience Research Institute
Peking University Health Science
  Center
38 Xue Yuan Road
100083 Beijing
Peoples Republic of China

Howard A. Heit, MD, FACP, FASAM
8316 Arlington Boulevard, Suite 232
Fairfax, VA 22031
USA

Fiona Hicks
Consultant in Palliative Medicine
St James's University Hospital
Becket Street
Leeds, W. Yorks LS9 7TF
United Kingdom

Anita Holdcroft, MB, ChB, MD, FRCA
Department of Anaesthesia
Chelsea and Westminster Hospital
369 Fulham Road
London SW10 9NH
United Kingdom

John H. Hughes, MB, BS, FRCA
Department of Pain Relief
James Cook University Hospital
Marton Road
Middlesbrough TS4 3BW
United Kingdom

Anne Hunt, RGN, PhD
Royal College of Nursing Institute
Radcliffe Infirmary
Woodstock Road
Oxford OX2 6HE
United Kingdom

Troels S. Jensen, MD, PhD
Department of Neurology
Aarhus University Hospital
8000 Aarhus
Denmark

Eija A Kalso, MD, PhD
Pain Relief Unit
Helsinki University
Haartmaninkatu 4
PO Box 340
0029 Helsinki
Finland

Dilip Kapur, MB, ChB, FRCA
Pain Management Unit
Flinders Medical Centre
Bedford Park, SA 5042
Australia

Francis J. Keefe, PhD
Box 3159
Department of Psychology
Duke University Medical Center
Durham, NC 27710
USA

Margaret M. Kotz, DO
Addiction Recovery Services
University Hospitals of Cleveland
Case Western Reserve Medical School
11100 Euclid Ave.
Cleveland, OH 44106
USA

Walter Ling, MD
16556 Park Lane Circle
Los Angeles, CA 90049
USA

Phillipe A. Lacoux, MD
Department of Anaesthesia
Ninewells Hospital
Dundee DD1 9SY
United Kingdom

John D. Loeser, MD
Department of Neurological Surgery
University of Washington
Box 356470
Seattle WA 98195
USA

Joyce H. Lowinson, MD
Department of Psychiatry
The Rockefeller University
1230 York Avenue
New York, NY 10021
USA

Pamela E. MacIntyre, MBBS,
  FANZCA
Acute Pain Service
University of Adelaide
Royal Adelaide Hospital
North Terrace
Adelaide, SA 5000
Australia

William A. Macrae, MB, ChB,
  DObstRCOG, FRCA
The Pain Service
Ninewells Hospital
Dundee DD1 9SY
United Kingdom

S. Malhotra, MBBS, FRCA
Magill Department of Anaesthesia,
  Intensive Care and Pain Management
Department of Anaesthesia
Chelsea and Westminster Hospital
369 Fulham Road
London SW10 9NH
United Kingdom

Gary J. McFarlane, MB, ChB, PhD
Chronic Disease Epidemiology Unit
Room 2-705
University of Manchester
Stopford Building
Oxford Road
Manchester M13 9PT
United Kingdom

Patricia A. McGrath, PhD
Chronic Pain Program
The Hospital for Sick Children
University of Toronto
555 University Avenue
Toronto, ON M5G 1X8
Canada

Patrick J. McGrath, PhD
Pain and Palliative Care Program
Dalhousie University and IWK Health
  Centre
Halifax, NS B3H 4H7
Canada

Ross McPherson, MBBS, FANZCA
Department of Anaesthesia and Pain
  Management
University of Sydney
Royal North Shore Hospital
St Leonards, NSW 2065
Australia

Henry J. McQuay, DM, FRCA,
  FRCP(Edin)
Oxford Pain Relief Unit
Churchill Hospital
Headington, Oxford OX3 7LJ
United Kingdom

George Mendelson, MBBS, MD,
  FRANZCP, FFPMANZCA
Suite 18, 33 Queens Road
Melbourne, VIC 3004
Australia

Henry R. Miyoshi, BS
Department of Pharmacy
Harborview Medical Center ZA-55
325 Ninth Avenue
Seattle, WA 98104
USA

Lénaïc Monconduit, PhD
INSERM E216 Neurobiologie de la
  Douleur Trigéminale
Faculté de Chirurgie Dentaire
11 Boulevard Charles de Gaulle
63000 Clermont-Ferrand
France

Turo J. Nurmikko, MD
Pain Research Institute
Clinical Sciences Building
University Hospital Aintree
Liverpool L9 7AL
United Kingdom

Tim F. Oberlander, MD, FRCPC
Division of Developmental Pediatrics
  and Centre for Community Child
  Health Research
University of British Columbia
4480 Oak Street
Vancouver, BC V6H 3V4
Canada

Akiko Okifuji, PhD
Pain Research and Management Center
University of Utah
615 Arapeen Drive #200
Salt Lake City, UT 84108
USA

Jes Olesen, MD
Department of Neurology
University of Copenhagen
Glostrup Hospital
57 Nordre Ringwej
2600 Glostrup
Denmark

Jon B. Olson, MD
11505 6th NW
Seattle, WA 98177
USA

Gayle G. Page, RN, DNSc
School of Nursing
Johns Hopkins University
525 North Wolfe Street
Baltimore, MD 21205
USA

Minha Rajput, ND, DO, BsC
The Pain Service
Ninewells Hospital
Dundee DD1 9SY
United Kingdom

Ke Ren, MD, PhD
666 West Baltimore Street, Room 5A26
University of Maryland Dental School
Baltimore, MD 21201
USA

Patricia A. Roche, MSc, PhD,
  CSP(Dip)
School of Health Sciences,
  Physiotherapy
Queen Margaret University College
Leith Campus
Edinburgh EH6 8HF
United Kingdom

Michael C. Rowbotham, MD
UCSF Pain Clinical Research Center
1701 Divisadero Street Suite 480
San Francisco, CA 94115
USA

Seddon R. Savage, MS, MD
Dartmouth Center on Addiction,
  Recovery and Education
40 North College Street
Hanover, NH 03755
USA

Sidney H. Schnoll, MD, PhD
Purdue Pharma L.P.
One Stamford Forum
Stamford, CT 06901
USA

Catherine J. Seers
Royal College of Nursing Institute
Radcliffe Infirmary
Woodstock Road
Oxford OX2 6HE
United Kingdom

Barry J. Sessle, MDS, PhD, DSc,
  FRSC
Faculty of Dentistry
University of Toronto
124 Edward Street Room 366
Toronto ON M5G 1G6
Canada

Karen H. Simpson, FRCA
Consultant in Anaesthesia and Pain
  Management
St James's University Hospital
Becket Street
Leeds, W. Yorks LS9 7TF
United Kingdom

Soren H. Sindrup, MD
Department of Clinical Pharmacology
Institute of Medical Biology
Odense University
5000 Odense
Denmark

R. William Stones, MD, FRCOG
Department of Gynaecology
University of Southampton
Level F (815) Princess Anne Hospital
Southampton SO16 5YA
United Kingdom

Karen L. Syrjala, PhD
Fred Hutchinson Cancer Research
  Center
D5-220
1100 Fairview Avenue North
Seattle, WA 98109
USA

Rolf-Detlef Treede, MD
Institute of Physiology
Duesbergweg 6
55128 Mainz
Germany

Dennis C. Turk, PhD
John and Emma Bonica Professor of
  Anesthesiology and Pain Research
Department of Anesthesiology
University of Washington
Seattle, WA 98195
USA

Luis Villanueva, DDS, PhD
INSERM, E216, Neurobiologie de la
  Douleur Trigéminale
Faculté de Chirurgie Dentaire
11, Boulevard Charles de Gaulle
63000 Clermont-Ferrand
France

Paul J. Watson, PhD, MSc, MCSP
Department of Anaesthesia and Pain
  Management
University of Leicester
Gwendolen Road
Leicester LE5 4PW
United Kingdom

Judith Watt-Watson, RN, PhD
Faculty of Nursing and Centre for the
  Study of Pain
University of Toronto
124 Edward Street, Room 374
Toronto, ON M5G 1G6
Canada

Amanda C. Williams, PhD
Clinical Health Psychology
University College London
Gower Street
London WC1E 6BT
United Kingdom

Harriet M. Wittink, PhD, PT, OCS
Scherpenburgerwaard 6
3984 PB Odijk
The Netherlands

S.M. Yentis, FRCA
Magill Department of Anaesthesia,
  Intensive Care and Pain Management
Department of Anaesthesia
Chelsea and Westminster Hospital
369 Fulham Road
London SW10 9NH
United Kingdom

Lonnie K. Zeltzer, MD
Pediatric Pain Program
UCLA School of Medicine
10833 Le Conte Avenue, #22-464
  MDCC
Los Angeles, CA 90095
USA

Foreword

The third revision of the International Association for the Study of Pain (IASP) *Core Curriculum* has been many years in gestation. It follows the very successful format used by Dr. Howard L. Fields, editor of the second edition. For the first time IASP proposes to make this core curriculum available both in printed form and via the IASP Web site (www.iasp-pain.org). Inevitably, the information in this curriculum is, to a greater or lesser degree, out of date before publication. In the future, the curriculum core group believes the Web to be an ideal way to bring timely and rapid updates of this curriculum to the widest possible audience. We hope that this resource can become a dynamic and freely available asset for anyone with an interest in pain.

Readers and users of the core owe the biggest debt of thanks to the many authors who have given their time and knowledge to this revision of the curriculum. The content has been expanded by over one-third; new chapters have been added, and virtually all the text and the references have been revised. It is hoped that members will find this a significantly improved resource for patient care and training purposes.

The completion of the third edition of the core would not have been possible without the huge amounts of hard work carried out by the editorial production team in the IASP office in Seattle: Elizabeth Endres (Production Editor), Kathy Havers (Programs Coordinator), and Dale Schmidt (Desktop Technician). In addition, three individuals have carried the majority of the workload of preparing and collating the material in the *Core Curriculum*. This group has seen this project through to its conclusion, and it is a pleasure to acknowledge the enormous contributions of Drs. Stephen Butler, Dil Kapur, and, in particular, Geoffrey Gourlay.

J. EDMOND CHARLTON

Part I
General

Core Curriculum for Professional Education in Pain, edited by J. Edmond Charlton, IASP Press, Seattle, © 2005.

1

Anatomy and Physiology

I. Peripheral mechanisms

A. Be aware of the existence of two kinds of nociceptors: lightly myelinated A-delta and unmyelinated C fibers. Know the structure and anatomical organization of peripheral and central endings of cutaneous and deep primary afferents (Willis and Coggeshall 1991; Byers and Bonica 2001; Kruger et al. 2003).

B. Know the cytoarchitectural organization of the dorsal horn and how the different laminae are related to the terminal location of primary afferents. Know that large, A-beta afferents terminate mainly in laminae III through V, whereas cutaneous A-delta and C fibers terminate in a highly topographic fashion, mainly within laminae I and II (Willis and Coggeshall 1991; Sugiura 1996; Byers and Bonica 2001). Be aware that primary afferents from the viscera terminate in a more diffuse fashion in laminae I, V, and X (Ness and Gebhart 1990; Byers and Bonica 2001).

C. Know the capabilities of nociceptors to detect different kinds of noxious stimuli and the difficulties of defining a nociceptor only by its threshold or by the fact that its activation elicits pain (Besson and Chaouch 1987; Handwerker and Kobal 1993, Raja et al. 1999). Know the molecular and biophysical mechanisms underlying mechanical, heat, cold, and chemical nociceptive transduction. Be aware that most nociceptors have the ability to detect a wide range of physical or chemical noxious stimuli. Know that the sensation of pain results from the integration of the signals traveling in different types of primary afferents, which, when stimulated alone, act as labeled lines (Waldmann and Lazdunski 1998; Hill 2001; Julius and Basbaum 2001; Belmonte et al. 2004; Wood et al. 2004).

D. Be aware that, compared to the nociceptors in skin, the primary afferents in corneal (Belmonte et al. 2004), dental (Byers and Närhi 1999), visceral (Ness and Gebhart 1990; Cervero and Laird 1999), and other deep tissues (Byers and Bonica 2001) have distinct protective functions that may account for their particular functional features and anatomical distribution.

E. Know that, in addition to signaling damaging stimuli, subpopulations of small-diameter afferent fibers convey inputs that elicit pleasant sensations of touch (Wessberg et al. 2003) and innocuous thermal (Green 2004), and itchy sensations (Ikoma et al. 2003). Be aware that nociceptors convey other inputs important for homeostatic functions including local metabolism, neuroendocrine, vascular, and trophic functions (Byers and Bonica 2001; Craig 2003).

F. Be aware that fine primary afferents, including "silent nociceptors," can be activated or become sensitized by substances released during inflammation, and actually participate in neurogenic inflammation. Know the mechanisms by which A-beta fibers and the nociceptors participate in neuropathic and inflammatory forms of hyperalgesia and allodynia. Be aware of the involvement of nociceptors in primary and secondary hyperalgesia (Levine and Reichling 1999; Handwerker and Schmelz 2004).

G. Know that sensitization is mediated by a number of substances, including inflammatory mediators, proteinases (Vergnolle et al. 2003), and neurotrophic factors released following tissue damage or by inflammatory cells (McMahon and Jones 2004), and that these in turn may regulate gene expression and affect sensory neuronal function (Woolf and Salter 2000). Be aware that several molecular mechanisms participate in sensitization phenomena, including G-protein-coupled receptors, ligand-gated ion channels, and Trk receptors (Hill 2001; Julius and Basbaum 2001; Wood et al. 2004).

3

H. Know of the existence of subpopulations of C fibers based on their neurochemical features. Know what peptides and excitatory amino acids are found in primary afferent nociceptors and understand their role in nociception and in neurogenic inflammation (Carlton 2001; Hill 2001).

I. Be aware of the interactions between the immune system and nociceptors. Know the substances that are synthesized in immune cells and the circumstances that elicit their release (Machelska and Stein 2002; Cunha and Ferreira 2003). Know the mechanisms by which the sympathetic nervous system alters nociceptor function (Baron and Jänig 2004).

J. Know that antidromic activation of nociceptors may occur following presynaptic interactions between primary afferents at the level of the dorsal horn (Wall 1995; Cervero et al. 2003).

II. Central mechanisms of nociceptive transmission: the spinal and medullary dorsal horns

A. Know Rexed's lamination scheme for the spinal and medullary dorsal horns, how it relates to the terminals of different types of primary afferents, and the location of superficial, noxious-specific and deep, wide-dynamic-range neurons (Willis and Coggeshall 1991; Byers and Bonica 2001).

B. Know the response properties, coding mechanisms, convergence of peripheral inputs, and differential projections to supraspinal centers of superficial and deep dorsal horn nociceptive neurons (Willis and Coggeshall 1991; Sessle 2000; Villanueva and Nathan 2000; Craig 2003; Price et al. 2003). Be aware that lamina I neurons modulate the excitability of deep spinal and medullary dorsal horn neurons through both local intraspinal pathways and pathways descending from the brainstem (Dallel et al. 1998; Dickenson et al. 2004).

C. Know that modulatory inputs subserved by inhibitory and excitatory cotransmission may change the intrinsic firing properties of dorsal horn neurons to several functional states (Jo and Schlichter 1999; Derjean et al. 2003). Be aware of the contribution of short-term (wind-up) and long-term (LTP) amplification mechanisms to synaptic plasticity in the dorsal horn following noxious stimulation (Herrero et al. 2000; Sandkühler 2000; Ji et al. 2003). Know that dorsal horn sensitization by noxious stimuli is mediated by several molecular signaling mechanisms including glutamate, neuropeptides, the expression of immediate early genes, and neurotrophic factors (Hill 2001; Hunt and Mantyh 2001; McMahon and Jones 2004).

D. Know that the anterolateral quadrant of the spinal cord contains the axons of both superficial and deep dorsal horn nociceptive neurons and the main ascending pathways giving rise to both cutaneous and visceral pain in animals and humans (Vierck et al. 1986; Gybels and Sweet 1989; Villanueva and Nathan 2000). Be aware that in addition to spinothalamic axons, the anterolateral quadrant contains two main nociceptive pathways that relay within the brainstem reticular formation and parabrachial nucleus (Craig and Dostrovsky 1999; Villanueva and Nathan 2000; Gauriau and Bernard 2002).

III. Central mechanisms of nociceptive transmission: segmental and brainstem pain modulation

A. Know that segmental inhibitions can be elicited by activity in large-diameter cutaneous afferent fibers and innocuous mechanical stimuli (Wall 1996). Be aware that stronger, longer-lasting segmental and extrasegmental analgesic effects can be obtained following percutaneous activation of fine-diameter fibers (Chung et al. 1984; Bouhassira et al. 1987; Sandkuhler 2000).

B. Know that sympathetically maintained spontaneous and evoked activity may generate a state of central sensitization (Baron and Jänig 2004). Be aware that dorsal column stimulation, which is usually termed spinal cord stimulation in human beings, may relieve ischemic pain and probably does so through central inhibitory mechanisms influencing sympathetic neurons (Linderoth and Meyerson 1995).

C. Know that several spino-brainstem-spinal pathways are activated simultaneously when a noxious stimulus occurs, providing widespread negative and positive feedback loops by which nociceptive signals may attenuate or increase their own magnitudes (Villanueva and Le Bars 1995; Porreca et al. 2002; Dickenson et al. 2004; Fields et al. 2005).

IV.   Central mechanisms of nociceptive transmission: thalamocortical mechanisms

  A.   Know that medial and lateral thalamic regions distribute nociceptive signals to a number of cortical areas. Be aware that these thalamic areas receive nociceptive inputs either indirectly via the brainstem (Craig and Dostrovsky 1999; Villanueva and Nathan 2000; Gauriau and Bernard 2002) or directly from superficially or deeply located parts of the dorsal horn (Willis and Coggeshall 1991; Apkarian and Shi 1994; Lenz and Dougherty 1997; Craig 2003). Know that thalamic activity is highly dependent on reciprocal interactions with its cortical targets (Villanueva and Fields 2004).

  B.   Know that a noxious stimulus activates not only several cortical areas, but also an increasing number of subcortical and cortical regions as the intensity of the stimulus increases (Derbyshire et al. 1997; Porro 2003). Be aware that powerful top-down, endogenous mechanisms of pain modulation originate in the cortex because almost all nociceptive relays within the central nervous system are under corticofugal modulation (Jasmin et al. 2003; Villanueva and Fields 2004). Know that a painful stimulus activates not only cortical and subcortical structures but also the endogenous mu-opioid system (Zubieta et al. 2001). Know that corticofugal modulation selectively alters pain perception following manipulation of a number of factors including attention, expectation, placebo and hypnotic manipulations, and the pain that can occur in the absence of detectable organic lesions (Ramachandran 1998; Harris 1999; Casey and Bushnell 2000; Peyron et al. 2000; Rainville 2002; Ploghaus et al. 2003).

REFERENCES

Apkarian AV, Shi T. Squirrel monkey lateral thalamus. I. Somatic nociresponsive neurons and their relation to spinothalamic terminals. *J Neurosci* 1994; 14:6779–6795.

Baron R, Jänig W. The role of the sympathetic nervous system in pain processing. In: Villanueva L, Dickenson AH, Ollat H (Eds). *The Pain System in Normal and Pathological States: A Primer For Clinicians,* Progress in Pain Research and Management, Vol. 31. Seattle: IASP Press, 2004, pp 193–210.

Belmonte C, Acosta MC, Gallar J. Neural basis of sensation in intact and injured corneas. *Exp Eye Res* 2004; 78:513–525.

Bouhassira D, Le Bars D, Villanueva L. Heterotopic activation of A-delta and C fibres triggers inhibition of trigeminal and spinal convergent neurones in the rat. *J Physiol (Lond)* 1987; 389:301–317.

Besson JM, Chaouch A. Peripheral and spinal mechanisms of pain. *Physiol Rev* 1987; 67:67–184.

Byers MR, Närhi MVO. Dental injury models: experimental tools for understanding neuroinflammatory interactions and polymodal nociceptor functions. *Crit Rev Oral Biol Med* 1999; 10:4–39.

Byers MR, Bonica JJ. Peripheral pain mechanisms and nociceptor plasticity. In: Loeser JD, Butler SH, Chapman CR, Turk DC (Eds). *Bonica's Management of Pain,* 3rd ed. Philadelphia: Lippincott, Williams & Wilkins, 2001, pp 26–72.

Carlton SM. Peripheral excitatory amino acids. *Curr Opin Pharmacol* 2001; 1:52–56.

Casey KL, Bushnell MC. *Pain Imaging,* Progress in Pain Research and Management, Vol. 18. Seattle: IASP Press, 2000.

Cervero F, Laird JM. Visceral pain. *Lancet* 1999; 353:2145–2148.

Cervero F, Laird JM, Garcia-Nicas E. Secondary hyperalgesia and presynaptic inhibition: an update. *Eur J Pain* 2003; 7:345–351.

Chung JM, Lee KH, Hori Y, Endo K, Willis WD. Factors influencing peripheral nerve stimulation produced inhibition of primate spinothalamic tract cells. *Pain* 1984; 19:277–293.

Craig AD. Pain mechanisms: labeled lines versus convergence in central processing. *Annu Rev Neurosci* 2003; 26:1–30.

Craig AD, Dostrovsky JO. Medulla to thalamus. In: Wall PD, Melzack R (Eds). *Textbook of Pain.* Edinburgh: Churchill Livingstone, 1999, pp 183–214.

Cunha FQ, Ferreira SH. Peripheral hyperalgesic cytokines. *Adv Exp Med Biol* 2003; 521:2–39.

Dallel R, Dualé C, Molat JL. Morphine administered in the substantia gelatinosa of the spinal trigeminal nucleus caudalis inhibits nociceptivie activities in the spinal trigeminal nucleus oralis. *J Neurosci* 1998; 18:3529–3536.

Derbyshire SW, Jones AK, Gyulai F, et al. Pain processing during three levels of noxious stimulation produces differential patterns of central activity. *Pain* 1997; 73:431–445.

Derjean D, Bertrand S, Le Masson G, et al. Dynamic balance of metabotropic inputs causes dorsal horn neurons to switch functional states. *Nat Neurosci* 2003; 6:274–281.

Dickenson AH, Suzuki R, Matthews EA, et al. Balancing excitations and inhibitions in spinal circuits. In: L. Villanueva, A. H. Dickenson and H. Ollat (Eds.) *The Pain System in Normal and Pathological States: A Primer for Clinicians,* Progress in Pain Research and Management, Vol. 31. Seattle: IASP Press, 2004, pp 79–106.

Fields HL, Basbaum AI, Heinricher MM. Central nervous system mechanisms of pain modulation. In: McMahon, Koltzenburg M (Eds). *Textbook of Pain.* Edinburgh: Churchill Livingstone, 2005, in press.

Gauriau C, Bernard JF. Pain pathways and parabrachial circuits in the rat. *Exp Physiol* 2002; 87:251–258.

Green BG. Temperature perception and nociception. *J Neurobiol* 2004; 61:13–29.

Gybels J, Sweet WH. *Neurosurgical Treatment of Persistent Pain.* Karger: Basel, 1989.

Handwerker HO, Kobal G. Psychophysiology of experimentally induced pain. *Physiol Rev* 1993; 73:639–671.

Handwerker HO, Schmelz M. Peripheral mechanisms of allodynia and other forms of hyperalgesia in human skin. In: Villanueva L, Dickenson AH, Ollat H (Eds). *The Pain System in Normal and Pathological States: A Primer for Clinicians,* Progress in Pain Research and Management, Vol. 31. Seattle: IASP Press, 2004, pp 45–56.

Harris AJ. Cortical origin of pathological pain. *Lancet* 1999; 354:1464–1466.

Herrero JF, Laird JMA, Lopez-Garcia JA. Wind-up of spinal cord neurones and pain sensation: much ado about something? *Prog Neurobiol* 2000; 61:169–203.

Hill RG. Molecular basis for the perception of pain. *Neuroscientist* 2001; 7:282–292.

Hunt SP, Mantyh PW. The molecular dynamics of pain control. *Nature Rev* 2001; 2:83–91.

Ikoma A, Rukwied R, Stander S, et al. Neurophysiology of pruritus: interaction of itch and pain. *Arch Dermatol* 2003; 139:1475–1478.

Jasmin L, Rabkin SD, Granato A, Boudah A, Ohara P. Analgesia and hyperalgesia from GABA-mediated modulation of the cerebral cortex. *Nature* 2003; 424:316–320.

Ji RR, Kohno T, Moore KA, Woolf CJ. Central sensitization and LTP: do pain and memory share similar mechanisms ? *Trends Neurosci* 2003; 26:696–705.

Jo YH, Schlichter R. Synaptic corelease of ATP and GABA in cultured spinal neurons. *Nat Neurosci* 1999; 2:241–245.

Julius D, Basbaum AI. Molecular mechanisms of nociception. *Nature* 2001; 413:203–210.

Kruger L, Light AR, Schweizer FE. Axonal terminals of sensory neurons and their morphological diversity. *J Neurocytol* 2003; 32:205–216.

Lenz FA, Dougherty PM. Pain processing in the human thalamus. In: Steriade M, Jones EG, McCormick DA (Eds). *Thalamus, vol II, Experimental and Clinical Aspects.* Amsterdam: Elsevier, 1997, pp 617–654.

Levine JD, Reichling DB. Peripheral mechanisms of inflammatory pain. In: Wall PD, Melzack R (Eds).Textbook of Pain. Edinburgh: Churchill Livingstone, 1999, pp 59–84.

Linderoth B, Meyerson BA. Dorsal column stimulation: modulation of somatosensory and autonomic function. *Sem Neurosci* 1995; 7:263–277.

Machelska H, Stein C. Immune mechanisms in pain control. *Anesth Analg* 2002; 95:1002–1008.

McMahon SB, Jones NG. Plasticity of pain signaling: Role of neurotrophic factors exemplified by acid-induced pain. *J Neurobiol* 2004; 61:72–87.

Ness TJ, Gebhart GF. Visceral pain : a review of experimental studies. *Pain* 1990; 41:167–234.

Peyron R, Laurent B, Garcia-Larrea L. Functional imaging of brain responses to pain. A review and meta-analysis. *Neurophysiol Clin* 2000; 30:263–288.

Ploghaus A, Becerra L, Borras C, Borsook D. Neural circuitry undelying pain modulation: expectation, hypnosis, placebo. *TICS* 2003; 7:197–200.

Porreca F, Ossipov MH, Gebhart GF. Chronic pain and medullary descending facilitation. *Trends Neurosci* 2002; 25:319–325.

Porro C. Functional imaging and pain: behavior, perception and modulation. *Neuroscientist* 2003; 9:354–369.

Price DD, Greenspan JD, Dubner R. Neurons involved in the exteroceptive function of pain. *Pain* 2003; 106:215–219.

Rainville P. Brain mechanisms of pain affect and pain modulation. *Curr Opin Neurobiol* 2002; 12:195–204.

Raja SN, Meyer RA, Ringkamp M, Campbell JN. Peripheral neural mechanisms of nociception. In: Wall PD, Melzack R (Eds). *Textbook of Pain,* 4th ed. Edinburgh: Churchill Livingstone, 1999, pp 11–57.

Ramachadran VS. Consciousness and body image: lessons from phantom limbs, Capgras syndrome and pain asymbolia. *Phil Trans R Soc Lond B* 1998; 353:1851–1859.

Sandkuhler J. Learning and memory in pain pathways. *Pain* 2000; 88:113–118.

Sessle BJ. Acute and chronic craniofacial pain: brainstem mechanisms of nociceptive transmission and neuroplasticity, and their clinical correlates. *Crit Rev Oral Biol Med* 2000; 11:57–91.

Sugiura Y. Spinal organization of C-fiber afferents related with nociception or non-nociception. *Prog Brain Res* 1996; 113:320–339.

Vergnolle N, Ferazzini M, D'Andrea MR, Buddenkotte J, Steinhoff M. Proteinase-activated receptors: novel signals for peripheral nerves. *Trends Neurosci* 2003; 26:496–500.

Vierck CJ, Greenspan JD, Ritz LA, Yeomans DC. The spinal pathways contributing to the ascending conduction and the descending modulation of pain sensations and reactions. In: Yaksh TL (Ed). *Spinal Afferent Processing.* New York: Plenum, 1986, pp 275–329.

Villanueva L, Le Bars D. The activation of bulbo-spinal controls by peripheral nociceptive inputs: diffuse noxious inhibitory controls (DNIC). *Biol Res* 1995; 28:113–125.

Villanueva L, Nathan PW. Multiple pain pathways. In: Devor M, Rowbotham MC, Wiesenfeld-Hallin Z (Eds). *Proceedings of the 9th World Congress on Pain,* Progress in Pain Research and Management, Vol. 16. 2000, pp 371–386.

Villanueva L, Fields HL. Endogenous central mechanisms pain modulation. In: Villanueva L, Dickenson AH, Ollat H (Eds). *The Pain System in Normal and Pathological States: A Primer for Clinicians,* Progress in Pain Research and Management, Vol. 31. Seattle: IASP Press, 2004, pp 223–246.

Waldmann, R., Lazdunski, M., H+-gated cation channels: neuronal acid sensors in the NaC/DEG family of ion channels. *Curr Opin Neurobiol* 1998; 8:418–424.

Wall PD. Do nerve impulses penetrate terminal arborizations? A Presynaptic control mechanism. *Trends Neurosci* 1995; 18:99–103.

Wall PD. Comments after 30 years of the gate-control theory. *Pain Forum* 1996; 5:12–22.

Wessberg J, Olausson H, Fernstrom Wiklund K, Vallbo AB. Receptive field properties of unmyelinated tactile afferents in the human skin. *J Neurophysiol* 2003; 89:1567–1575.

Willis WD, Coggeshall RE. *Sensory Mechanisms of the Spinal Cord,* 2nd ed. New York: Plenum Press, 1991.

Wood JN, Boorman JP, Okuse K, Baker MD. Voltage-gated sodium channels and pain pathways. *J Neurobiol* 2004; 61:55–71.

Woolf CJ, Salter MW. Neuronal plasticity: increasing the gain in pain. *Science* 2000; 288:1765–1769.

Zubieta JK, Smith YR, Bueller JA, Xu Y, Kilbourn MR, et al. Regional mu opioid receptor regulation of sensory and affective dimensions of pain. *Science* 2001; 293:311–315.

Core Curriculum for Professional Education in Pain, edited by J. Edmond Charlton, IASP Press, Seattle, © 2005.

2

Pharmacology of Pain Transmission and Modulation

I. General issues

A. Pain can only be studied fully in integrated systems. Pain is a conscious experience that emerges from brain activity. The word "pain" does not equate with nociception, which is a preconscious neural activity that is normally necessary, but not sufficient, for pain. When we speak of "pain transmission," we are referring to nociceptive transmission, since pain per se cannot be communicated by animals.

B. Drug actions may be highly selective, but rarely specific, and effects may be seen in animals at doses that are not possible in patients.

C. Be aware that animal studies, although extremely valuable in modeling clinical conditions, generally provide information on efficacy and may not affect cognitive and affective aspects of human pain.

D. Know that behavioral studies in animals generally study threshold responses but can reveal secondary effects of drugs, whereas electrophysiological studies can provide information on suprathreshold responses yet often not side effects.

E. Molecular approaches have been valuable in the identification of channels and receptors in pain pathways, and approaches such as the use of knockout mice are a very powerful means of identifying function. However, the interpretation of data may be complicated by the effects of changes other than those to the receptor/channel that was deleted.

F. Many of the transmitter and receptor systems in the central nervous system undergo developmental changes, and therefore infants should not be viewed simply as small adults (Alvares and Fitzgerald 1999; Hunt and Mantyh 2001; Carpenter and Dickenson 2002).

II. Peripheral mechanisms

A. Know that the nociceptor is composed of a number of sensory and chemical receptors that result in the polymodal nature of nociceptive sensory neurons (Besson and Chaouch 1987; Dray and Perkins 1993; Eglen et al. 1999; Millan 1999).

B. Be aware that a large number of chemical mediators such as ATP, prostanoids, bradykinin, serotonin, histamine, and hydrogen ions (acid pH) can activate nociceptors (Eglen et al. 1999; Millan 1999). Heat responses involve the capsaicin-activated vanilloid receptor family and the transient receptor potential V (TRPV) receptors. ATP acts on a large family of PX receptors, hydrogen ions act on acid-sensing ion channels (ASICs) and TRPV1, and the receptors for all these chemicals are invariably multiple (Dray and Perkins 1993; Dray et al. 1994; Dray 1997; Hill 1999; Julius and Basbaum 2001).

C. Know that these chemicals and also neuropeptides (e.g., substance P and calcitonin gene related peptide [CGRP] through the axon reflex) and prostaglandins participate in peripheral events leading to hyperalgesia and edema in inflammation, including increased blood flow (Besson and Chaouch 1987; Dray and Perkins 1993; Millan 1999).

D. Be aware of the difference between activation and sensitization of the peripheral terminals of primary afferent nociceptors. Be aware that some compounds do both (e.g., bradykinin), whereas others are primarily sensitizing (e.g., prostaglandins). Sensitization leads to a drop in the threshold for activation of nociceptors.

E. Be aware that there are several classes of anti inflammatory agents. Be aware that cyclooxygenase (COX), the key enzyme for the production of prostaglandins in inflammatory exudates, exists in at least two forms, so that inhibitors of the inducible COX-2 have similar efficacy to other NSAIDs but have reduced gastrointestinal side effects, although there is an increased risk of cardiovascular and renal side effects (Appleton 1997; Fitzgerald 2003; Kiefer and Dannhardt 2004).

F. Know that populations of silent nociceptors may become active during inflammation (Millan 1999).

G. Neuropathic pain involves changes in the peripheral and central nervous systems (Suzuki and Dickenson 2000). The former changes involve clustering and other changes in sodium channels that promote ectopic activity (Waxman 1999). The effects of local anesthetics and anticonvulsants such as carbamazepine in neuropathic pain are probably partly due to their blocking of these sodium channels. Novel sodium channels in C fibers have been described that may provide novel drug targets. Cross-talk between damaged fibers can also occur, as can changes in expression and redistribution of channels and other proteins (Suzuki and Dickenson 2000).

H. Be aware that there are growth factors, for example nerve growth factor (NGF), which are produced by neural and non-neural tissue, that may influence the responsiveness, phenotype, and regrowth of sensory neurons in states of both inflammation and nerve injury (McMahon at al. 1993; Millan 1999).

I. Be aware that cytokines and changes in the peptide content of sensory neurons have an impact upon inflammation and neuropathy (Sommer 2001).

J. Know the basis for the involvement of the sympathetic nervous system in certain pain states including nerve injury (Jänig and Baron 2001).

III. Synaptic transmission in the dorsal horn

A. Understand the importance of N- and P-type calcium channels in the mechanisms of transmitter release from nerve terminals. Agents that block these voltage-dependent calcium channels (VDCCs) may include gabapentin (Vanegas and Schaible 2000; Matthews and Dickenson 2001). Other means of modulation of release can occur through activation of receptors that reduce Ca^{2+} influx or cause hyperpolarization, such as opioid receptors. Realize that the expression and function of VDCCs can change in different pain models (Dickenson 1994b; Price et al. 1994).

B. Be aware that C fibers contain and release glutamate, and whereas a proportion also contain substance P and CGRP, others are nonpeptide (the isolectin B_4 population). The peptide content and phenotype are altered by tissue and nerve damage.

C. Know that glutamate, the excitatory amino acid (EAA) implicated in transmission from primary afferent nociceptors to dorsal horn neurons, has a number of receptors (AMPA, kainate, *N* methyl D aspartate [NMDA], and metabotropic), and that various combinations of these receptors exist on neurons in various laminae of the dorsal horn. The activation of these receptors determines the time course of the responses of dorsal horn cells to noxious stimuli and their different susceptibilities to pharmacological agents (Dickenson 1995; Millan 1999).

D. Know that some neuropeptides present in primary afferent nociceptors are excitatory (e.g., including substance P and CGRP; Hunt and Mantyh 2001), while others are inhibitory (e.g., somatostatin) to dorsal horn neurons.

E. Understand the processes that underlie wind-up and central hyperalgesia. Be aware of the pivotal role of the NMDA-type of EAA receptor in these processes (Dickenson 1994b). Understand how central mechanisms can change in pathological events such as neuropathy (Dickenson et al. 2001).

F. Understand the importance of postsynaptic modulation of transmission by drugs that block the receptors for the peptides and glutamate (Fields et al. 1991). Know that ketamine, memantine, and dextromethorphan block the NMDA-receptor complex (Dickenson 1994b; Price et al. 1994). Know that there are many sites for modulation of the NMDA receptor (glycine site, polyamine site, channel) and that drugs that antagonize subtypes of the receptor may have fewer side effects than existing drugs (Chizh et al. 2001).

G. Be aware that prostaglandins, generated by spinal COX, affect synaptic transmission in the spinal cord as well as contributing to inflammatory pain in peripheral tissues; therefore, cyclooxygenase inhibitors such as aspirin and NSAIDs may have both peripheral and central nervous system actions relevant to analgesia (Yaksh and Malmberg 1994). COX-2 now appears to be constitutive in the spinal cord.

IV. Central sensitization

A. Know that prolonged firing of unmyelinated primary afferents can initiate glutamate-receptor mediated, prolonged enhancement of excitatory synaptic transmission to dorsal horn nociceptive neurons and in the brainstem rostroventral medulla.

B. Be aware that NMDA-mediated wind-up like mechanisms underlie this central hypersensitivity, but that intracellular changes, the generation of nitric oxide and prostanoids, highly diffusible mediators, and other mediators are all important downstream mechanisms (Meller and Gebhart 1993). Know the broad classes of agents capable of blocking the development of central sensitization, which include VDCC blockers, NMDA-receptor antagonists, nitric oxide synthase inhibitors, and agents that increase inhibitions (McQuay and Dickenson 1990; McMahon et al. 1993; Dickenson 1994b; Dickenson et al. 2001).

C. Be aware that central sensitization is more susceptible to inhibitory or analgesic agents when they are administered before, rather than after, the initiating afferent barrage. Know that this is the rationale used to justify preemptive analgesia, but that this is difficult to study in clinical settings (McQuay and Dickenson 1990; Coderre et al. 1993; Dickenson 1994b; Woolf 1994).

D. Be aware that central sensitization has been observed in laboratory models of inflammation and neuropathic pain and can be demonstrated in human psychophysical studies (Woolf and Doubell 1994).

E. Know that pain signaling transmitters can activate the expression of certain intracellular agents and genes that may contribute to central sensitization (Dubner and Ruda 1992; Meller and Gebhart 1993; Dray et al. 1994; Petersen-Zeitz and Basbaum 1999).

F. Be aware that anticonvulsants and excitability blockers may have actions at both central and peripheral sites (Dray et al. 1994).

G. Know that there is increasing evidence for roles of non-neuronal cells such as glia in spinal events that lead to persistent pain (Watkins and Maier 2003).

V. Neurotransmitters in pain modulation

A. Know that a number of receptor systems can be activated by transmitters and drugs to produce analgesic effects. These include opioid receptors, alpha-2 adrenoceptors, some of the 5-HT receptors (5-HT$_1$ in particular), the adenosine A$_1$ receptor, and cannabinoids (Yaksh and Malmberg 1994; Dickenson 1994a, 1995; Millan 1999; Chapman and Iversen 2002).

B. Know the four main types of opioid receptors (mu, delta, kappa, and ORL-1) and the various opioid peptides and, in the case of the mu receptor, the major classes of clinically used drugs acting on this receptor (Yaksh and Noueihed 1985; Dickenson 1994a). Be aware that molecular studies of the opioid receptors have led to detailed knowledge of their structure, their mechanism, and their precise location in the nervous system (Dickenson 1994a; Uhl et al. 1994; Darland et al. 1998).

C. Subtypes, interactions, and changes in expression of the opioid receptors have been shown in neurons, but as yet, the basic findings are difficult to relate to the clinical use of opioids (Dickenson and Suzuki 1999).

D.   Understand that numerous factors, such as nerve injury and inflammation, can reduce and enhance opioid analgesia (Dickenson 1994; Rowbotham 2001). Be aware of proposed mechanisms of opioid tolerance that include NMDA receptors, cholecystokinin, and dynorphin (Basbaum 1995). Also realize that opioid analgesia will depend on various factors that include route of administration, formulation, type of opioid, type of pain state, and symptoms (Dickenson and Suzuki 1999; Rowbotham 2001).

E.   Know that opioid agonists act in the central nervous system at both spinal and supraspinal sites involved in pain transmission and modulation (Yaksh and Noueihed 1985; Besson and Chaouch 1987; Meller and Gebhart 1993). After inflammation, peripheral sites of action of opioids can contribute (Machelska et al. 1999, Stein et al. 2003).

F.   Know that at the spinal cord level, opioids act predominantly presynaptically to inhibit transmitter release from nociceptive sensory neurons and postsynaptically to inhibit activity of dorsal horn neurons (Dickenson 1994a).

G.   Be aware that several neurotransmitters are involved in descending pain modulation and facilitation from brainstem and midbrain centers (e.g., norepinephrine, serotonin, glutamate, NMDA, and gamma-aminobutyric acid) (Yaksh and Noueihed 1985; Besson and Chaouch 1987; Fields et al. 1991; Dickenson 1994a; Hunt and Mantyh 2001). Understand that these neurotransmitters bind to different receptor classes so that some will mediate inhibition and others, facilitation, of pain. Some systems can interact synergistically, and others will interact antagonistically (Dickenson and Sullivan 1993). The role of descending facilitations in spinal cord function is gaining prominence, whereas many previous studies have concentrated on inhibitions.

H.   Realize that the supraspinal monoamine systems are also modulated by opioid receptors, and that this mechanism forms an important component of opioid analgesia (Millan 1999). Antidepressants, alpha-2 adrenoceptor agonists such as clonidine, and the triptans all interact in some way with norepinephrine and serotonin transmission.

I.   Understand the use of adjuncts to enhance opioid analgesia based on the principle that drugs can either increase inhibitions or decrease excitations; thus, combinations of appropriate agents are logical when single agents are insufficient (Dickenson and Sullivan 1993; Dickenson 1994a; Yaksh and Malmberg 1994).

REFERENCES

Alvares D, Fitzgerald M. Building blocks of pain: the regulation of key molecules in spinal sensory neurones during development and following peripheral axotomy. *Pain* 1999; Suppl 6:S71–S85.

Appleton I. Non-steroidal anti-inflammatory drugs and pain. In: Dickenson AH, Besson JM (Eds). *The Pharmacology of Pain,* Handbook of Experimental Pharmacology, Vol. 130. Springer-Verlag, 1997, pp 43–60.

Basbaum AI. Insights into the development of opioid tolerance. *Pain* 1995; 61:349-52.

Besson J M, Chaouch A. Peripheral and spinal mechanisms of nociception. *Physiol Rev* 1987; 67:67–186.

Carpenter K, Dickenson AH. Molecular aspects of pain. *Pharmacogenomics J* 2002; 2:87–95.

Chapman V, Iversen L. Cannabinoids: a real prospect for pain relief. *Curr Opin Pharmacol* 2002; 2:50–55.

Chizh BA, Headley PM, Tzschentke TM. NMDA receptor antagonists as analgesics: focus on the NR2B subtype. *Trends Pharmacol Sci* 2001; 22:636–642.

Coderre TJ, Katz J, Vaccarino AL, Melzack R. Contribution of central neuroplasticity to pathological pain: review of clinical and experimental evidence. *Pain* 1993; 52:259–285.

Darland T, Heinricher MM, Grandy DK. Orphanin FQ/nociceptin; a role in pain and analgesia, but so much more. *Trends Neurosci* 1998; 21:215–221.

Dickenson AH. Where and how opioids act. In: Gebhart GF, Hammond DL, Jensen T (Eds). *Proceedings of the 7th World Congress on Pain,* Progress in Pain Research and Management, Vol. 2. Seattle: IASP Press, 1994a, pp 525–552.

Dickenson AH. NMDA receptor antagonists as analgesics. In: Fields HL, Liebeskind JC (Eds). *Pharmacological Approaches to the Treatment of Pain: New Concepts and Critical Issues,* Progress in Pain Research and Management, Vol. 1. Seattle: IASP Press, 1994b, pp 173–187.

Dickenson AH. Spinal cord pharmacology of pain. *Br J Anaesth* 1995; 75:193–200.

Dickenson AH, Sullivan AF. Combination therapy in analgesia: seeking synergy. *Curr Opin Anaesthesiol* 1993; 6:861–865.

Dickenson AH, Suzuki R. Function and dysfunction of opioid receptors in the spinal cord. In: Kalso E, McQuay HJ, Wiesenfeld-Hallin Z (Eds). *Opioid Sensitivity of Chronic Noncancer Pain,* Progress in Pain Research and Management, Vol. 14. Seattle: IASP Press, 1999, pp 77–74.

Dickenson AH, Matthews EA, Suzuki R. Central nervous system mechanisms of pain in peripheral neuropathy. In: Hansson PT, Fields HL, Hill RG, Marchettini P (Eds). *Neuropathic Pain: Pathophysiology and Treatment,* Progress in Pain Research and Management, Vol. 21. Seattle: IASP Press, 2001, pp 85–106.

Dray A. Peripheral mediators of pain. In: Dickenson AH, Besson JM (Eds). *The Pharmacology of Pain,* Handbook of Experimental Pharmacology, Vol. 130. Springer-Verlag, 1997, pp 21–42.

Dray A, Perkins MN. Bradykinin and inflammatory pain. *Trends Neurosci* 1993; 16:99–104.

Dray A, Urban L, Dickenson AH. Pharmacology of chronic pain. *Trends Pharmacol Sci* 1994; 15:190–197.

Dubner R, Ruda MA. Activity dependent neuronal plasticity following tissue injury and inflammation. *Trends Neurosci* 1992; 15:96–103.

Eglen RM, Hunter JC, Dray A. Ions in the fire: recent ion-channel research and approaches to pain therapy. *Trends Pharmacol Sci* 1999; 20:337–342.

Fields HL, Heinricher MM, Mason P. Neurotransmitters in nociceptive modulatory circuits. *Annu Rev Neurosci* 1991; 14:219–245.

Fitzgerald GA. COX-2 and beyond: approaches to prostaglandin inhibition in human disease. *Nat Rev Drug Discov* 2003; 2:879–890.

Hill RG. Peripheral analgesic pharmacology. In: Max M (Ed). *Pain 1999—An Updated Review.* Seattle: IASP Press, 1999, pp 391–395.

Hunt SP, Mantyh PW. Molecular basis of pain control. *Nat Rev* 2001; 2:83–91.

Jänig W, Baron R. The role of the sympathetic nervous system in neuropathic pain: clinical observations and animal models. In: Hansson PT, Fields HL, Hill RG, Marchettini P (Eds). *Neuropathic Pain: Pathophysiology and Treatment,* Progress in Pain Research and Management, Vol. 21. Seattle: IASP Press, 2001, pp 125–149.

Julius D, Basbaum AI. Molecular mechanisms of nociception. *Nature* 2001; 413(6852):203–210.

Kiefer W, Dannhardt G. Novel insights and therapeutical applications in the field of inhibitors of COX-2. *Curr Med Chem* 2004; 11:3147–3161.

Machelska H, Binder W, Stein C. Opioid receptors in the periphery. In: Kalso, E, McQuay, HJ, Wiesenfeld-Hallin, Z (Eds). *Opioid Sensitivity of Chronic Noncancer Pain,* Progress in Pain Research and Management, Vol. 14. Seattle: IASP Press, 1999, pp 45–58.

Matthews EA, Dickenson AH. Effects of spinally delivered N- and P-type voltage-dependent calcium channel antagonists on dorsal horn neuronal responses in a rat model of neuropathy. *Pain* 2001; 92:235–246.

McMahon SB, Lewin GR, Wall PD. Central excitability triggered by noxious inputs. *Curr Opin Neurobiol* 1993; 3:602–610.

McQuay HJ, Dickenson AH. Implications of nervous system plasticity for pain management. *Anaesthesia* 1990; 45:101–102.

Meller ST, Gebhart GF. Nitric oxide (NO) and nociceptive processing in the spinal cord. *Pain* 1993; 52:127–136.

Millan MJ. The induction of pain: an integrative review. *Prog Neurobiol* 1999; 57:1–164.

Petersen-Zeitz KR, Basbaum AI. Second messengers the substantia gelatinosa and injury-induced persistent pain. *Pain* 1999; 6(Suppl):S5–S12.

Price DD, Mao J, Mayer DJ. Central neural mechanisms of normal and abnormal pain states. In: Fields HL, Liebeskind LC (Eds). *Pharmacological Approaches to the Treatment of Pain: New Concepts and Critical Issues,* Progress in Pain Research and Management, Vol. 1. Seattle: IASP Press, 1994, pp 61–84.

Rowbotham MC. Efficacy of opioids in neuropathic pain. In: Hansson PT, Fields HL, Hill RG, Marchettini P (Eds). *Neuropathic Pain: Pathophysiology and Treatment,* Progress in Pain Research and Management, Vol. 21. Seattle: IASP Press, 2001, pp 203–213.

Sommer C. Cytokines and neuropathic pain. In: Hansson PT, Fields HL, Hill RG, Marchettini P (Eds). *Neuropathic Pain: Pathophysiology and Treatment,* Progress in Pain Research and Management, Vol. 21. Seattle: IASP Press, 2001, pp 37–62.

Stein C, Schäfer M, Machelska H: Attacking pain at its source: new perspectives on opioids. *Nat Med* 2003; 9:1003–1008.

Suzuki R, Dickenson AH. Neuropathic pain: nerves bursting with excitement. *Neuroreport* 2000; 11:R17–21.

Uhl GR, Childers S, Pasternak G. An opiate receptor gene family reunion. *Trends Neurosci* 1994; 17:89–93.

Vanegas H, Schaible H. Effects of antagonists to high-threshold calcium channels upon spinal mechanisms of pain, hyperalgesia and allodynia. *Pain* 2000; 85:9–18.

Watkins LR, Maier SF. Glia: a novel drug discovery target for clinical pain. *Nat Rev* 2003; 2:973–985.

Waxman S. The molecular pathophysiology of pain: abnormal expression of sodium channel genes and its contribution to hyperexcitability of primary sensory neurons. *Pain* 1999; 6:S133–140.

Woolf CL. A new strategy for the treatment of inflammatory pain. *Drugs* 1994; (Suppl)5:1–9.

Woolf CJ, Doubell TP. The pathophysiology of chronic pain: increased sensitivity to low threshold alpha beta fibre inputs. *Curr Opin Neurobiol* 1994; 4:525–534.

Yaksh TL, Malmberg AB. Interaction of spinal modulatory systems. In: Fields HL, Liebeskind JC (Eds). *Pharmacological Approaches to the Treatment of Pain: New Concepts and Critical Issues,* Progress in Pain Research and Management, Vol. 1. Seattle: IASP Press, 1994, pp 151–171.

Yaksh TL, Noueihed R. The physiology and pharmacology of spinal opiates. *Annu Rev Pharmacol Toxicol* 1985; 25:433–462.

Core Curriculum for Professional Education in Pain, edited by J. Edmond Charlton, IASP Press, Seattle, © 2005.

3

The Development of Pain Systems

I. The development of pain behavior

   A. Know the features of early reflex responses to tactile and noxious stimulation of the body surface in the fetus (Narayanan and Fox 1971) and newborn (Ekholm 1967; Fitzgerald 1999).

   B. Be aware of how cutaneous reflex thresholds, magnitudes, and durations to noxious mechanical and heat stimuli differ in neonates and adults (Fitzgerald 1999; Andrews 2003) and how the response to formalin changes with postnatal age (Teng and Abbott 1998). Understand that prolonged cutaneous sensitization or hyperalgesia lasting days and weeks can be measured in infant rats and humans using cutaneous reflexes (Fitzgerald et al. 1989; Andrews and Fitzgerald 2002; Andrews et al. 2002).

   C. Understand that the inability of human infants to report pain necessitates the use of indirect physiological and behavioral methods to assess the existence and severity of pain, and recognize that there is a lot of individuality of response even at very young ages (Morison et al. 2001; Stevens and Franck 2001). Have a good understanding of the range of methods used to measure human infant pain, including hormonal responses (Giannakoulopoulos et al. 1994); physiological measures such as heart rate variability, crying and palmar sweating, and facial expression or grimaces (Craig et al. 2002); and neurophysiological methods such as flexion reflexes (Andrews 2003). Understand that reflex responses have the advantage of direct parallels with laboratory studies (Fitzgerald and De Lima 2001).

   D. Be aware that such physiological measures are mediated largely subcortically (Oberlander et al. 2002) and cannot be equated with true "pain experience," which requires functional maturation of higher brain centers. Stronger reflexes do not necessarily mean more perceived pain but may be protective and beneficial to the organism.

II. The development of peripheral mechanisms

   A. Know that dorsal root ganglion (DRG) neurons including nociceptors arise from neural crest cells, are committed to their lineages at an early embryonic stage (Anderson 1999; Zirlinger et al. 2002), and are therefore specified independently of their peripheral or central targets. Know that the majority of lumbar DRG cells in the rodent are born before birth in a rostrocaudal wave from E12 (embryonic day 12; gestation period of a rat = 21.5 days) onwards, the peak of large A-cell birth occurring before that of small C cells (Altman and Bayer 1984).

   B. Understand that DRG cell development and the pattern and density of sensory innervation are regulated by access to target-derived neurotrophic factors. Know the effect of neurotrophic factors, nerve growth factor (NGF), neurotrophin-3 (NT-3), brain-derived neurotrophic factor (BDNF), and glial-derived growth factor (GDNF) and their receptor proteins upon the survival and development of sensory neurons (Snider 1994; Lindsay 1996; Ernfors 2001).

   C. Understand that, in the newborn, most nociceptor sensory neurons are dependent on nerve growth factor (NGF) for survival, but that trk expression and neurotrophin dependence change markedly with postnatal age (Bennett et al. 1996). Be aware that independent of cell survival, neurotrophins also regulate axon outgrowth (Davies 2000; Markus et al. 2002), physiological receptor properties (Koltzenburg 1999), and target innervation density (Albers et al. 1994; LeMaster et al. 1999).

D. Understand the timing and pattern of peripheral and central outgrowth and target innervation of DRG cell processes (Jackman and Fitzgerald 2000; Wang and Scott 2000). Know that from the outset each DRG innervates characteristic skin dermatomes and projects in a precise somatotopic pattern in the dorsal horn using a number of extracellular molecular cues (Dickson 2002). Understand that DRGs are not matched to particular skin targets and that while the peripheral target skin influences the pattern of central nervous system projections, it does not direct cutaneous axons to specific populations of neurons in the dorsal horn (Wang and Scott 2002). Know that skin is initially hyperinnervated and that the exuberant epidermal innervation gradually retracts with postnatal age (Jackman and Fitzgerald 2000; Peters et al. 2002).

E. Understand the process of postnatal physiological maturation of nociceptors and other cutaneous sensory terminals. Know that changes in conduction velocity of afferent fibers, action potential shape, receptor transduction, firing frequencies, and receptive field properties take place over the postnatal period (Fitzgerald 1987b; Fitzgerald and Fulton 1992; Koltzenburg et al. 1997; Woodbury and Koerber 2003).

F. Know that many channels, receptors, and neurotransmitters expressed by DRG cells are developmentally regulated (Alvares and Fitzgerald 1999), such as vanilloid (TRPV1) receptors, TTX-resistant Na channels, and opioid receptors (Beland et al. 2001; Benn et al. 2001; Guo et al. 2001), and be aware of the potential functional consequences of such regulation.

III. The development of central dorsal horn mechanisms

A. Know that the postnatal period is a time of considerable synaptic growth and reorganization in the dorsal horn of the spinal cord. Be aware that some immature A fibers extend dorsally up into laminae II and I, a feature that is not seen in adults, and that over the first three postnatal weeks these fibers gradually withdraw to deeper laminae (Beggs et al. 2002; Woodbury and Koerber 2003). Understand that C fibers grow specifically to laminae I and II (Fitzgerald 1987a), and so for a considerable postnatal period these laminae are occupied by both A- and C-fiber terminals. Understand that this postnatal laminar reorganization of primary afferent terminals involves a competitive interaction between A and C fibers (Torsney et al. 2000) and is an NMDA-mediated, activity-dependent process (Beggs et al. 2002).

B. Know the pattern and timing of the birth and maturation of projection neurons and interneurons in the dorsal horn, and be aware that projection neurons are born and mature in advance of local interneurons (Altman and Bayer 1994; Bice and Beal 1997a,b). Know that the neurogenesis of supraspinal projection neurons depends upon axon length such that neurons with the longest axons projecting to rostral brain centers complete neurogenesis before neurons with shorter axons, which project only to the caudal brainstem (Bice and Beal 1997a,b). Understand that the specification of these neurons is under homeobox gene control (Gross et al. 2002).

C. Understand how the properties of cutaneous afferent evoked spike activity in the dorsal horn evoked by electrical or natural stimulation alter with development (Fitzgerald and Jennings 1999; Bardoni 2000; Torsney and Fitzgerald 2002; Baccei et al. 2003) and how afferent terminal reorganization may influence these physiological responses (Park et al. 1999; Beggs et al. 2002). Be aware that A-fiber activity produces sensitization and c-fos activation in the neonatal but not the adult dorsal horn (Jennings and Fitzgerald 1996, 1998). Understand that while C-fiber-evoked responses are present from birth, they mature over the postnatal period (Torsney and Fitzgerald 2002; Baccei et al. 2003). Understand that convergence of responses in dorsal horn cells increases and that the size of the peripheral cutaneous receptive field of dorsal horn cells decreases with age (Fitzgerald and Jennings 1999, Torsney and Fitzgerald 2002).

D. Know that some inhibitory mechanisms in the dorsal horn are immature at birth and that descending inhibition does not begin to become functionally effective until postnatal day 10 in the rat (Fitzgerald and Koltzenburg 1986; Boucher et al. 1998; van Praag and Frenk 1991). Understand how this delayed inhibitory maturation might influence central pain processing (Fitzgerald 1999).

E. Be aware that many neurotransmitter receptor systems involved in pain pathways are developmentally regulated (Fitzgerald 1997; Alvares and Fitzgerald 1999; Bardoni 2000). Know that spinal cord NMDA receptors change their expression pattern, affinity for NMDA, and subunit composition during spinal cord development. Understand that "silent synapses" are found in the immature dorsal horn. These are NMDA-only synapses with limited function at resting membrane potentials; they disappear with age with the onset of colocalization of AMPA and NMDA receptors (Baba et al. 2001). Be aware that expression and distribution of dorsal horn neuropeptide receptors, including NK1 receptors, changes over the postnatal period (Kar and Quirion 1995). Know that dorsal horn GABA receptors undergo considerable postnatal alterations, switching from depolarizing to hyperpolarizing effects (Reichling et al. 1994; Ben-Ari 2002) and shifting their co-release properties with glycine (Keller et al. 2001).

IV. Development of nociceptive connections in higher centers

A. Know the pattern and timing of growth of axon projections to the thalamus in rodents and humans (Bicknell and Beal 1984; Fitzgerald 1999). Understand that many neonatal thalamocortical synapses are silent, consisting of NMDA receptors only, and are converted to functional synapses (NMDA and AMPA receptors) by activity-dependent mechanisms at days 8–9 (Isaac et al. 1997).

B. Understand that cortical synaptic circuitry develops rapidly in the second postnatal week (O'Leary et al. 1994; Stern et al. 2001). Know that neonatal somatosensory cortical cells have larger receptive fields than adults and that evoked potentials from the forepaw in the rat somatosensory cortex are not mature until 2 weeks.

C. Understand that the development of neural circuits is influenced by sensory experience during restricted critical periods early in life and that this phenomenon is especially evident in the developing cortex (O'Leary et al. 1994; Fox 2002; Kaas and Catania 2002). Understand that the delayed maturation of inhibitory processes, occurring several weeks after excitatory connections, may be a general pattern in the developing brain.

D. Be aware of how little we know of the developing cortex in relation to pain and of the development of attention, memory, and cognitive factors in relation to the perception of pain in infants and children (Anand and Carr 1989; Fitzgerald 1999). Understand that analogous to the experience-driven development of sensory systems, the functional maturation of limbic circuits is significantly influenced by early socio-emotional experience, which will also affect pain perception (Pryce et al. 2002).

V. Mechanisms of persistent pain in infants

A. Understand that the mechanisms of chronic inflammatory and neuropathic pain in infancy and childhood will be superimposed upon a nervous system that is still immature and where sensory pathways are still undergoing synaptogenesis and tuning of connections, as described above (Fitzgerald and Beggs 2001; Fitzgerald and Howard 2003).

B. Be aware of the value of studying immature animal models of persistent inflammatory pain. Know that behavioral studies suggest that inflammatory hyperalgesia is less pronounced in young animals (Jiang and Gebhart 1998; Marsh et al. 1999). Understand the underlying developmental neurobiology of central sensitization and recognize that the ability of dorsal horn cells to display enlargement of receptive fields, increased spontaneous activity, and enhanced responses to mechanical, thermal, and electrical stimulation differs in the newborn and adult cord (Torsney and Fitzgerald 2002).

C. Understand that the epidemiology of neuropathic pain in infants and children is not well understood (Olsson and Berde 1993; Anand and Birch 2002). Be aware that the effects of nerve injury differ in neonates and adults. Know that peripheral nerve injury during a critical neonatal period causes extensive death of axotomized DRG cells, which can be temporarily prevented by access to neurotrophins (Alvares and Fitzgerald 1999; Ernfors 2001), and has been linked with low levels of heat shock proteins, such as Hsp27 (Lewis et al. 1999).

    D.   Understand that neonatal axotomy also results in substantial alterations within the spinal cord, such as withdrawal of the central terminals of damaged axons and sprouting of adjacent, intact axon collaterals into the denervated region (Fitzgerald 1999), which disrupts the somatotopic organization of central terminals within the dorsal horn (Shortland and Fitzgerald 1991). Know that the resulting rearrangement of connections in the developing rat nervous system is not confined to dorsal horn cells but is found in higher levels of the nervous system including the cortex (Kaas et al. 1983). Understand that although this phenomenon could be a useful compensatory device to restore sensory input from an area of the body surface in which it has been lost, the effects may be detrimental and may trigger chronic pain.

VI.   Long-term effects of neonatal pain

    A.   Know about the animal models in which tissue injury or repeated noxious stimuli applied in infancy lead to changes in later sensory behavior and spinal cord connections (Fitzgerald and Walker 2003). Be aware that neonatal skin wounding leads to local sprouting of cutaneous sensory axons and a long-lasting expansion of dorsal horn cell receptive fields (Torsney and Fitzgerald 2003). Understand that while these neural changes may support reports of long-term effects of human infant pain, the complexity of these effects in humans and the need for careful design and interpretation have been emphasized (Grunau 2000).

REFERENCES

Albers KM, Wright DE, Davis BM. Overexpression of nerve growth factor in epidermis of transgenic mice causes hypertrophy of the peripheral nervous system. *J Neurosci* 1994; 14:1422–1432.

Altman J, Bayer SA. The development of the rat spinal cord. *Adv Anat Embryol Cell Biol* 1984; 85:1–164.

Alvares D, Fitzgerald M. Building blocks of pain: the regulation of key molecules in spinal sensory neurones during development and following peripheral axotomy. *Pain* 1999; 6(Suppl):S71–85.

Anand KJ, Carr DB. The neuroanatomy, neurophysiology, and neurochemistry of pain, stress, and analgesia in newborns and children. *Pediatr Clin North Am* 1989; 36:795–822.

Anand P, Birch R. Restoration of sensory function and lack of long-term chronic pain syndromes after brachial plexus injury in human neonates. *Brain* 2002; 125:113–122.

Anderson DJ. Lineages and transcription factors in the specification of vertebrate primary sensory neurons *Curr Opin Neurobiol* 1999; 9:517–524

Andrews K. Neurophysiological measures of infant pain. In: Schechter N, Berde C, Yaster M (Eds). *Pain in Children and Adolescents.* Lippincott, Williams & Wilkins, 2003.

Andrews K, Fitzgerald M. Wound sensitivity as a measure of analgesic effects following surgery in human neonates and infants. *Pain* 2002; 99:185–192.

Andrews KA, Desai D, Dhillon HK, Wilcox DT, Fitzgerald M. Abdominal sensitivity in the first year of life: comparison of infants with and without prenatally-diagnosed unilateral hydronephrosis. *Pain* 2002; 100:35–46.

Baba H, Doubell TP, Moore KA, Woolf CJ. Silent NMDA receptor-mediated synapses are developmentally regulated in the dorsal horn of the rat spinal cord. *J Neurophysiol* 2000; 83:955–962.

Baccei ML, Bardoni R, Fitzgerald M. Development of nociceptive synaptic inputs to the neonatal dorsal horn: glutamate release by capsaicin and menthol. *J Physiol* 2003; 549(Pt 1):231–242.

Bardoni R. Excitatory synaptic transmission in neonatal dorsal horn: NMDA and ATP receptors. *News Physiol Sci* 2000; 16:95–100.

Beggs S, Torsney C, Drew LJ, Fitzgerald M. The postnatal reorganization of primary afferent input and dorsal horn cell receptive fields in the rat spinal cord is an activity-dependent process. *Eur J Neurosci* 2002; 16:1249–1258.

Beland B, Fitzgerald M. Mu- and delta-opioid receptors are downregulated in the largest diameter primary sensory neurons during postnatal development in rats. *Pain* 2001; 90:143–150.

Ben-Ari Y. Excitatory actions of GABA during development: the nature of the nurture (review). *Nat Rev Neurosci* 2002; 3(9):728–739.

Benn SC, Costigan M, Tate S, Fitzgerald M, Woolf CJ. Developmental expression of the TTX-resistant voltage-gated sodium channels $Na_v1.8$ (SNS) and $Na_v1.9$ (SNS2) in primary sensory neurons. *J Neurosci* 2001 21:6077–6085.

Bennett DL, Averill S, Clary DO, Priestley JV, McMahon SB. Postnatal changes in the expression of the trkA high-affinity NGF receptor in primary sensory neurons. *Eur J Neurosci* 1996; 8:2204–2208.

Bice TN, Beal JA. Quantitative and neurogenic analysis of the total population and subpopulations of neurons defined by axon projection in the superficial dorsal horn of the rat lumbar spinal cord. *J Comp Neurol* 1997a; 388:550–564

Bice TN, Beal JA. Quantitative and neurogenic analysis of neurons with supraspinal projections in the superficial dorsal horn of the rat lumbar spinal cord. *J Comp Neurol* 1997b; 388:565–574.

Bicknell HRJ, Beal JA. Axonal and dendritic development of substantia gelatinosa neurons in the lumbosacral spinal cord of the rat. *J Comp Neurol* 1984; 226:508–522.

Boucher T, Jennings E, Fitzgerald M. The onset of diffuse noxious inhibitory controls (DNIC) in postnatal rat pups—a c-Fos study. *Neurosci Lett* 1998; 257:9–12.

Craig KD, Korol CT, Pillai RR, et al. Challenges of judging pain in vulnerable infants. *Clin Perinatol* 2002; 29(3):445–457.

Davies AM. Neurotrophins: neurotrophic modulation of neurite growth. *Curr Biol* 2000; 10:R198–200.

Dickson BJ. Molecular mechanisms of axon guidance. *Science* 2002; 298:1959–1964.

Ekholm J. Postnatal changes in cutaneous reflexes and in the discharge pattern of cutaneous and articular sense organs. *Acta Physiol Scand* 1967; (Suppl 297):1–130.

Ernfors P. Local and target-derived actions of neurotrophins during peripheral nervous system development. *Cell Mol Life Sci* 2001; 58:1036–1044.

Fitzgerald M. The prenatal growth of fine diameter afferents into the rat spinal cord—a transganglionic study *J Comp Neurol* 1987a; 261:98–104.

Fitzgerald M. Cutaneous primary afferent properties in the hindlimb of the neonatal rat. *J Physiol* 1987b; 383:79–92.

Fitzgerald M. Neonatal pharmacology of pain. In: Besson J-M, Dickenson AH (Eds). *Handbook of Experimental Pharmacology.* Heidelberg: Springer-Verlag, 1997, pp 447–465.

Fitzgerald M. The developmental neurobiology of pain. In: *Textbook of Pain,* 4th ed. Wall PD, Melzack R (Eds). Churchill Livingstone, 1999, pp 235–252.

Fitzgerald M, Beggs S. The neurobiology of pain: developmental aspects. *Neuroscientist* 2001; 7:246–257.

Fitzgerald M, De Lima J. Hyperalgesia and allodynia in infants. In: Finley GA, McGrath PJ, (Eds). *Acute and Procedure Pain in Infants and Children,* Progress in Pain Research and Management, Vol. 20. Seattle: IASP Press, 2001, pp 1–12.

Fitzgerald M, Fulton BP. The physiological properties of developing sensory neurons. In: Scott SA (Ed). *Sensory Neurons: Diversity, Development and Plasticity.* Oxford: Oxford University Press, 1992; pp 287–306.

Fitzgerald M, Howard R. The neurobiological basis of pediatric pain. In: Schechter N, Berde C, Yaster (Eds). *Pain in Children and Adolescents,* 2nd ed. Lippincott, Williams & Wilkins, 2003.

Fitzgerald M, Jennings E. The postnatal development of spinal sensory processing. *Proc Natl Acad Sci USA* 1999; 96:7719–7722.

Fitzgerald M, Koltzenburg M. The functional development of descending inhibitory pathways in the dorsolateral funiculus of the newborn rat spinal cord. *Dev Brain Res* 1986; 24:261–270.

Fitzgerald M, Walker S. The role of activity in developing pain pathways. In: Dostrovsky JO, Carr DB, Koltzenburg M (Eds). *Proceedings of the 10th World Congress on Pain,* Progress in Pain Research and Management, Vol. 24. IASP Press, 2003, pp 185–196.

Fitzgerald M, Millard C, MacIntosh N. Cutaneous hypersensitivity following peripheral tissue damage in newborn infants and its reversal with topical anaesthesia. *Pain* 1989; 39:31–36.

Fox K. Anatomical pathways and molecular mechanisms for plasticity in the barrel cortex. *Neuroscience* 2002; 111(4):799–814.

Giannakoulopoulos X, Sepulveda W, Kourkis P, Glover V, Fisk NM. Fetal plasma cortisol and beta-endorphin response to intrauterine needling. *Lancet* 1994; 344:77–81.

Gross MK, Dottori M, Goulding M. Lbx1 specifies somatosensory association interneurons in the dorsal spinal cord. *Neuron* 2002; 34:535–549.

Grunau RE. Long-term consequences of pain in human neonates. *Pain Res Clin Manage* 2000; 10:101–134.

Guo A, Simone DA, Stone LS, et al. Developmental shift of vanilloid receptor 1 (VR1) terminals into deeper regions of the superficial dorsal horn: correlation with a shift from TrkA to Ret expression by dorsal root ganglion neurons. *Eur J Neurosci* 2001; 14:293–304.

Isaac, JT, Crair MC, Nicoll RA, Malenka RC. Silent synapses during development of thalamocortical inputs. *Neuron* 1997; 18:269–280.

Jackman A, Fitzgerald M. Development of peripheral hindlimb and central spinal cord innervation by subpopulations of dorsal root ganglion cells in the embryonic rat. *J Comp Neurol* 2000; 418:281–298.

Jennings E, Fitzgerald M. C-fos can be induced in the neonatal rat spinal cord by both noxious and innocuous peripheral stimulation. *Pain* 1996; 68:301–306.

Jennings E, Fitzgerald M. Postnatal changes in responses of rat dorsal horn cells to afferent stimulation: a fibre-induced sensitization. *J Physiol (Lond)* 1998; 509:859–868.

Jiang MC, Gebhart GF. Development of mustard oil-induced hyperalgesia in rats. *Pain* 1998; 77:305–313.

Kaas JH, Catania KC. How do features of sensory representations develop? *Bioessays* 2002; 24:334–343.

Kaas JH, Merzenich MM, Killackey HP. The reorganization of somatosensory cortex following peripheral nerve damage in adult and developing mammals. *Annu Rev Neurosci* 1983; 6:325–356.

Kar S, Quirion R. Neuropeptide receptors in developing and adult rat spinal cord: an in vitro quantitative autoradiography study of calcitonin gene-related peptide, neurokinins, mu-opioid, galanin, somatostatin, neurotensin and vasoactive intestinal polypeptide receptors. *J Comp Neurol* 1995; 354:253–281.

Keller AF, Coull JA, Chery N, Poisbeau P, De Koninck Y. Region-specific developmental specialization of GABA-glycine cosynapses in laminas I–II of the rat spinal dorsal horn. *J Neurosci* 2001; 21:7871–7880.

Koltzenburg M. The changing sensitivity in the life of the nociceptor. *Pain* 1999; (Suppl 6):S93–S102.

Koltzenburg M, Stucky CL, Lewin GR. Receptive properties of mouse sensory neurons innervating hairy skin. *J Neurophysiol* 1997; 78:1841–1850.

LeMaster AM, Krimm RF, Davis BM, et al. Overexpression of brain-derived neurotrophic factor enhances sensory innervation and selectively increases neuron number. *J Neurosci* 1999; 19:5919–5931.

Lewis SE, Mannion RJ, White FA, et al. A role for HSP27 in sensory neuron survival. *J Neurosci* 1999; 19:8945–8953.

Lindsay RM. Role of neurotrophins and trk receptors in the development and maintenance of sensory neurons: an overview. *Philos Trans R Soc Lond B Biol Sci* 1996; 351:365–374.

Markus A, Patel TD, Snider WD. Neurotrophic factors and axonal growth. *Curr Opin Neurobiol* 2002; 12:523–531.

Marsh D, Dickenson A, Hatch D, Fitzgerald M. Epidural opioid analgesia in infant rats. II: Responses to carrageenan and capsaicin. *Pain* 1999; 82:33–38.

Morison SJ, Grunau RE, Oberlander TF, Whitfield MF. Relations between behavioral and cardiac autonomic reactivity to acute pain in preterm neonates. *Clin J Pain* 2001; 17:350–358.

Narayanan CH, Fox MV, Hamburger V. Prenatal development of spontaneous and evoked activity in the rat. *Behaviour* 1971; 40:100–134.

Oberlander TF, Grunau RE, Fitzgerald C, Whitfield MF. Does parenchymal brain injury affect biobehavioral pain responses in very low birth weight infants at 32 weeks' postconceptional age? *Pediatrics* 2002; 110:570–576.

O'Leary DD, Ruff NL, Dyck RH. Development, critical period plasticity, and adult reorganizations of mammalian somatosensory systems. *Curr Opin Neurobiol* 1994; 4:535–544.

Olsson G, Berde CB. Neuropathic pain in children and adolescents. In: Schechter N, Berde CB, Yaster M (Eds). *Pain in Infants, Children and Adolescents*. Baltimore: Williams and Wilkins, 1993; 473–494.

Park JS, Nakatsuka T, Nagata K, Higashi H, Yoshimura M. Reorganization of the primary afferent termination in the rat spinal dorsal horn during post-natal development. *Brain Res Dev Brain Res* 1999; 113:29–36.

Peters EM, Botchkarev VA, Muller-Rover S, et al. Developmental timing of hair follicle and dorsal skin innervation in mice. *J Comp Neurol* 2002; 448:28–52.

Pryce CR, Ruedi-Bettschen D, Dettling AC, Feldon J. Early life stress: long-term physiological impact in rodents and primates. *News Physiol Sci* 2002; 17:150–155

Reichling DB, Kyrozis A, Wang J, MacDermott A. Mechanisms of GABA and glycine depolarization induced calcium transients in rat dorsal horn neurons. *J Physiol* 1994; 476:411–421.

Shortland P, Fitzgerald M. Functional connections formed by saphenous nerve terminal sprouts in the dorsal horn following neonatal sciatic nerve section. *Eur J Neurosci* 1991 3:383–396.

Snider WD. Functions of neurotrophins during nervous system development: what the knockouts are teaching us. *Cell* 1994; 77:627–638.

Stern EA, Maravall M, Svoboda K. Rapid development and plasticity of layer 2/3 maps in rat barrel cortex in vivo. *Neuron* 2001; 31(2):305–315.

Stevens BJ, Franck LS. Assessment and management of pain in neonates. *Paediatr Drugs* 2001; 3:539–558.

Teng CJ, Abbott FV. The formalin test: a dose-response analysis at three developmental stages. *Pain* 1998; 76:337–347.

Torsney C, Fitzgerald M. Age-dependent effects of peripheral inflammation on the electrophysiological properties of neonatal rat dorsal horn neurons. *J Neurophysiol* 2002; 87:1311–1317.

Torsney C, Fitzgerald M. Spinal dorsal horn cell receptive field size is increased in adult rats following neonatal hindpaw skin injury. *J Physiol* 2003; 550(Pt 1):255–261.

Torsney C, Meredith-Middleton J, Fitzgerald M. Neonatal capsaicin treatment prevents the normal postnatal withdrawal of A fibres from lamina II without affecting fos responses to innocuous peripheral stimulation. *Brain Res Dev Brain Res* 2000; 121:55–65.

Van Praag H, Frenk H. The development of stimulation-produced analgesia (SPA) in the rat. *Dev Brain Res* 1991; 64:71–76.

Wang G, Scott SA. The "waiting period" of sensory and motor axons in early chick hindlimb: its role in axon pathfinding and neuronal maturation. *J Neurosci* 2000; 20:5358–5366.

Wang G, Scott SA. Development of "Normal" dermatomes and somatotopic maps by "Abnormal" populations of cutaneous neurons. *Dev Biol* 2002; 251:424–433.

Woodbury CJ, Koerber HR. Widespread projections from myelinated nociceptors throughout the substantia gelatinosa provide novel insights into neonatal hypersensitivity. *J Neurosci* 2003; 23:601–610.

Zirlinger M, Lo L, McMahon J, McMahon AP, Anderson DJ. Transient expression of the bhlh factor neurogenin-2 marks a subpopulation of neural crest cells biased for a sensory but not a neuronal fate. *Proc Natl Acad Sci* 2002; 99:8084–8089.

Core Curriculum for Professional Education in Pain, edited by J. Edmond Charlton, IASP Press, Seattle, © 2005.

4

Designing, Reporting, and Interpreting Clinical Research Studies about Treatments for Pain: Evidence-Based Medicine

I. Understand the basics of critical appraisal of the literature and evidence-based medicine.

  A. Evidence-based medicine (Moore et al. 2003, Straus et al. 2005)

   1. Formulate an answerable question.
   2. Track down the best evidence.
   3. Critically appraise the evidence.
   4. Integrate with clinical expertise and patient values.
   5. Know the levels of evidence, and the advantages and disadvantages of each (Oxford University 2001).

    Level 1a—Multiple RCTs (with narrow confidence intervals)
    Level 1b—Individual RCT (with narrow confidence interval)
    Level 2a—Multiple cohort studies (including low-quality RCT; e.g., <80% follow-up)
    Level 2b—Individual cohort study (including low-quality RCT; e.g., <80% follow-up)
    Level 3a—Multiple case-control studies
    Level 3b—Individual case-control study
    Level 4—Case series (and poor quality cohort and case-control studies)
    Level 5—Expert opinion

    Note: Population-based cross-sectional studies measure only a single point in time and cannot be used to estimate the effect of therapy.

   6. Critical evaluation of actual practice.

  C. Criteria for RCT quality (Jadad and McQuay 1993)

   1. Does it include the use of words such as randomly, random, and randomization?
   2. Was the study described as double-blind?
   3. Was there a description of withdrawals and dropouts?

  D. Meta-analysis (Berlin et al. 1989)

   1. Advantages and pitfalls of these analyses
   2. Concept of effect size and confidence intervals
   3. Effect of study design on the results

  E. Systematic reviews (Cochrane Collaboration 2005)

II. Understand general principles of valid clinical research.

  A. Epidemiology (Rothman 2002; Coggon et al. 2003)

   1. Study designs: advantages and disadvantages of each type (survey, case-control, cohort, RCT)
   2. Risks in any analysis

    a. Bias
    b. Confounding
    c. Interaction of effects (effect modification)

    3. Control groups

       a. Placebo control group
       b. Active comparator
       c. No treatment control group

    4. Prospective vs. retrospective research designs
    5. Outcomes

       a. Final measured value
       b. Change in value (final minus baseline value)
       c. Percentage change in value (change divided by baseline value)
       d. Odds ratio
       e. Relative risk
       f. Absolute risk difference

B. Measurement and questionnaires (Streiner and Norman 2003)

    1 What do you want to learn?
    2. Conceptual framework, types of questions, type of scale
    3. Reliability, validity, responsiveness
    4. Sensitivity and specificity
    5. Positive and negative predictive value

C. Biostatistics (Rosner 1999)

    1. Probability

       a. Binomial distribution
       b. Sample size and power analysis

    2. Summary values

       a. Measures of effect size

          i.   Group means or medians
          ii. Proportion of responders (e.g. 30% death rate)

       b. Statistical significance

          i.   95% confidence intervals (best choice)
          ii. *P* value (most common but not as useful)
          iii. Other terms: standard deviation, standard error

       c. Attributing meaning to the results

          i.   Statistical significance (i.e., *P* value) is necessary, but it only tells you if it happened by chance, not how big the effect is.
          ii. The size of the effect tells you if the finding is important or trivial (e.g., How much change was there in pain score? Is the patient better or not? How many patients can we expect to get better?).

III. Understand that the analysis will affect the clinical applicability of a study.

A. Continuous vs. count or proportions statistics

B. Chi-square analysis

C. *t*-test analysis

D. Logistic and linear regression

E. Additive vs. synergistic effects of combination treatments

F. Multiple endpoints and the problem of "multiplicity"

IV.   Understand basic components of a clinical trial (Pocock 1983, Piantadosi 1997; Max and Lynn 2004).

  A.   Types of clinical trial designs

    1.   Structure

        a.   Parallel group designs with two or more groups
        b.   Crossover designs with two or more treatment periods (or *N*-of-1 designs within an individual), usually with a washout period between exposures to reduce the influence of carryover effects
        c.   Factorial designs
        d.   Sequential designs
        e.   Assay sensitivity: need a treatment that is known to work (i.e., an active comparator)
        f.   Dose-response relationships
        g.   Testing superiority vs. equivalence of treatments

    2.   Phases of clinical trials:

        a.   Phase I: Initial safety-toxicity trial; usually done in normals, except for cancer chemotherapy trials
        b.   Phase II: Dose-finding trials, in normals or in those with disease
        c.   Phase III: A pivotal clinical trial in the target population allows for regulatory approval; usually more than one pivotal Phase III trial is required
        d.   Phase IV: Post-marketing safety or secondary use trials

    3.   Efficacy vs. effectiveness

        a.   Efficacy: Does the treatment work in the tightly controlled clinical trial setting? Can have a homogenous group of likely responders.
        b.   Effectiveness: Does the treatment work in the real world, where the patient population and dosing may vary?

  B.   Important components of the study methods

    1.   Randomization
    2.   Control groups
    3.   Blinding and threats to the integrity of the blinding (e.g. from side effects)
    4.   Patient selection: inclusion and exclusion criteria
    5.   Informed consent
    6.   Single vs. multiple sites
    7.   Primary vs. secondary endpoints
    8.   Duration of the trial: treatment period, follow-up period
    9.   Subgroup analyses; covariates
    10. Dropouts
    11. Assessment of adverse effects
    12. Rescue therapy
    13. Concomitant treatments
    14. Data and safety monitoring plan
    15. Role of the funding source and potential biases introduced
    16. General ethical considerations
    17. Analysis (general issues to consider)

        a.   Much more than a statistical question; depends on the underlying biology, not just the data values
        b.   Biology leads to a question, which leads to a hypothesis, which leads to an analysis
        c.   Must do an intention-to-treat analysis for unbiased estimate of outcome

V.   Understand special features of the study of pain (Farrar and Halpern 2003).

  A.   Pain is always a subjective experience

B. Behavior and function do not always match pain report and are important features (Fordyce et al 1984; Turk and Okifuji 1997)

C. Multiple components of pain: intensity, unpleasantness, specific qualities (e.g. burning, allodynia), location, relief, and temporal aspects (e.g., onset of relief, duration of relief) (Backonja and Galer 1998)

D. Controversies in the determinants of abnormality in sensation (Verdugo et al. 2004)

E. How to determine if an effect is clinically important to patients (Farrar 2000)

F. Understand that factors other than pain can affect the report of pain

G. Common symptoms associated with the report of pain (e.g., sleep disturbance, fatigue, depression, and anxiety) and their influence on the study of pain

H. Outcome domains and measures that are important in pain studies (IMMPACT 2005): not only pain, but also, for example, physical and emotional functioning

I. Differences in the study requirements of medications, procedures, and other therapies

J. Studies of acute and chronic pain must be designed differently

K. Placebo effect (Feinstein 2002; Hrobjartsson 2002)

   1. Uses of inert vs. active placebos

   2. Ethical aspects of using placebos in pain clinical trials

      a. Special issues in acute pain trials
      b. Special issues in nonpharmacological trials (e.g., placebo and other comparison groups)
      c. Special methods for study

   3. Complementary and alternative therapies
   4. Enrichment studies
   5. Add-on designs
   6. Mechanism-based treatments

REFERENCES

Backonja MM, Galer BS. Pain assessment and evaluation of patients who have neuropathic pain. *Neurol Clin* 1998; 16:775–790.

Berlin JA, Laird NM, Sacks HS, Chalmers TC. A comparison of statistical methods for combining event rates from clinical trials. *Stat Med* 1989; 8:141–151.

Cochrane Collaboration. 2005. Available at: www.cochrane.org/reviews/index.htm. Accessed May 31, 2005.

Coggon D, Rose GA, Barker DJP. *Epidemiology for the Uninitiated,* 5th ed. London: BMJ Publishing Group, 2003.

Farrar JT. What is clinically meaningful? Outcome measures in pain clinical trials. *Clin J Pain* 2000; 16S:106–110.

Farrar JT, Halpern SD. Understanding clinical trials in pain research. In: Bruera E, Portenoy RK (Eds). *Cancer Pain: Assessment and Management.* Cambridge: Cambridge University Press, 2003.

Feinstein AR. Post-therapeutic response and therapeutic "style": re-formulating the "placebo effect." *J Clin Epidemiol* 2002; 55:427–429.

Fordyce WE, Lansky D, Calsyn DA, et al. Pain measurement and pain behavior. *Pain* 1984; 18:53–69.

Hrobjartsson A. What are the main methodological problems in the estimation of placebo effects? *J Clin Epidemiol* 2002; 55:430–435.

IMMPACT. *Initiative on Methods, Measurement, and Pain Assessment in Clinical Trials.* Available at: www.immpact.org. Accessed May 31, 2005.

Jadad AR, McQuay HJ. A high-yield strategy to identify randomized controlled trials for systematic reviews. *Online J Curr Clin Trials* 1993; No. 33.

Max M, Lynn J (Eds). *Symptoms Research: Methods and Opportunity.* Available at: painconsortium.nih.gov/symptomresearch. Accessed August 11, 2005.

Moore A, Edwards J, Barden J, McQuay H. *Bandolier's Little Book of Pain.* Oxford: Oxford University Press, 2003.

Oxford University. *Oxford Centre for Evidence-based Medicine Levels of Evidence, 2001.* Available at: www.cebm.net/levels_of_evidence.asp#top. Accessed May 31, 2005.

Piantadosi S. *Clinical Trials: A Methodologic Perspective,* Vol. 323. Hoboken, NJ: Wiley & Sons, 1997.

Pocock S J. *Clinical Trials: A Practical Approach.* Chichester; New York: John Wiley & Sons, 1983.

Rosner B. *Fundamentals of Biostatistics.* Pacific Grove, CA: Duxbury Press, 1999.

Rothman KJ. *Epidemiology: An Introduction.* New York: Oxford University Press, 2002.

Straus SE, Richardson WS, Glasziou P, Haynes RB. *Evidence-Based Medicine: How to Practice and Teach EBM.* Edinburgh: Churchill Livingstone, 2005.

Streiner D, Norman GH. *Health Measurement Scales: A Practical Guide to Their Development and Use.* New York: Oxford University Press, 2003.

Turk DC, Okifuji A. Evaluating the role of physical, operant, cognitive, and affective factors in the pain behaviors of chronic pain patients. *Behav Modif* 1997; 21:259–280.

Verdugo RJ, Bell LA, Campero M, et al. Spectrum of cutaneous hyperalgesias/allodynias in neuropathic pain patients. *Acta Neurol Scand* 2004; 110:368–376.

Core Curriculum for Professional Education in Pain, edited by J. Edmond Charlton, IASP Press, Seattle, © 2005.

5

Animal Models of Pain and Ethics of Animal Experimentation

I.   Animal models of pain (Le Bars et al. 2001)

    A.   Know criteria that define useful and ethical animal models of pain.

    B.   Know the characteristics and uses of the following animal models of pain:

        1.   Tail or paw withdrawal to thermal stimulation (e.g., tail flick test)
        2.   Hot plate test
        3.   Assessing mechanical sensitivity (e.g., von Frey filament stimulation, Randall-Selitto test)
        4.   Tooth pulp stimulation
        5.   Paw or intra articular injections of yeast, formalin, carrageenan, adjuvant, etc.
        6   Intramuscular injection of irritant
        7.   Intraperitoneal injections of irritant solutions
        8.   Intramedullary injection of osteolytic sarcoma cells into bone
        9.   Hollow organ distension
        10. Skin incision
        11. Constriction or compression of peripheral or spinal nerves or roots
        12. Partial or complete transection of peripheral or spinal nerves or roots

    C.   Know which tests measure changes in reflexes and which measure changes in behavior; know the central nervous system (CNS) level of organization of the response and the extent to which sensory and motor components contribute to interpretation of results.

    D.   Know which tests model tonic pain, phasic pain, visceral pain, neuropathic pain, inflammation, or other pain conditions (Mason et al. 1985; Bennett and Xie 1988; Ness and Gebhart 1988; Hargreaves et al. 1988).

    E.   Know the extent to which the model and pathology (if present) replicate a pain condition in humans, and the extent to which treatments predict application to humans. Know whether the model conforms to ethical guidelines for animal use, and why or why not (see below).

II. Ethics of animal experimentation (IASP 1983; Caplan 1986; Fox and Mickley 1987; Dubner and Ren 1999).

    A.   Understand moral and ethical issues and arguments associated with the use of animals for experimentation.

    B.   Understand and subscribe to the need to justify the use of animals to both the scientific and nonscien-tific communities.

    C.   Know how to design experiments that minimize the numbers of animals used (know how to deter-mine the required number), that maximize statistical inferences, and that maximize the recording of variables relevant to the assessment of pain experienced by the animals.

    D.   Know how to employ a nociceptive stimulus or condition (e.g., inflammation) that is minimal in in-tensity and duration (tested on the investigator when possible) so as to shorten the duration of an ex-periment consistent with the attainment of justifiable, ethical research objectives.

E.   Know reasons why unanesthetized animals should not be minimally exposed to nociceptive stimuli from which they cannot escape, or which they cannot avoid or terminate, and why pharmacologically paralyzed animals also should be anesthetized or rendered neurosurgically insensate.

F.   Know the International Association for the Study of Pain (1983) guidelines establishing ethical standards for animal experimentation.

REFERENCES

Bennett GJ, Xie Y K. A peripheral mononeuropathy in rat that produces disorders of pain sensation like those seen in man. *Pain* 1988; 33:87–108.

Caplan A. Moral community and the responsibility of scientists. *Acta Physiol Scand Suppl* 1986; 128:(554)78–90.

Dubner R, Ren K. Assessing transient and persistent pain in animals. In: Wall PD, Melzack R (Eds). *Textbook of Pain.* Edinburgh: Churchill Livingstone, 1999, pp 359–369.

Fox MW, Mickley LD (Eds). *Advances in Animal Wel-fare Science.* Dordrecht: Kluwer Academic Publishers, 1987.

Hargreaves K, Dubner R, Brown F, Flores C, Joris J. A new and sensitive method for measuring thermal nociception in cutaneous hyperalgesia. *Pain* 1988; 32:77–88.

International Association for the Study of Pain. Ethical guidelines for investigations of experimental pain in conscious animals. *Pain* 1983; 16:109–110.

Le Bars D, Gozariu M, Cadden SW. Animal models of nociception. *Pharmacol Rev* 2001; 53:597-652.

Mason P, Strassman A, Maciewicz R. Is the jaw opening reflex a valid model of pain? *Brain Res Rev* 1985; 10:137–146.

Ness TJ, Gebhart GF. Colorectal distension as a noxious visceral stimulus: physiologic and pharmacologic characteri-zation of pseudaffective reflexes in the rat. *Brain Res* 1988; 450:153–169.

ADDITIONAL READING

Anseloni VC, Ennis M, Lidow MS. Optimization of the mechanical nociceptive threshold testing with the Randall-Selitto assay. *J Neurosci Methods* 2003; 131:93–97.

Brennan TJ, Vandermeulen EP, Gebhart GF. Characterization of a rat model of incisional pain. *Pain* 1996; 64:493–501.

Chaplan SR, Bach FW, Pogrel JW, Chung JM, Yaksh TL. Quantitative assessment of tactile allodynia in the rat paw. *J Neurosci Methods* 1994; 53:55–63.

Committee on Pain and Distress in Laboratory Animals, Institute of Laboratory Animal Resources, Commission on Life Sci-ences, National Research Council. *Recognition and Allevia-tion of Pain and Distress in Laboratory Animals.* Washington, DC: National Academy Press, 1992.

Decosterd I, Woolf CJ. Spared nerve injury: an animal model of persistent peripheral neuropathic pain. *Pain* 2000; 87:149–158.

Kim SH, Chung JM. An experimental model for peripheral neuropathy produced by segmental spinal nerve ligation in the rat. *Pain* 1992; 50:355–363.

Ren K. An improved method for assessing mechanical allodynia in the rat. *Physiol Behav* 1999; 67:711–716.

Schwei MJ, Honore P, Rogers SD, et al. Neurochemical and cellular reorganization of the spinal cord in a murine model of bone cancer pain. *J Neurosci* 1999; 19:10886–10897.

Seltzer Z, Dubner R, Shir Y. A novel behavioral model of neuropathic pain disorders produced in rats by partial sciatic nerve injury. *Pain* 1990; 43:205–218.

Sluka KA, Kalra A, Moore SA. Unilateral intramuscular injections of acidic saline produce a bilateral, long-lasting hyperalgesia. *Muscle Nerve* 2001; 24:37–46.

Vonvoigtlander PF. Pharmacological alteration of pain: the discovery and evaluation of analgetics in animals. In: Lednicer D (Ed). *Central Analgetics.* New York: John Wiley & Sons, 1982, pp 51–79.

Wood PL. Animal models in analgesic testing. In: Kuhar M, Pasternak G (Eds). *Analgesics: Neurochemical, Behavioral and Clinical Perspectives.* New York: Raven Press, 1984, pp 175–194.

Core Curriculum for Professional Education in Pain, edited by J. Edmond Charlton, IASP Press, Seattle, © 2005.

6

Ethical Standards in Pain Management and Research

I. General

Know the basic ethical standards in pain management and research (United Nations Office of the High Commissioner for Human Rights 1948; International Association for the Study of Pain 1983, 1995; American Medical Association, Council on Ethical and Judicial Affairs 2001; National Comprehensive Cancer Network 2001; Council for International Organizations of Medical Sciences 2002; Institute of Medicine 2002; World Medical Association 2004).

A. Philosophical concepts

1. Understand the concepts of subjective experience of pain and objective assessment of pain, and ways these confusions have contributed to problems in research and practice (Vrancken 1989; Rollin 1990; Max 1992; Cunningham 1993; Rich 2000).
2. Understand the distinction between the concepts of pain and suffering, and ways this distinction may or may not give scientific and moral status to the emotional component of pain (Roy 1992; Shapiro 1995).
3. Be aware of ways in which scientific and clinical attention to individual and group differences in the intensity and meaning of pain may conflict with the scientific ideal of predictable, universal causes and markers of pain (Vrancken 1989; Rich 2000).

B. Ethical obligations

1. Be aware of the importance of individual cultures, basic human rights and responsibilities, and the need for constant review of current practices (Council for International Organizations of Medical Sciences 2002).
2. Understand that witnesses to patients' suffering of unnecessary pain have a moral responsibility to those patients, even if the witnesses are not clinically responsible for that pain (Hilberg 1992). Understand the potential moral difficulties associated with professionals' development of emotional distance from patients in pain (Shapiro and Ferrell 1992; Cunningham 1993; Shapiro 1995; Rich 2000).
3. Understand that any pain above moderate levels can be physically and psychologically harmful. Preventing or alleviating such pain is not merely a matter of charity or doing good (beneficence), but carries a duty to prevent harm (nonmaleficence) (Melzack 1988; Carr 1993; Walco et al. 1994).
4. Be aware that patients in pain may be at great risk for injury to their dignity, as well as to their autonomy; patients whose pain has been ignored, especially iatrogenic pain, may experience their pain in the same way as do victims of torture (Randall and Lutz 1991). International declarations proscribe torture or other degrading treatment (United Nations Office of the High Commissioner for Human Rights 1948).
5. Understand the principle of justice as it may apply to all individuals and groups of patients in areas of pain prevention, assessment, and treatment (Foley 1995). Defending current practice merely by pointing to historical or current standard practice may be a form of false justice (Cunningham 1993; Walco et al. 1994; International Association for the Study of Pain 1995).

II. Clinical care

A. Professional power and responsibility

1. Be aware of the power professionals may have over patients and families, including physical, bureaucratic, psychological, informational, political, and economic. Understand the moral sensitivity required to use this power in a supportive manner, rather than an indifferent or abusive one (Roy 1992; Shapiro and Ferrell 1992; Porter 1994).

2. Know whether determinations of concepts, such as appropriate pain behavior, patients' tolerance levels, and advantages and disadvantages of treatment alternatives, speak primarily to the needs of patients and their families or primarily to the needs of clinicians (Roy 1992; Qiu 1993; Walco et al. 1994; Shapiro 1995).

3. Be aware of the ways in which the social history of attitudes about pain and the medical history of assessment, treatment, and value of pain can affect current lay and professional attitudes about patients with pain (Vrancken 1989; Macrae et al. 1992; Max 1992; Cunningham 1993; Porter 1994; Walco et al. 1994).

4. Understand the difference between informed consent in clinical treatment and in research, as well as the moral importance of both. Be aware of effective ways to involve patients and their families in the pain assessment and treatment process (National Comprehensive Cancer Network 2001; McGrath et al. 1994).

B. Vulnerable groups

1. Understand the full range of conditions (e.g., dementia, developmental disabilities, severe head injury, stroke) that can lead to limitations in ability to communicate due to cognitive impairment (Hadjistavropoulos et al. 2001; Breau et al. 2004). Understand the use of nonverbal methods to assess pain (Melding 1992; Shapiro and Ferrell 1992; Cunningham 1993; Shapiro 1995).

2. Understand the vulnerability of patients with diseases such as cancer or conditions such as burns, where there has been a historical, professional acceptance of severe, unremitting pain (Max 1992). Know the difference between psychological dependence, physical dependence, and tolerance. Understand common fears and confusions about opioid pain control (Walco et al. 1994; see Chapter 44).

3. Understand the vulnerability of dying patients or others with serious conditions, who prefer death over life because their pain is not adequately controlled. Be aware that the acceptability of physician-assisted suicide may be related to lack of knowledge and availability of effective means of pain control (Foley 1995). Understand the ethical principle of "double effect," as it applies to pain control (it is acceptable to provide medication for pain control, which has as a secondary effect hastening death, when the primary intention is to provide adequate pain control that can be provided in no other manner) (American Medical Association 2001).

4. Understand the vulnerability of chronic pain patients, especially as it may be related to the mystery and complexity of the condition, and the clinician's wish for simple diagnoses and treatment (Vrancken 1989; Melding 1992; Roy 1992; Shapiro 1995).

5. Understand the vulnerability of patients who live in locations where laws or economic factors restrict the availability and use of effective treatments, even to patients in need.

C. Quality assurance

1. Be aware of the moral responsibility for providing appropriate pain care, and the consequent need for an interdisciplinary, system-wide approach that acknowledges the physiological and psychological complexity of pain (Max 1992). This responsibility applies to institutions as well as to units and individuals.

2. Understand that standards of care change and will need constant and regular review. This review must involve changes in moral awareness and commitment, as well as changes in the technical education of professionals.

III. Research

A. Statements of research ethics

1. Know the standards provided in international, national, and professional statements of biomedical research ethics, including instances where standards conflict with one another (McNeill 1993; International Association for the Study of Pain 1995; Council for International Organizations of Medical Sciences 2002; World Medical Association 2004).

2. Understand that laws or rules, traditions, and resources within particular societies and medical cultures may make these standards only partly applicable, or difficult to apply (Council for International Organizations of Medical Sciences 2002; Qiu 2004).

B. Research design, review, and implementation

1. Understand that ethical research requires sound methods, but sound methods do not guarantee ethical research. Researchers are responsible for the well-being of subjects even when subjects or their proxies have given consent (McGrath 1993; Rothman and Michels 1994; International Association for the Study of Pain 1995; Council for International Organizations of Medical Sciences 2002; World Medical Association 2004).

2. Understand philosophical arguments for and against randomized, controlled trials, including the use of placebo controls, when effective forms of pain prevention or control are already scientifically proven (Rothman and Michels 1994).

3. Understand the ethical issues in specific areas of research such as at the extremes of age and in palliative and intensive care. Know that these are legitimate areas for research but that scrupulous care must be taken at all times of the needs of the patient.

4. Be aware that the requirement not to exceed the subject's tolerance limit applies equally to situations of experimentally induced pain and to situations of research about pain that is consequent to disease, injury, or medical procedures (International Association for the Study of Pain 1995).

5. Understand benefits, appropriate use, standard methodologies, and ethical concerns of qualitative research about pain.

6. Know that clinical trials should be registered with a public trials registry before patient enrolment (De Angelis et al 2004).

7. Be aware that the complex nature of pain and the common use of interdisciplinary teams for clinical practice do not contradict the ethical requirement that particular research projects be carried out only by appropriately qualified persons.

8. Be aware that independent review is always necessary. Ethical review committees must ensure that research permission is never adversely affected by factors such as reputation of proposed principal investigators, traditional medical acceptability of certain levels of pain in subjects, funding needs of the research institution, or lack of adequate subject representation on the committee.

9. Be aware of potential problems of unfair profit or scientific bias due to the priorities of the research funding source, whether that source is institutional, commercial, private nonprofit, or government (McNeill 1993; Council for International Organizations of Medical Sciences 2002).

C. Informed consent (Council for International Organizations of Medical Sciences 2002)

1. Understand informed consent. This must be legally competent, voluntary, informed, and with understanding (International Association for the Study of Pain 1995).

2. Be aware that, in some countries, the dignity and autonomy of the subject, which researchers protect with informed consent, cannot be separated from that of the family or community (Qiu 2004).

3. Be aware that those groups of persons who are vulnerable in the clinical context may also be vulnerable in the research context because they cannot give voluntary consent. Additional groups might include prisoners, the mentally ill, students, research center employees, or those who generally have limited access to health care.

4. Be aware that some groups, such as children or pregnant women, are vulnerable to unfair exclusion from pain research.

5. Understand that some groups may be exploitable, in addition to or instead of vulnerable, because they can be misused. Subjects in externally sponsored research projects may be at special risk (Qiu 2004).

6. Know that patients or their proxies need full information about any proposed research including benefits, risks, costs, and side effects. This information must include options for pain reduction or control. Those taking part in any study must consider all factors from both the patient's and the professional view, giving equal weight to both. The patient or their proxy must be made aware that it is possible to opt out of the study without penalty (Rothman and Michels 1994; International Association for the Study of Pain 1995).

D. Animals (International Association for the Study of Pain 1983; see Chapter 5)

1. Know the ethical standards for animal pain research.
2. Know the standards for sound animal pain research, including attention to the animals' physiological and mental health.

REFERENCES

American Medical Asso-ciation, Council on Ethical and Judicial Affairs. *Principles of Medical Ethics.* Available at: www.amaassn.org/ama/pub/category/2512.html. Accessed June 15, 2005.

Breau LM, Camfield CS, McGrath PJ, Finley GA. Risk factors for pain in children with severe neurological impairments. *Dev Med Child Neurol* 2004; 46(6):364–371.

Carr DB. Pain control: the new "whys" and "hows." *Pain: Clin Updates* 1993; I:1–4.

Council for International Organizations of Medical Sciences (CIOMS) and World Health Organization (WHO). *International Ethical Guidelines for Biomedical Research Involving Human Subjects.* Geneva: CIOMS, 2002. Available at: www.cioms.ch/frame_guidelines_nov_2002.htm. Accessed June 15, 2005.

Cunningham N. Moral and ethical issues in clinical practice. In: Anand KJS, McGrath PJ (Eds). *Pain in Neonates.* Amsterdam: Elsevier Science, 1993, pp 255–273.

De Angelis C, Drazen JM, Frizelle FA, et al. Clinical trial registration: a statement from the International Committee of Medical Journal Editors. *New Engl J Med* 2004; 351:1250–1251.

Foley KM. Pain, physician assisted suicide and euthanasia. *Pain Forum* 1995; 4:163–178.

Hadjistavropoulos T, von Baeyer C, Craig KD. Pain assessment in persons with limited ability to communicate. In Turk D, Melzack R (Eds). *Handbook of Pain Assessment,* 2nd ed. New York: Guilford Press, 2001, pp 134–149.

Hilberg R. *Perpetrators, Victims, Bystanders: The Jewish Catastrophe 1933–1945.* New York: Aaron Asher Books, 1992.

Institute of Medicine. *Responsible Research: A Systems Approach to Protecting Research Participants,* 2002. Available at: www.nap.edu/catalog/10508.html.

International Association for the Study of Pain. Ethical guidelines for investigations of experimental pain in conscious animals. *Pain* 1983; 16:109–110.

International Association for the Study of Pain. Guidelines for pain research in humans. Report of the Committee on Ethical Issues. *Pain* 1995; 63:277–278.

Macrae WA, Davies HTO, Crombie IK. Pain: paradigms and treatments. *Pain* 1992; 49:289–291.

Max MB. Improving outcomes of analgesic treatment: is education enough? *IASP Newsletter* 1992: Nov/Dec:2–6.

McGrath PA. Inducing pain in children: a controversial issue. *Pain* 1993; 52:255–257.

McGrath PJ, Finley GA, Ritchie J. *Pain, Pain, Go Away: Helping Children with Pain.* Bethesda, MD: Association for the Care of Chil-dren's Health, 1994.

McNeill PM. *The Ethics and Politics of Human Experimenta-tion.* Cambridge: Cambridge University Press, 1993.

Melding PS. Psychosocial aspects of chronic pain and the eld-erly. *IASP Newsletter* 1992; Jan/Feb: 2–4.

Melzack R. The tragedy of needless pain: a call for social action. In: Dubner R, Gebhart GF, Bond MR (Eds). *Proceedings of the Vth World Congress on Pain,* Pain Research and Clinical Management, Vol. 3. Amsterdam: Elsevier, 1988, pp 1–11.

National Comprehensive Cancer Network. *Cancer Pain. Treatment Guidelines for Patients,* Version I, January 2001. Available at: www.nccn.org/patients/patient_gls/_english/_pain/contents.asp. Accessed June 15, 2005.

Porter R. Pain and history in the western world. In: Djite-Bruce FA (Trans). *The Puzzle of Pain.* East Roseville, NSW: Gordon and Breach Arts International, 1994, pp 98–119.

Qiu RZ. Conflict of interests in research ethics: a Chinese perspective. *J Clin Ethics* 2004; 15:48–50.

Randall GR, Lutz EL. *Serving Survivors of Torture: A Practical Manual for Health Professionals and Other Service Providers.* Washington, DC: American Association for the Advancement of Science, 1991.

Rich B. An ethical analysis of the barriers to effective pain relief. *Camb Q Healthc Ethics* 2000; 9:54–70.

Rollin BE. *The Unheeded Cry: Animal Consciousness, Animal Pain and Science.* Oxford: Oxford University Press, 1990.

Rothman KJ, Michels KB. The continuing unethical use of placebo controls. *N Engl J Med* 1994; 331:394–398.

Roy R. *The Social Context of the Chronic Pain Sufferer.* Toronto: Uni-versity of Toronto Press, 1992.

Shapiro BS. The suffering of children and their families. In: Ferrell BR (Ed). *Suffering: Human Dimensions of Pain and Illness.* Boston: Jones & Bartlett, 1995.

Shapiro BS, Ferrell BR. Pain in children and the frail eld-erly: similarities and implications. *APS Bull* 1992; Oct/Nov:11–13.

United Nations. Office of the High Commissioner for Human Rights. *Universal Declaration of Human Rights,* 1948. Available at: www.ohchr.org/english/issues/education/training/udhr.htm. Accessed June 15, 2005

Vrancken MAE. Schools of thought on pain. *Pain* 1989; 29:435–444.

Walco GA, Cassidy RC, Schechter NL. Pain, hurt, and harm: the ethics of pain control in infants and children. *N Engl J Med* 1994; 331:541–544.

World Medical Association. *World Medical Association Declaration of Helsinki: Recommendations Guiding Physicians in Biomedical Research Involving Human Subjects,* 1964, revised in Tokyo 2004. Available at: www.wma.net/e/policy/b3.htm. Accessed June 15, 2005.

Part II
Assessment and Psychology of Pain

Core Curriculum for Professional Education in Pain, edited by J. Edmond Charlton, IASP Press, Seattle, © 2005.

7

Pain Measurement in Humans

I. Know that pain is a subjective, multidimensional experience unique to the individual (Clark et al. 2002; Kumar et al. 2002).

   A. Understand the distinction between pain and nociception.

      1. Appreciate that pain is a conscious, aversive aspect of somatic awareness, the product of complex, central, nociception-induced processing, and not a primitive sensation.
      2. Appreciate that nociception is never conscious and engages sensory, emotional, and cognitive processing areas of the brain.

   B. Understand that pain is multidimensional.

      1. Appreciate that the pain experience may have sensory, emotional, and cognitive aspects.
      2. Appreciate the potential impact of pain on function, affective status, and quality of life.

II. Know the basic concepts of introspection and measurement of subjective experience (Nakamura and Chapman 2002).

   A. Understand pain measurement as the product of selective introspection, self-scaling by number or descriptor assignment, and reporting.

      1. Appreciate the importance of training or carefully instructing patients/subjects.

         a. Comprehend the difficulty patients/subjects face in separating pain from concomitant somatic sensations and emotions (paresthesias, dysesthesias, and anxiety).
         b. Comprehend the difficulty patients/subjects have in assigning numbers to a dynamic, complex experience.
         c. Comprehend that pain measurement often requires patients to draw upon memory for assessment or comparison.
         d. Comprehend that patients reporting pain need to distinguish pain at rest from pain with activity or pain during stress.

      2. Appreciate that not everyone can or will generate a meaningful pain score upon demand.

         a. Comprehend that some reluctant patients, if pressed to report pain, may produce a number without properly scaling their subjective experience.

   B. Understand a pain score as a number that can never measure pain perfectly.

      1. Appreciate that the goal of measurement is to capture true pain with as little measurement error as possible.
      2. Appreciate that the pain score reflects both measurement error and systematic individual differences.

   C. Understand validity and reliability and their importance for pain measurement.

      1. Appreciate that reliability is precision or consistency of measurement and validity is the accuracy of measurement.

         a. Comprehend that reliability and validity are *continua* rather than dichotomies, with coefficients ranging from 0 to 1.0.

2. Appreciate that reliability is the upper limit for validity.
3. Appreciate that useful assessment of individuals requires high reliabilities (≥ 0.90).

III. Know the challenges and limitations of measuring pain in special populations (Herr and Mobily 1991; McGrath and Brigham 2001).

A. Understand the challenges of developmentally sensitive instruments in children.

1. Appreciate that nociception produces an aversive, unpleasant experience in young neonates and infants.

a. Comprehend the challenges and problems of measuring pain in neonates and infants.
b. Comprehend the importance of simple observational and self-report scoring methods and category scales.
c. Comprehend the place of surrogate ratings of pain for neonates and infants.

2. Appreciate that pain expression differs across developmental stages.
3. Appreciate that pain behavior can be a function of many influences in addition to pain.

B. Understand that temporary or permanent inability to communicate does not mean that pain is absent.

C. Understand the problems of measuring pain in cognitively compromised patients, including those with dementia, poststroke syndromes, and mental illness.

1. Appreciate that pain expression may vary from normal when the central nervous system is damaged.
2. Appreciate that in some circumstances, conventional approaches based on introspection may not yield valid or reliable scores in cognitively compromised patients.

a. Comprehend the value of observational pain assessment tools for cognitively compromised patients.

IV. Know the options available for measuring pain directly by self-report (Melzack 1975; Kerns et al. 1985; Jensen et al. 1986, 1989; Chapman and Syrjala 2001; Cleeland and Syrjala 2001; Turk and Melzack 2001).

A. Understand the use of simple unidimensional pain scales.

1. Appreciate and be able to administer numerical rating scales, visual analogue scales, and category rating scales.

a. Comprehend the advantages of these tools in efficiency and minimization of responder burden.
b. Comprehend the limitations of these tools, including ambiguous upper anchors and reliabilities that may be too low for useful individual assessment.

B. Understand the use of complex unidimensional pain scales.

1. Appreciate the nature, advantages and limitations of magnitude estimation, cross-modality matching, and verbal descriptor scaling.

C. Understand the use of complex instruments for multidimensional scaling of pain.

1. Appreciate that some instruments such as the McGill Pain Questionnaire may permit the scaling of multiple dimensions of subjective experience.
2. Appreciate that some instruments such as the Brief Pain Inventory assess both pain and the subjective impact of pain on activity and functional capability.

V. Know the options available for measuring pain indirectly by observation (Craig et al. 2001; Keefe and Williams 2001).

A. Understand that methods exist for observing and scoring facial pain expression in children and others who cannot perform introspection and produce verbal reports.

B. Understand the concept of pain behavior (Hadjistavropoulos and Craig 2002).

1. Appreciate the use of simple pain behavior ratings in specific situations.
2. Appreciate the availability of complex formal inventories that relate activities to pain report.

a. Comprehend the concept of scoring and interpreting complex behavior patterns.

3. Appreciate the availability of wearable electronic motion loggers that can chart 24-hour activity levels in persons living with pain.
4. Appreciate the advantages and limitations of pain behavior assessment versus subjective report measures.

VI. Know the basic issues surrounding pain measures as outcomes in clinical studies (Stone and Shiffman 1994; Kane 1997).

A. Understand the advantages and limitations of simple unidimensional scales for outcome evaluation.

1. Appreciate the advantages of rapid, simple assessment.
2. Appreciate that chronic pain requires greater complexity of assessment.
3. Appreciate that simple unidimensional scales have limited breadth for the assessment of functioning.
4. Appreciate the advantages of assessing pain at variable times and in varied settings (ecological momentary assessment).

B. Understand the value of multiple measures and correlational techniques for improving the capture of true pain.

C. Understand the value of repeated measurement for outcomes research.

1. Appreciate that average outcomes may not apply to all individuals under study.

VII. Know the importance of including strong outcome measures in studies of the impact of pain (Dworkin and Whitney 2001).

A. Understand the importance of measures such as activity level, functional capability, quality of life, costs of care, and disability.

B. Understand the value of including such measures with pain measures in studies of pain interventions.

REFERENCES

Chapman CR, Syrjala KL. Measurement of pain. In: Loeser JD, Butler SH, Chapman CR, Turk DC (Eds). *Bonica's Management of Pain*. Philadelphia: Lippincott, Williams and Wilkins, 2001, pp 310–328.

Clark WC, Yang JC, Tsui SL, Ng KF, Bennett Clark S. Unidimensional pain rating scales: a multidimensional affect and pain survey (MAPS) analysis of what they really measure. *Pain* 2002; 98:241–247.

Cleeland CS, Syrjala KL. How to assess cancer pain. In: Turk DC, Melzack R (Eds). *Handbook of Pain Assessment*, 2nd ed. New York: Guilford Press, 2001, pp 362–390.

Craig KD, Prkachin KM, Grunau RE. The facial expression of pain. In: Turk DC and Melzack R (Eds). *Handbook of Pain Assessment,* 2nd ed. New York: Guilford Press, 2001, pp 153–169.Dworkin SF, Whitney CW. Relying on objective and subjective measures of chronic pain. In: Turk DC, Melzack R (Eds). *Handbook of Pain Assessment*, 2nd ed. New York: Guilford Press, 2001, pp 429–446.

Hadjistavropoulos T, Craig KD. A theoretical framework for understanding self-report and observational measures of pain: a communications model. *Behav Res Ther*2002; 40:551–570.

Herr KA, Mobily PR. Pain assessment in the elderly: clinical considerations. *J Gerontol Nurs* 1991; 17:12–19.

Jensen MP, Karoly P, Braver S. The measurement of clinical pain intensity: a comparison of six methods. *Pain* 1986; 27:117–126.

Jensen MP, Karoly P, O'Riordan EF, Bland F Jr, Burns RS. The subjective experience of acute pain: an assessment of the utility of 10 indices. *Clin J Pain* 1989; 5:153–159.

Kane RL. *Understanding Health Care Outcomes Research*. New York: Aspen, 1997.

Keefe FJ, Williams DA. Assessment of pain behaviors. In: Turk DC, Melzack R (Eds). *Handbook of Pain Assessment*, 2nd ed. New York: Guilford Press, 2001, pp 257–274.

Kerns RD, Turk DC, Rudy TE. The West Haven-Yale Multidimensional Pain Inventory (WHYMPI). *Pain* 1985; 23:345–356.

Kumar S, Tandon OP, Mathur R. Pain measurement: a formidable task. *Ind J Physiol Pharmacol* 2002; 46:396–406.

McGrath PA, Brigham M. Pain assessment in children and adolescents. In: Turk DC, Melzack R (Eds). *Handbook of Pain Assessment,* 2nd ed. New York: Guilford Press, 2001, pp 97–118.

Melzack R. The McGill Pain Questionnaire: major properties and scoring methods. *Pain* 1975; 1:277–299.

Nakamura Y, Chapman CR. Measuring pain: an introspective look at introspection. *Conscious Cogn* 2002; 11:582–592.

Stone AA, Shiffman S. Ecological momentary assessment (EMA) in behavioral medicine. *Ann Behav Med* 1994; 16:199–202.

Turk DC, Melzack R (Eds). *Handbook of Pain Assessment,* 2nd ed. New York: Guilford Press, 2001, pp 295–314.

Core Curriculum for Professional Education in Pain, edited by J. Edmond Charlton, IASP Press, Seattle, © 2005.

8

Placebo and Pain

Be aware that the placebo effect in pain is a product of many factors.

I.   Know definitions of placebo, observed from various points of view with special reference to placebo analgesia (Wall 1992, 2003).

II.   Be aware of placebo as a phenomenon in a wide variety of clinical and scientific settings (Shapiro and Shapiro 1997).

III. Be aware of historical aspects of placebo, explaining prescientific concepts and ideas that linger on within the medical profession, in the public at large, and in folk medicine (Beecher 1955; Brody 2000).

IV.   Placebo effect: Be able to formulate definition and discussion items (Price 2000).

V.   Be aware of the variety of described placebo mechanisms; know the basic scientific publications on various concepts:

   A.   Expectation, desire (Kirsch 1985; Voudouris et al. 1990)

   B.   Learning, conditioned reflex (Montgomery and Kirsch 1997)

   C.   Cognitive modulation (Villemure and Bushnell 2002)

   D.   Neurotransmitter reactions (Amanzio and Benedetti 1999; ter Riet et al. 1998)

   E.   Context mechanisms (Di Blasi et al. 2001)

   F.   Most appropriate action of the organism to find relief from pain (Wall 2000)

VI.   Be aware of the various ways of interpreting aspects of the placebo response as a phenomenon (Kleijnen et al. 1994; Price 2001).

VII. Be aware of placebo as a methodological instrument in randomized controlled trials in pain research (Kleijnen et al. 1994).

VIII. Be aware of the role of expectancies in clinical trial design, as the power of the patient's expectations underscores the importance of perceived assignment rather than actual assignment in clinical trial design (Finniss and Benedetti 2005).

IX.   Be aware of the observation of placebo as a controversial "noise" factor, or response bias in the analysis of scientific data (Hróbjartsson and Gótzsche 2001; Vase et al. 2002).

X.   Be aware of the ethical aspects in relation to the application of placebo both in scientific and clinical practice (World Medical Association 2000; Lewis et al. 2002).

XI.   Be aware of the open-hidden paradigm as a way of demonstrating and investigating the nonspecific factors (similar or identical to placebo factors) and as an ethical alternative to the administration of a placebo (Finniss and Benedetti 2005).

XII. Be aware of the recognition of placebo as a treatment modality, either intended or by coincidence (Brody and Brody 2000).

XIII. Be aware of the relationship of placebo and psychological mechanisms in pain and its treatment; the "doctor" as placebo (Brody 2000; Price and Bushnell 2004).

XIV. Be aware of the terminology and the area of relevance of the nocebo effect (Wall 2000).

REFERENCES

Amanzio M, Benedetti F. Neuropharmacological dissection of placebo analgesia: expectation-activated opioid systems versus conditioning-activated subsystems. *J Neurosci* 1999; 19(1):484–494.

Beecher HK. The powerful placebo. *JAMA* 1955; 159:1602–1607.

Brody H. *The Placebo Response.* New York: Cliff Street Books, 2000.

Brody H, Brody D. *The Placebo Response: How You Can Release the Body's Inner Pharmacy for Better Health.* Cliff Street Books, 2000.

Di Blasi Z, Harkness E, Ernst E, Georgiou A, Kleijnen J. Influence of context effects on health outcomes: a systematic review. *Lancet* 2001; 57:757–762.

Fields HL, Price DD. Toward a neurobiology of placebo analgesia. In: Harrington A (Ed). *The Placebo Effect: An Interdisciplinary Exploration.* Cambridge, MA: Harvard University Press, 1997, pp 93–115.

Finniss DG, Benedetti F. Mechanisms of the placebo response and their impact on clinical trials and clinical practice. *Pain* 2005; 114:3–6.

Hróbjartsson A, Gótzsche PC. Is the placebo powerless? An analysis of clinical trials comparing placebo treatment with no treatment. *N Engl J Med* 2001; 344:1594–1602.

Kirsch I. Response expectancy as a determinant of experience and behaviour. *Am Psychol* 1985; 40:151–160.

Kleijnen J, Craen AJM de, Everdingen J van, Krol L. Placebo effect in double-blind clinical trials: a review of interactions with medications. *Lancet* 1994; 344:1347–1349.

Lewis JA, Jonsson B, Kreutz G, Sampaio C, van Zwieten-Boot B. Placebo controlled trials and the Declaration of Helsinki. *Lancet* 2002; 359:1337–1340.

Montgomery GH, Kirsch I. Classical conditioning and the placebo effect. *Pain* 1997; 72:107–113.

Price DD. Factors that determine the magnitude and presence of placebo analgesia. In: Devor M, Rowbotham MC, Wiesenfeld-Hallin Z (Eds). *Proceedings of the 9th World Congress on Pain,* Progress in Pain Research and Management, Vol. 16. Seattle: IASP Press, 2000.

Price DD. Assessing placebo effects without placebo groups: an untapped possibility? *Pain* 2001; 90:201–203.

Price DD, Bushnell MC. Overview of pain dimensions and their psychological modulation. In: Price DD, Bushnell MC (Eds). *Psychological Methods of Pain Control: Basic Science and Clinical Perspectives,* Progress in Pain Research and Management, Vol. 29. Seattle: IASP Press, 2004.

ter Riet G, de Craen AJM, de Boer A , Kessels A. Is placebo analgesia mediated by endogenous opioids? A systematic review. *Pain* 1998; 76:273–275.

Shapiro AK, Shapiro E. The placebo: is it much ado about nothing? In: Harrington A (Ed). *The Placebo Effect: An Interdisciplinary Exploration.* Cambridge, MA: Harvard University Press, 1997.

Vase L, Riley III JL, Price DD. A comparison of placebo effects in clinical analgesic trials versus studies of placebo analgesia. *Pain* 2002; 99:433–452.

Villemure C, Bushnell MC. Cognitive modulation of pain: How do attention and emotion influence pain processing? *Pain* 2002; 95:195–199.

Voudouris NJ, Peck CL, Coleman G. The role of conditioning and expectancy in the placebo response. *Pain* 1990; 43:121–128.

Wall PD. The placebo effect: an unpopular topic. *Pain* 1992; 51:1–3.

Wall PD. *The Science of Suffering.* London: Orion Books, 2000, pp 131–145.

Wall PD. The placebo and the placebo response. In: Wall PD, Melzack R (Eds). *Textbook of Pain.* Edinburgh: Churchill Livingstone, 2003, pp 1297–1308.

World Medical Association. *World Medical Association Declaration of Helsinki: Ethical Principles for Medical Research Involving Human Subjects.* Ferney-Voltaire: World Medical Association, 2000.

Core Curriculum for Professional Education in Pain, edited by J. Edmond Charlton, IASP Press, Seattle, © 2005.

9

Clinical Nerve Function Studies and Imaging

I.   General considerations for the use of nerve function and imaging studies

    A.   Be aware that no objective measure of ongoing pain is available. The gold standard for assessing pain is the subjective report of the individual. This can be supplemented by observation of facial expression, posture, and other behavioral indices.

    B.   Laboratory tests, however, can provide objective evidence for positive and negative sensory phenomena and differential involvement of nociceptive and non-nociceptive afferents (Cruccu et al. 2004).

II.   Electrical nerve stimulation (Kimura et al. 1994; Nuwer et al. 1994; Treede 2003; Cruccu et al. 2004)

    A.   Be aware that the large myelinated afferents of the tactile system have the lowest threshold to electrical stimuli and hence are predominantly assessed with standard methods of clinical neurophysiology.

    B.   Know that the measurement of sensory nerve conduction velocity can demonstrate the loss of A-beta afferent fibers, but is insensitive to selective loss of A-delta and C fibers.

    C.   Know that somatosensory evoked potential studies can provide detailed information on the location of a lesion along the somatosensory pathways of the lemniscal system, but are insensitive to selective lesions of the nociceptive system.

    D.   Know that some trigeminal (Blink reflex, masseter inhibitory reflex) and spinal reflexes (withdrawal reflex) have both nociceptive and non-nociceptive components that can be exploited in the differential assessment of some lesions.

III.   Laser-evoked potentials (Bromm and Treede 1991; Kakigi et al. 2000; Lorenz and Garcia-Larrea 2003; Plaghki and Mouraux 2003; Treede et al. 2003; Cruccu et al. 2004)

    A.   Be aware that large myelinated afferents of the tactile system are insensitive to heat stimuli and that rapidly rising heat stimuli are an appropriate tool to assess the function of nociceptive pathways.

    B.   Know that laser evoked potentials have been validated as sensitive tools to assess deficits of small-fiber function, the spinothalamic tract, and other parts of the nociceptive system in individual patients.

    C.   Be aware that laser evoked potentials are sensitive to changes in attentional state.

IV.   Quantitative sensory testing (Gracely et al. 1988; Arezzo et al. 1993; Yarnitsky et al. 1995; Ziegler et al. 1999; Greenspan 2001; LeBars et al. 2001; Cruccu et al. 2004)

    A.   Know that quantitative sensory testing can be used to test large and small nerve fiber function.

    B.   Know that vibration and brushing detection is mediated by A-beta fibers.

    C.   Know that cool detection thresholds depend primarily on A-delta-fiber function.

    D.   Know that warm detection thresholds depend primarily on C-fiber function.

    E.   Know that pain evoked by pinpricks depends primarily on A-delta-fiber function.

    F.   Know that heat pain thresholds depend on A-delta and C-fiber function, but that slowly increasing temperature changes preferentially recruit C fibers and rapidly increasing temperatures recruit A-delta fibers.

G.   Know that cold pain threshold primarily depends on C-fiber function.

V.   Skin biopsies (McArthur et al. 1998; Nolano et al. 1999; Cruccu et al. 2004)

A.   Be aware that innervation density by sensory nerves, including C fibers, can be assessed in skin punch biopsies.

B.   Know that skin biopsies are more sensitive and less invasive than nerve biopsies.

VI.   Magnetic resonance imaging (May et al. 1999; Davis 2000; Tracey 2001; Grachev and Apkarian 2002)

A.   Be aware that functional magnetic resonance imaging (fMRI) can provide indirect information on brain activity through hemodynamic measures.

B.   Know that fMRI provides better temporal resolution than positron emission tomography (PET).

C.   Know that structural MRI can be used to examine morphometric changes in the brain related to chronic pain conditions.

D.   Know that magnetic resonance spectroscopy can be used to examine brain chemistry.

VII.   Positron emission tomography (Jones et al. 1991; Talbot et al. 1991; Tölle et al. 1999; Casey et al. 2000; Zubieta et al. 2001)

A.   Be aware that PET can provide indirect information on brain activity (hemodynamic or metabolic imaging) and neuropharmacology (receptor imaging).

B.   Know that radioligands can be used to image availability of neurotransmitter binding sites, and thus potentially assess degeneration, receptor internalization, and endogenous ligand occupation in the presence and absence of different types of pain.

C.   Be aware that PET has poor temporal resolution.

VIII.   Electro- and magnetoencephalography (Anogianakis et al. 1992; Schnitzler and Ploner 2000; Garcia-Larrea et al. 2003; Schlereth et al. 2003)

A.   Know that electroencephalography (EEG) and magnetoencephalography (MEG) reflect the synaptic activity in the brain.

B.   Be aware that EEG- and MEG-source analysis has a limited spatial precision of about 10 mm, but unsurpassed temporal resolution.

IX.   What imaging reveals about pain (Devinsky et al. 1995; Coghill et al. 1998, 2003; Bushnell et al. 1999; Gelnar et al. 1999; Ploghaus et al. 1999; Treede et al. 1999, 2000; Baron et al. 2000; Peyron et al. 2000; Gracely et al. 2002; Frot and Mauguière 2003; Lorenz et al. 2003; Strigo et al. 2003; Wager et al. 2004; Wise et al. 2004; Apkarian et al 2005)

A.   Know that the basic pattern of brain activation with acute painful stimuli includes thalamus, primary somatosensory cortex, operculo-insular cortex, cingulate cortex, prefrontal cortex, and cerebellum.

B.   Be aware that certain aspects of the brain activation patterns may differ among pain states (e.g., cutaneous vs. visceral; acute vs. chronic) and may be modulated under hyperalgia or allodynia.

C.   Know that brain imaging can be used to examine the basis of pain modulation by psychological factors such as attention, emotion, and expectancy.

D.   Know that brain imaging can be used to examine the forebrain mechanisms of analgesia (e.g., opioid analgesia, placebo analgesia).

E.   Be aware that PET and fMRI analyses involve statistical tests and therefore can prove the presence but not the absence of activation in a given region.

REFERENCES

Anogianakis G, Badier JM, Barrett G, et al. A consensus statement on relative merits of EEG and MEG. *Electroenceph Clin Neurophysiol* 1992; 82:317–319.

Apkarian AV, Bushnell MC, Treede RD, Zubieta JK. Human brain mechanisms of pain perception and regulation in health and disease. *Eur J Pain* 2005; 9:463–484.

Arezzo JC, Bolton CF, Boulton A, et al. Quantitative sensory testing: a consensus report from the Peripheral Neuropathy Association. *Neurology* 1993; 43:1050–1052.

Baron R, Baron Y, Disbrow E, Roberts TPL. Activation of the somatosensory cortex during A-beta-fiber mediated hyperalgesia—a MSI study. *Brain Res* 2000; 871:75–82.

Bromm B, Treede R-D. Laser-evoked cerebral potentials in the assessment of cutaneous pain sensitivity in normal subjects and patients. *Rev Neurol (Paris)* 1991; 147:625–643.

Bushnell MC, Duncan GH, Hofbauer RK, et al. Pain perception: is there a role for primary somatosensory cortex? *Proc Natl Acad Sci USA* 1999; 96:7705–7709.

Casey KL, Svensson P, Morrow TJ, et al. Selective opiate modulation of nociceptive processing in the human brain. *J Neurophysiol* 2000; 84:525–533.

Coghill RC, Sang CN, Berman KF, Bennett GJ, Iadarola MJ. Global cerebral blood flow decreases during pain. *J Cereb Blood Flow Metab* 1998;18:141–147.

Coghill RC, McHaffie JG, Yen YF. Neural correlates of interindividual differences in the subjective experience of pain. *Proc Natl Acad Sci USA* 2003; 100:8538–8542.

Cruccu G, Anand P, Attal N, et al. EFNS guidelines on neuropathic pain assessment. *Eur J Neurol* 2004;11:153–162.

Davis KD. The neural circuitry of pain as explored with functional MRI. *Neurol Res* 2000; 22:313–317.

Devinsky O, Morrell MJ, Vogt BA. Contributions of anterior cingulate cortex to behaviour. *Brain* 1995; 118:279–306.

Frot M, Mauguière F. Dual representation of pain in the operculo-insular cortex in humans. *Brain* 2003; 126:438–450.

Garcia-Larrea L, Frot M, Valeriani M. Brain generators of laser-evoked potentials: from dipoles to functional significance. *Neurophysiol Clin* 2003; 33:279–292.

Gelnar PA, Krauss BR, Sheehe PR, et al. A comparative fMRI study of cortical representations for thermal painful, vibrotactile, and motor performance tasks. *Neuroimage* 1999; 10:460–482.

Gracely RH, Lota L, Walter DJ, Dubner R. A multiple random staircase method of psychophysical pain assessment. *Pain* 1988; 32:55–63.

Gracely RH, Petzke F, Wolf JM, Clauw DJ. Functional magnetic resonance imaging evidence of augmented pain processing in fibromyalgia. *Arthritis Rheum* 2002; 46:1333–1343.

Grachev ID, Apkarian AV. Multi-chemical networking profile of the living human brain: potential relevance to molecular studies of cognition and behavior in normal and diseased brain. *J Neural Transm* 2002; 109:15–33.

Greenspan JD. Quantitative assessment of neuropathic pain. *Curr Pain Headache Rep* 2001; 5:107–113.

Jones AKP, Qi LY, Fujirawa T, et al. In vivo distribution of opioid receptors in man in relation to the cortical projections of the medial and lateral pain systems measured with positron emission tomography. *Neurosci Lett* 1991; 126:25–28.

Kakigi R, Watanabe S, Yamasaki H. Pain-related somatosensory evoked potentials. *J Clin Neurophysiol* 2000; 17:295–308.

Kimura J, Daube J, Burke D, et al. Human reflexes and late responses. Report of an IFCN committee. *Electroenceph Clin Neurophysiol* 1994; 90:393–403.

Le Bars D, Gozariu M, Cadden SW. Animal models of nociception. *Pharmacol Rev* 2001; 53:597–652.

Lorenz J, Garcia-Larrea L. Contribution of attentional and cognitive factors to laser evoked brain potentials. *Neurophysiol Clin* 2003; 33:293–301.

Lorenz J, Minoshima S, Casey KL. Keeping pain out of mind: the role of the dorsolateral prefrontal cortex in pain modulation. *Brain* 2003; 126:1079–1091.

May A, Ashburner J, Büchel C, et al. Correlation between structural and functional changes in brain in an idiopathic headache syndrome. *Nat Med* 1999; 5:836–838.

McArthur JC, Stocks EA, Hauer P, et al. Epidermal nerve fiber density: normative reference range and diagnostic efficiency. *Arch Neurol* 1998; 55:1513–1520.

Nolano M, Simone DA, Wendelschafer-Crabb G, et al. Topical capsaicin in humans: parallel loss of epidermal nerve fibers and pain sensation. *Pain* 1999; 81:135–145.

Nuwer MR, Aminoff M, Desmedt J, et al. IFCN recommended standards for short latency somatosensory evoked potentials. Report of an IFCN committee. *Electroenceph Clin Neurophysiol* 1994; 91:6–11.

Peyron R, Laurent B, García-Larrea L. Functional imaging of brain responses to pain. A review and meta- analysis. *Neurophysiol Clin* 2000; 30:263–288.

Plaghki L, Mouraux A. How do we selectively activate skin nociceptors with a high power infrared laser? Physiology and biophysics of laser stimulation. *Neurophysiol Clin* 2003; 33:269–277.

Ploghaus A, Tracey I, Gati JS, et al. Dissociating pain from its anticipation in the human brain. *Science* 1999; 284:1979–1981.

Schlereth T, Baumgärtner U, Magerl W, et al. Left-hemisphere dominance in early nociceptive processing in the human parasylvian cortex. *Neuroimage* 2003; 20:441–454.

Schnitzler A, Ploner M. Neurophysiology and functional neuroanatomy of pain perception. *J Clin Neurophysiol* 2000; 17:592–603.

Strigo IA, Duncan GH, Boivin M, Bushnell MC. Differentiation of visceral and cutaneous pain in the human brain. *J Neurophysiol* 2003; 89:3294–3303.

Talbot JD, Marrett S, Evans AC, et al. Multiple representations of pain in human cerebral cortex. *Science* 1991; 251:1355–1358.

Tölle TR, Kaufmann T, Siessmeier T, et al. Region-specific encoding of sensory and affective components of pain in the human brain: a positron emission tomography correlation analysis. *Ann Neurol* 1999; 45:40–47.

Tracey I. Prospects for human pharmacological functional magnetic resonance imaging (phMRI). *J Clin Pharmacol* 2001; 41:21S–28S.

Treede R-D. Neurophysiological studies of pain pathways in peripheral and central nervous system disorders. *J Neurol* 2003 250:1152–1161.

Treede R-D, Kenshalo DR, Gracely RH, Jones AKP. The cortical representation of pain. *Pain* 1999; 79:105–111.

Treede R-D, Apkarian AV, Bromm B, et al. Cortical representation of pain: functional characterization of nociceptive areas near the lateral sulcus. *Pain* 2000; 87:113–119.

Treede R-D, Lorenz J, Baumgärtner U. Clinical usefulness of laser-evoked potentials. *Neurophysiol Clin* 2003; 33:303–314.

Wager TD, Rilling JK, Smith EE, et al. Placebo-induced changes in FMRI in the anticipation and experience of pain. *Science* 2004; 303:1162–1167.

Wise RG, Williams P, Tracey I. Using fMRI to quantify the time dependence of remifentanil analgesia in the human brain. *Neuropsychopharmacology* 2004; 29:626–635.

Yarnitsky D, Sprecher E, Zaslansky R, Hemli JA. Heat pain thresholds: normative data and repeatability. *Pain* 1995; 60:329–332.

Ziegler EA, Magerl W, Meyer RA, Treede R-D. Secondary hyperalgesia to punctate mechanical stimuli: central sensitization to A-fibre nociceptor input. *Brain* 1999; 122:2245–2257.

Zubieta J-K, Smith YR, Bueller JA, et al. Regional mu opioid receptor regulation of sensory and affective dimensions of pain. *Science* 2001; 293:311–315.

Core Curriculum for Professional Education in Pain, edited by J. Edmond Charlton, IASP Press, Seattle, © 2005.

10

Epidemiology

I.   Appreciate the uses of data from epidemiological studies of pain

   A. Measuring burden in a population.

   B. Investigating etiology.

   C. Determining natural history and identifying predictors of outcome.

   D. Informing studies of management and policy.

II. Measuring burden in a population

   A. Understand the epidemiological measures of occurrence.

      1. Prevalence: in particular to appreciate the distinction between prevalence measured at a single point in time (point prevalence) and over a longer period (period prevalence).
      2. Incidence: in particular to appreciate the distinction between the first-ever onset of pain (first-ever incidence), onset of an episode (episode incidence) and the proportion of a population who have experienced at least one episode over a defined period of time (cumulative incidence).

      In general, in large-scale population-based epidemiological studies of pain it is difficult to measure episode incidence.

   B. Appreciate the potential contribution of different types of data such as population studies of self-reported pain, social and occupational statistics (e.g., disability benefit, work loss), and health services data (e.g., prescription for analgesic, visits to general practice, hip replacement operation) in measuring burden.

   C. Know the prevalence and, where available, the incidence of common pain syndromes in general populations (Crombie et al. 1999; Macfarlane et al. 2004).

III Investigating etiology

   A. Understand the different observational study designs used to investigate etiology, and understand the strengths, weaknesses, and appropriate uses of each of these designs.

      1. Ecological: comparing, at a population level, the occurrence of pain.
      2. Case-control: comparing people with and without pain with respect to potential risk factors.
      3. Cohort: comparing people with and without risk factors with respect to subsequent occurrence of pain.

   B. Understand how epidemiological studies measure the strength of association between a risk factor and pain. These measures include odds ratios (case-control studies) and relative risks (cohort studies) (Silman and Macfarlane 2002). Understand how the precision of these estimates is expressed through confidence intervals.

   C. Know the major types of risk factor for the development of common pain syndromes (Crombie et al. 1999). Appreciate the possible interaction between these types of risk factor (e.g., the influence of adverse psychological factors and the social environment).

      1. Demographic (age, gender)

   2. Biological

      a. Constitutional and lifestyle (e.g., weight)
      b. Mechanical (including injury)
      c. Disease pathology
      d. Genetic

   3. Psychological
   4. Social and cultural environment

IV.   Determining natural history and identifying predictors of outcome

   A.   Appreciate the application of cohort study methodology to the investigation of the natural history of pain. Understand the application of data from such studies in predicting the outcome in individuals. This may be expressed as predictive value and absolute risk.

   B.   Know the major influences on the outcome of an episode of pain

      1. Demographic (e.g., age, gender)
      2. Clinical factors (prior history of pain, duration of episode, pain severity, and disability level).
      3. Biological (constitutional and lifestyle, e.g., weight)
      4. Psychological
      5. Social and cultural environment

V.   Informing studies of management and policy

   A.   Appreciate that risk factors identified by etiological studies can inform interventions. This can be at the level of:

      1. The individual (e.g., mechanical lifting in the workplace)
      2. Populations at high risk (e.g., screen and intervene in those with high levels of psychological distress)
      3. General population (e.g., levels of fitness)

REFERENCES

Crombie IK, Croft PR, Linton S, LeResche L, von Korff M (Eds). *The Epidemiology of Pain.* Seattle: IASP Press, 1999.

Macfarlane GJ, Jones GT, McBeth J. The epidemiology of pain. In: *Melzack and Wall's Textbook of Pain.* Amsterdam: Elsevier, 2005, in press.

Silman AJ, Macfarlane GJ. *Epidemiological Studies: A Practical Guide.* Cambridge University Press, 2002.

Core Curriculum for Professional Education in Pain, edited by J. Edmond Charlton, IASP Press, Seattle, © 2005.

11

Psychosocial and Cultural Aspects of Pain

I. Definition and measurement of pain

    A. Know the definition of pain as a biopsychosocial experience. Understand that pain is a subjective experience with important affective, cognitive, and behavioral as well as sensory components. Appreciate what is known and not known about the influences of development, environment, and genetics on pain components (Merskey and Bogduk 1994; Turk and Gatchel 1999; Edwards et al. 2001a; Flores et al. 2002; Sufka and Price 2002; Flor and Hermann 2004; Mogil and Devor 2004; Price and Bushnell 2004; Riley and Wade 2004).

    B. Know that pain measurement is fundamentally inferential. Thus, the objective is to evaluate and relieve the subjective experience. This can be accomplished only through the interpretation of a variety of verbal (self-report) and nonverbal behaviors, including treatment-related behaviors. These must be considered in a context of communication influences as well as physiological differences (Melzack and Katz 1999; Jensen and Karoly 2001; Turk and Melzack 2001; Hadjistavropoulos and Craig 2002).

    C. Distinguish between pain as a subjective experience; pain behavior as a pattern of audible or observable actions (e.g., posture, facial expression, verbalizations); and physical, emotional, and disability functioning (Keefe and Block 1982; Hadjistavropoulos and Craig 1994; Melzack and Katz 1999; Turk and Melzack 2001; Gatchel 2004).

    D. Describe the major psychological and behavioral consequences of acute pain, progressive disease-related pain, chronic nonprogressive pain, and end-of-life care (Abresch et al. 2002; Breitbart and Payne 2004; A.C. Williams 2004; D.A. Williams 2004).

    E. Understand the potential shifts in goals, approaches, and legal issues for pain associated with terminal illness (Meisel et al. 2000; Steinhauser et al. 2000; Breitbart and Payne 2004).

    F. Identify psychosocial developmental issues that must be considered in evaluating and treating pain (Turk and Melzack 2001; Turner and Romano 2001; Farrell and Gibson 2004; McGrath 2004; von Baeyer and Spagrun 2005).

    G. Recognize that verbal reports provide unique access to subjective experiences but have limitations, including response biases, and are complemented by observed nonverbal behaviors and self-reported or observed functional activities. Also, recognize that inferences of the observer can be erroneous or biased (Turk and Flor 1987; Labus et al. 2003).

    H. Understand measurement methods and their strengths and weaknesses for assessing these multiple dimensions of pain (Jensen and Karoly 2001; Turner and Romano 2001; Jensen 2003a,b; see also Chapter 43).

    I. Be familiar with the psychometric concepts of reliability, validity, sensitivity, specificity, usability, standardization, and norms (Jensen 2003a,b; Bolton 2004; Herr et al. 2004).

    J. Understand which self-report and psychological tests have been validated and standardized on chronic pain populations and thus can be utilized with appropriate conclusions (Turk and Melzack 2001; Turner and Romano 2001; Dworkin et al. 2005).

II.   Individual differences

    A.   Recognize fundamental individual differences in affective, cognitive, and behavioral responses to pain and understand their interactions with physiology (Turk and Monarch 2002).

        1.   Affective processes

            a.   Understand the various emotional reactions to actual or potential tissue damage, including anxiety, fear, depression, and anger (Romano and Turner 1985; Vlaeyen and Linton 2000; Rainville 2004; Symreng and Fishman 2004).

            b.   Distinguish affective states associated with acute, recurrent, progressive, and chronic pain (Gallagher and Verma 2004; Holder-Perkins and Wise 2004).

            c.   Know that anticipatory anxiety, distress, and fear may exacerbate pain or predict pain severity (Syrjala and Chapko 1995; Linton 2004).

        2.   Cognitive processes

            a.   Be able to describe basic cognitive processes that determine the nature of painful experience, including beliefs, meaning, appraisal, expectancy, attention, distraction, somatic preoccupation, labeling/reinterpretation, and observational learning (Kotarba 1983; Barkwell 1991; Moerman and Jonas 2002; Bushnell et al. 2004; Hadjistavropoulos and Craig 2004; Holder-Perkins and Wise 2004).

            b.   Describe the major interactions between cognitive appraisals and affective reactions (e.g., the role of catastrophizing, helplessness, and other maladaptive patterns of thinking, or the consequences of self-efficacy and personal control) (Rosenstiel and Keefe 1983; Turner et al. 2000; Sullivan et al. 2001; Tan et al. 2002).

        3.   Behavioral processes

            a.   Understand the principles of operant theory as they relate to the acquisition and maintenance of pain behavior and their role in devising intervention strategies (i.e., primary and secondary reinforcement, punishment, extinction, schedules of reinforcement, shaping, avoidance learning, stimulus control, modeling, and observational learning) (Fordyce 1976; Sanders 2002).

            b.   Know the distinction between operant and respondent conditioning (Fordyce 1976; Sanders 2002).

            c.   Understand that function, activity level, and disability are associated with, but are not the same as, pain (Robinson 2001).

        4.   Integrated psychophysiological model

            a.   Recognize the substantial variability in response to actual tissue damage or potential tissue damage as reflected in the modest correlations among physical damage, pain, and disability for acute, progressive, and chronic pain (Syrjala and Chapko 1995; Flor and Hermann 2004; Manning 2004).

            b.   Understand the basic neurochemical and neurologic mechanisms through which emotion, cognition, and behavior influence each other and are influenced by physiology (Geden et al. 1984; Rainville et al. 1997; Turk and Flor 1999; Wolfe 1999; Price 2000; Bushnell et al. 2004; Chapman and Okifuji 2004).

III.   Coping

    A.   Know the basic coping styles and how they influence pain experience and responses to treatment (e.g., problem solving/active coping, information seeking, support seeking, reappraisal or reframing, distraction, praying/hoping, catastrophizing, avoidance or escape) (Fernandez and Turk 1989; Jordon et al. 1998; Keefe et al. 2000; Jensen et al. 2001; Skinner et al. 2003; Spinhoven et al. 2004).

    B.   Understand theoretical frameworks for coping that have demonstrated relevance to outcomes for pain and pain treatment.

1. Describe the transtheoretical model and current research on applicability of this model to pain treatment (Prochaska and DiClemente 1998; Kerns and Rosenberg 1999; Jensen et al. 2000; Dijkstra 2005).
2. Describe the concepts of catastrophizing and avoidance in relation to pain (Sullivan et al. 2001; Turner and Aaron 2001; Rosenberger et al. 2004; Severeijns et al. 2004).
3. Explain the concept of self-efficacy and its relationship to coping with pain (Jensen et al. 1991; Allegrante and Marks 2003).
4. Explain how motivation, coping style, social support, and social environment responses to pain can influence pain and treatment outcome (Jensen et al. 2001; Jensen et al. 2002; Hanly et al. 2004; Montoya et al. 2004; Nielson and Jensen 2004).

IV. Psychosocial and cultural factors in expectations and in access and adherence to treatment

A. Recognize the internal and exogenous barriers that impact access to and implementation of pain evaluation and treatment (e.g., individual motivation, beliefs, side effects, availability of opioids or other prescribed treatment) (Ward et al. 1993; Breitbart et al. 1998; Miaskowski et al. 2001; Jensen 2002).

B. Be familiar with how individual differences in both patients and health professionals affect adherence to treatment recommendations (DiMatteo et al. 2000; DiMatteo 2004).

C. Understand how expectations, coping, cultural factors, and environmental factors influence disability, treatment outcome, and maintenance of treatment effects (Gatchel and Epker 1999; Severeijns et al. 2001; Goossens et al. 2005).

V. Sociocultural, economic, and racial variation

A. Know that there are cultural, environmental, and racial variations in pain experience and expression and in health care seeking and treatment (Bonham 2001; Edwards et al. 2001b; LeResche 2001; Green et al. 2003; Linton 2004; Sullivan 2004).

B. Understand the contributions and limitations of race, ethnicity, economics, and genetics to pain experience, pain expression, and treatment access (Morrison et al. 2000; Edwards et al. 2001a; McCracken et al. 2001; Carey and Garrett 2003; Green et al. 2003; Fillingim 2004).

C. Recognize that racial, cultural, and gender differences in pain expression and treatment may reflect differences in health care professionals' responses (Todd et al. 2000; Bonham 2001; Hahn 2001; Carey and Garrett 2003; Green et al. 2003).

D. Describe some aspects of communication related to cultural and religious variation that health care professionals should consider when assessing and managing pain (Morris 1999; Flores et al. 2002; Davidhizar and Giger 2004).

E. Know that pain behaviors and complaints are best understood in the context of social transactions among the individual, spouse, employers, and health professionals and in the context of community, governmental, or legal procedures (Romano et al. 1995, 2000; Gatchel and Epker 1999; Main 1999; Robinson 2001; Linton 2004).

F. Recognize that social environment factors, including beliefs about the origins and nature of pain and how one should access health care, influence both experiential and expressive features of pain (Green et al. 2004; Linton 2004).

G. Understand that the workplace and the employee's appraisal of the work environment are potential sources of variation in pain, illness behavior, and disability (Feuerstein et al. 1999; Garofalo and Polatin 1999; Gatchel and Epker 1999; Robinson 2001).

VI. The family and pain

    A. Describe the potential role of the family in promoting illness or well behavior (Romano et al. 1995; Kerns 1999; Otis et al. 2004).

        1. Describe the role of familial models of pain complaint and disability as predisposing factors for maladaptive responses and disability (Romano et al. 1995).

    B. Be aware of the significance of stress, trauma (e.g., family violence, sexual abuse), and marital discord as predisposing, exacerbating, or maintaining factors in pain complaints and disability (Kerns 1999; McGrath and Dade 2004).

    C. Appreciate that communications of pain, distress, and suffering by patients elicit responses from health care providers and significant others, particularly family caregivers (Romano et al. 1995, 2000; Giardino et al. 2003; Smith et al. 2004).

VII. Emotional problems and psychiatric disorders associated with pain (Gatchel 2005).

    A. With regard to pain and depression:

        1. Be aware that pain and depression, as well as anxiety, are associated with each other. Know that chronic pain is not masked depression, nor is there evidence for the concept of a pain-prone personality disorder (Keefe et al. 1986; Averill et al. 1996; Gureje et al. 1998).

        2. Be aware that depression in chronic pain patients is more likely to be a consequence than a cause of chronic pain; but that psychosocial factors, may increase risk for the development of chronic pain, particularly anxiety, catastrophizing, alcohol or other use substance disorders, and occupational impairment (Atkinson et al. 1991; Polatin et al. 1993; Gatchel and Dersh 2002; Main 2002; Picavet et al. 2002; Boersma and Linton 2005).

        3. Understand that depression may be a predictor of pain severity, pain behavior, disability or adherence to pain treatment, and that the presence of pain may be a predictor of depression severity. However, be aware that these are associations not causal statements (Averill et al. 1996; DiMatteo et al. 2000; Lin et al. 2003).

        4. Recognize that early intervention is increasingly seen as central to the prevention of long term disability. Be able to evaluate psychosocial risk factors that influence the onset and maintenance of disability and understand interventions for their management (Picavet et al. 2002; Boersma and Linton 2005).

    B. Understand the complex interaction of pain expression with the following psychological factors:

        1. Recognize that personality disorders and maladaptive coping styles are frequently found in chronic pain patients, but it is uncertain whether the prevalence of personality disorders or of subtypes of personality disorders is greater in chronic pain patients than in the general population (Polatin et al. 1993; Weisberg and Keefe 1999; Geisser 2004).

        2. Describe the DSM-IV diagnostic concepts of somatoform disorders (e.g., somatization, conversion, pain hypochondriasis, body dysmorphic disorders, factitious disorders, and malingering). Understand the contradictions between this classification and the scientific research described in this chapter, particularly in section A above (American Psychiatric Association 2000).

        3. Be aware that chronic pain patients can present with signs and symptoms that are incongruent with medical expectations based upon anatomical and physiological knowledge. Appreciate that these cases cannot be considered malingering. While they may predict limited success with conventional medical treatment, they cannot be used to make a reliable psychiatric diagnosis (Craig and Badali 2004).

        4. Recognize that malingering and deception are possible, and identify factors that increase this likelihood as well as the limitations in our capacities to accurately assess malingering (Craig and Badali 2004).

REFERENCES

Abresch RT, Carter GT, Jensen MP, Kilmer DD. Assessment of pain and health-related quality of life in slowly progressive neuro-muscular disease. *Am J Hosp Palliat Care* 2002; 19:29–48.

Allegrante JP, Marks R. Self-efficacy in management of osteoarthritis. *Rheum Dis Clin N Am* 2003; 29:747–768.

American Psychiatric Association. *Diagnostic and Statistical Manual of Mental Disorders* (DSM-IV-TR). Washington, DC: American Psychiatric Association, 2000.

Atkinson JH, Slater MA, Patterson TL, Grant I, Garfin SR. Prevalence, onset, and risk of psychiatric disorders in men with chronic low back pain: a controlled study. *Pain* 1991; 45(2):111–121.

Averill PM, Novy DM, Nelson DV, Berry LA. Correlates of depression in chronic pain patients: a comprehensive examination. *Pain* 1996; 65:93–100.

Barkwell DP. Ascribed meaning: a critical factor in coping and pain attenuation in patients with cancer related pain. *J Palliat Care* 1991; 7:5–14.

Boersma K, Linton SJ. Screening to identify patients at risk: profiles of psychological risk factors for early interventions. *Clin J Pain* 2005; 21:38–43.

Bolton JE. Sensitivity and specificity of outcome measures in patients with neck pain: detecting clinically significant improvement. *Spine* 2004; 29:2410–2417.

Bonham VL. Race, ethnicity, and pain treatment: striving to understand the causes and solutions to the disparities in pain treatment. *J Law Med Ethics* 2001; 29:52–68.

Breitbart W, Passik S, McDonald MV, et al. Patient-related barriers to pain management in ambulatory AIDS patients. *Pain* 1998; 76:9–16.

Breitbart WS, Payne DK. Psychological and psychiatric dimensions of palliative care. In: Dworkin RH, Breitbart WS (Eds). *Psychosocial Aspects of Pain: A Handbook for Health Care Providers,* Progress in Pain Research and Management, Vol. 27. Seattle: IASP Press, 2004, pp 427–462.

Bushnell MC, Villemure C, Duncan GH. Psychophysical and neurophysiological studies of pain modulation by attention. In: Price DD, Bushnell MC (Eds). *Psychological Methods of Pain Control: Basic Science and Clinical Perspectives,* Progress in Pain Research and Management, Vol. 29, Seattle: IASP Press, 2004, pp 99–167.

Carey TS, Garrett JM. The relation of race to outcomes and the use of health care services for acute low back pain. *Spine* 2003; 28:390–394.

Chapman CR, Okifuji A. Pain: basic mechanisms and conscious experience. In: Dworkin RH, Breitbart WS (Eds). *Psychosocial Aspects of Pain: A Handbook for Health Care Providers.* Progress in Pain Research and Management, Volume 27. Seattle: IASP Press, 2004, pp 3–28.

Craig KD, Badali MA. Introduction to the special series on pain deception and malingering. *Clin J Pain* 2004; 20:377–382.

Davidhizar R, Giger JN. A review of the literature on care of clients in pain who are culturally diverse. *Int Nurs Rev* 2004; 51:47–55.

Dijkstra A. The validity of the Stages of Change model in the adoption of the self-management approach in chronic pain. *Clin J Pain* 2005; 21:27–37.

DiMatteo MR. Variations in patients' adherence to medical recommendations: a quantitative review of 50 years of research. *Med Care* 2004; 42:200–209.

DiMatteo MR, Lepper HS, Croghan TW. Depression is a risk factor for noncompliance with medical treatment: meta-analysis of the effects of anxiety and depression on patient adherence. *Arch Intern Med* 2000; 160:2101–2107.

Dworkin RH, Turk DC, Farrar JT, et al. Core outcome measures for chronic pain clinical trials: IMMPACT recommendations. *Pain* 2005; 113:9–19.

Edwards CL, Fillingim RB, Keefe F. Race, ethnicity and pain. *Pain* 2001a; 94:133–137.

Edwards RR, Doleys DM, Fillingim RB, Lowery D. Ethnic differences in pain tolerance: clinical implications in a chronic pain population. *Psychosom Med* 2001b; 63:316–323.

Farrell MJ, Gibson SJ. Psychosocial aspects of pain in older people. In: Dworkin RH, Breitbart WS (Eds). *Psychosocial Aspects of Pain: A Handbook for Health Care Providers,* Progress in Pain Research and Management, Vol. 27. Seattle: IASP Press, 2004, pp 495–518.

Fernandez E, Turk DC. The utility of cognitive coping strategies for altering pain perception: a meta-analysis. *Pain* 1989; 38:123–135.

Feuerstein M, Huang GD, Pransky G. Workstyle and work-related upper extremity disorders. In: Gatchel RJ, Turk DC (Eds). *Psychosocial Factors in Pain: Critical Perspectives.* New York: Guilford Press, 1999, pp 175–192.

Fillingim RB. Social and environmental influences on pain: implications for pain genetics. In: Mogil JS (Ed). *The Genetics of Pain,* Progress in Pain Research and Management, Vol. 28. Seattle: IASP Press, 2004, pp 283–304.

Flor H, Hermann C. Biopsychosocial models of pain. In: Dworkin RH, Breitbart WS (Eds). *Psychosocial Aspects of Pain: A Handbook for Health Care Providers,* Progress in Pain Research and Management, Vol. 27. Seattle: IASP Press, 2004, pp 47–76.

Flores G, Rabke-Verani J, Pine W, Sabharwal A. The importance of cultural and linguistic issues in the emergency care of children. *Pediatr Emerg Care* 2002; 18:271–284.

Fordyce WE. *Behavioral Methods for Chronic Pain and Illness.* St. Louis, MO: Mosby, 1976.

Gallagher RM, Verma S. Mood and anxiety disorders in chronic pain. In: Dworkin RH, Breitbart WS (Eds). *Psychosocial Aspects of Pain: A Handbook for Health Care Providers,* Progress in Pain Research and Management, Vol. 27. Seattle: IASP Press, 2004, pp 139–178.

Garofalo JP, Polatin P. Low back pain: an epidemic in industrialized countries. In: Gatchel RJ, Turk DC (Eds). *Psychosocial Factors in Pain: Critical Perspectives.* New York: Guilford Press, 1999, pp 164–174.

Gatchel RJ. Psychosocial factors that can influence the self-assessment of function. *J Occup Rehabil* 2004; 14:197–206.

Gatchel RJ. Comorbidity of chronic pain and mental health disorders: the biopsychological perspective. *Am Psychol* 2005; 59:795–805.

Gatchel RJ, Dersh J. Psychological disorders and chronic pain: Are there cause-and-effect relationships? In: Turk DC, Gatchel RJ (Eds). *Psychological Approaches to Pain Management: A Practitioner's Handbook.* New York: Guilford Press, 2002, pp 30–51.

Gatchel RJ, Epker J. Psychosocial predictors of chronic pain and response to treatment. In: Gatchel RJ, Turk DC (Eds). *Psychosocial Factors in Pain: Critical Perspectives.* New York: Guilford Press, 1999, pp 412–434.

Geden E, Beck N, Hauge G, Pohlman S. Self-report and psychophysiological effects of five pain-coping strategies. *Nurs Res* 1984; 33:260–265.

Geisser ME. The influence of coping styles and personality traits on pain. In: Dworkin RH, Breitbart WS (Eds). *Psychosocial Aspects of Pain: A Handbook for Health Care Providers,* Progress in Pain Research and Management, Vol. 27. Seattle: IASP Press, 2004, pp 521–546.

Giardino ND, Jensen MP, Turner JA, Ehde DD. Social environment moderates the association between catastrophizing and pain among persons with a spinal cord injury. *Pain* 2003; 106:19–25.

Goossens MEJB, Vlaeyen JWS, Hidding A, Kole-Snijders A, Evers SMAA. Treatment expectancy affects the outcome of cognitive-behavioral interventions in chronic pain. *Clin J Pain* 2005; 21:18–26.

Green CR, Anderson KO, Baker TA, et al. The unequal burden of pain: confronting racial and ethnic disparities in pain. *Pain Med.* 2003; 4:277–294.

Green CR, Baker TA, Ndao-Brumblay SK. Patient attitudes regarding healthcare utilization and referral: a descriptive comparison in African- and Caucasian-Americans with chronic pain. *J Nat Med Assoc* 2004; 96:31–42.

Gureje O, Von Korff M, Simon GE, Gater R. Persistent pain and well-being: a World Health Organization study in primary care. *JAMA* 1998; 280:147–151.

Hadjistavropoulos HD, Craig KD. Acute and chronic low back pain: cognitive, affective, and behavioral dimensions. *J Consult Clin Psychol* 1994; 62:341–349.

Hadjistavropoulos T, Craig KD. A theoretical framework for understanding self-report and observational measures of pain: a communications model. *Behav Res Ther* 2002; 40:551–570.

Hadjistavropoulos T, Craig KD. Social influences and the communication of pain.. In: Hadjistavropoulos T, Craig KD (Eds). *Pain: Psychological Perspectives.* New York: Lawrence Erlbaum, 2004, pp 87–112.

Hahn SR. Physical symptoms and physician-experienced difficulty in the physician-patient relationship. *Ann Intern Med* 2001; 134:897–904.

Hanly MA, Jensen MP, Ehde DM, Hoffman AJ, Patterson DR, Robinson LR. Psychosocial predictors of long-term adjustment to lower-limb amputation and phantom limb pain. *Disabil Rehabil* 2004; 26:882–893.

Herr KA, Spratt K, Mobily PR, Richardson G. Pain intensity assessment in older adults: use of experimental pain to compare psychometric properties and usability of selected pain scales with younger adults. *Clin J Pain* 2004; 20:207–219.

Holder-Perkins V, Wise T. Somatoform disorders and pain complaints. In: Dworkin RH, Breitbart WS (Eds). *Psychosocial Aspects of Pain: A Handbook for Health Care Providers,* Progress in Pain Research and Management, Vol. 27. Seattle: IASP Press, 2004, pp 179–194.

Jensen MP. Enhancing motivation to change in pain treatment. In: Turk DC, Gatchel R (Eds). *Psychological Approaches to Pain Management: A Practitioner's Handbook.* New York: Guilford Press, 2002, pp 71–93.

Jensen MP. Questionnaire validation: a brief guide for readers of the research literature. *Clin J Pain* 2003a; 19:345–352.

Jensen MP. The validity and reliability of pain measures in adults with cancer. *J Pain* 2003b; 4:2–21.

Jensen MP, Karoly P. Self-report scales and procedures for assessing pain in adults. In: Turk DC, Melzack R (Eds). *Handbook of Pain Assessment.* New York: Guilford Press, 2001, pp 15–34.

Jensen MP, Turner JA, Romano JM. Self-efficacy and outcome expectancies: relationship to chronic pain coping strategies and adjustment. *Pain* 1991; 44:263–269.

Jensen MP, Nielson WR, Romano JM, Hill ML, Turner JA. Further evaluation of the pain stages of change questionnaire: is the transtheoretical model of change useful for patients with chronic pain? *Pain* 2000; 86:255–264.

Jensen MP, Turner JA, Romano JM. Changes in beliefs, catastrophizing, and coping are associated with improvement in multidisciplinary pain treatment. *J Consult Clin Psychol* 2001; 69:655–662.

Jensen MP, Ehde DM, Hoffman AJ, et al. Cognitions, coping and social environment predict adjustment to phantom limb pain. *Pain* 2002; 95:133–142.

Jordon MS, Lumley MA, Leisen JC. The relationships of cognitive coping and pain control beliefs to pain and adjustment among African-American and Caucasian women with rheumatoid arthritis. *Arthritis Care Res* 1998; 11:80–88.

Keefe FJ, Block AR. Development of an observation method for assessing pain behavior in chronic low back pain patients. *Behav Ther* 1982; 13:363–375.

Keefe FJ, Wildins RH, Cook WA, Crisson JE, Muhlbaier LH. Depression, pain and pain behavior. *J Consult Clin Psychol* 1986; 54:665–669.

Keefe FJ, Lefebvre JC, Egan JR, Affleck G, Sullivan MJ, Caldwell D. The relationship of gender to pain, pain behavior, and disability in osteoarthritis patients: the role of catastrophizing. *Pain* 2000; 87:325–334.

Kerns RD. Family therapy for adults with chronic pain. In: Gatchel RJ, Turk DC (Eds). *Psychosocial Factors in Pain: Critical Perspectives.* New York: Guilford Press, 1999, pp 445–456.

Kerns RD, Rosenberg R. Predicting responses to self-management treatments for chronic pain: application to the pain stages of change model. *Pain* 1999; 84:49–56.

Kotarba JA. Perceptions of death, belief systems, and the process of coping with chronic pain. *Soc Sci Med* 1983; 17:681–689.

Labus JS, Keefe FJ, Jensen M.P. Self-reports of pain intensity and direct observations of pain behavior: when are they correlated? *Pain* 2003; 102:109–124.

LeResche L. Gender, cultural, and environmental aspects of pain. In: Loeser JD, Butler SH, Chapman CR, Turk DC (Eds). *Bonica's Management of Pain.* Philadelphia: Lippincott Williams & Wilkins, 2001, pp 191–195.

Lin EHB, Katon W, Von Korff M, et al. Effect of improving depression care on pain and functional outcomes among older adults with arthritis. *JAMA* 2003; 290:2428–2434.

Linton SJ. Environmental and learning factors in the development of chronic pain and disability. In: Price DD, Bushnell MC (Eds). *Psychological Methods of Pain Control: Basic Science and Clinical Perspectives,* Progress in Pain Research and Management, Vol. 29, Seattle: IASP Press, 2004, pp 143–168.

Main CJ. Medicolegal aspects of pain: the nature of psychological opinion in cases of personal injury. In: Gatchel RJ, Turk DC (Eds). *Psychosocial Factors in Pain: Critical Perspectives.* New York: Guilford Press, 1999, pp 132–147.

Main C. Concepts of treatment and prevention in musculoskeletal disorders. In: Linton S (Ed). *New Avenues for the Prevention of Chronic Musculoskeletal Pain and Disability.* Amsterdam: Elsevier, 2002.

Manning BH. Preclinical studies of pain modulation: lessons learned from animals. In: Price DD, Bushnell MC (Eds). *Psychological Methods of Pain Control: Basic Science and Clinical Perspectives,* Progress in Pain Research and Management, Vol. 29. Seattle: IASP Press, 2004, pp 43–72.

McCracken LM, Matthews AK, Tang TS, Cuba SL. A comparison of blacks and whites seeking treatment for chronic pain. *Pain* 2001; 17:249–255.

McGrath PA, Dade LA. Strategies to decrease pain and minimize disability. In: Price DD, Bushnell MC (Eds). *Psychological Methods of Pain Control: Basic Science and Clinical Perspectives,* Progress in Pain Research and Management, Vol. 29. Seattle: IASP Press, 2004, pp 73–96.

McGrath PJ. Psychosocial and psychiatric aspects of pain in children. In: Dworkin RH, Breitbart WS (Eds). *Psychosocial Aspects of Pain: A Handbook for Health Care Providers,* Progress in Pain Research and Management, Vol. 27. Seattle, IASP Press, 2004, pp 479–494.

Meisel A, Snyder L, Quill T, for the American College of Physicians-American Society of Internal Medicine End-of-Life Care Consensus Panel. Seven legal barriers to end-of-life care: myths, realities, and grains of truth. *JAMA* 2000; 284:2495–2501.

Melzack R, Katz J. Pain management in persons in pain. In: Wall PD, Melzack R (Eds). *Textbook of Pain.* Edinburgh: Churchill Livingstone, 1999.

Merskey H, Bogduk N. *Classification of Chronic Pain: Descriptions of Chronic Pain Syndromes and Definition of Pain Terms,* 2nd ed. Seattle: IASP Press, 1994.

Miaskowski C, Dodd MJ, West C, et al. Lack of adherence with the analgesic regimen: a significant barrier to effective cancer pain management. *J Clin Oncol* 2001; 19:4275–4279.

Moerman DE, Jonas WB. Deconstructing the placebo effect and finding the meaning response. *Ann Intern Med* 2002; 136:471–476.

Mogil JS, Devor M. Introduction to pain genetics. In: Mogil JS (Ed). *The Genetics of Pain,* Progress in Pain Research and Management, Vol. 28. Seattle: IASP Press, 2004, pp 1–18.

Montoya P, Larbig W, Braun C, Preissl H, Birbaumer N. Influence of social support and emotional context on pain processing and magnetic brain responses in fibromyalgia. *Arthritis Rheum* 2004; 50:4035–4044.

Morris DB. Sociocultural and religious meanings of pain. In: Gatchel RJ, Turk DC (Eds). *Psychosocial Factors in Pain: Critical Perspectives.* New York: Guilford Press, 1999, pp 118–131.

Morrison RS, Wallenstein S, Natale DK, Senzel RS, Huang LL. "We don't carry that": failure of pharmacies in predominantly non-white neighborhoods to stock opioid analgesics. *N Engl J Med* 2000; 342:1023–1026.

Nielson WR, Jensen MP. Relationship between changes in coping and treatment outcome in patients with fibromyalgia syndrome. *Pain* 2004; 109:233–241.

Otis JD, Cardella LA, Kerns RD. The influence of family and culture on Pain. In: Dworkin RH, Breitbart WS (Eds). *Psychosocial Aspects of Pain: A Handbook for Health Care Providers,* Progress in Pain Research and Management, Vol. 27. Seattle: IASP Press, 2004, pp 29–46.

Picavet HS, Vlaeyen JW, Schouten JS. Pain catastrophizing and kinesiophobia: predictors of chronic low back pain. *Am J Epidemiol* 2002; 156:1028–1034.

Polatin PB, Kinney RK, Gatchel RJ, Lillo E, Mayer TG. Psychiatric illness and chronic low-back pain. The mind and the spine: which goes first? *Spine* 1993; 18:66–71.

Price DD. Psychological and neural mechanisms of the affective dimension of pain. *Science* 2000; 288:1769–1772.

Price DD, Bushnell MC. Overview of pain dimensions and their psychological modulation. In: Price DD, Bushnell MC (Eds). *Psychological Methods of Pain Control: Basic Science and Clinical Perspectives,* Progress in Pain Research and Management, Vol. 29. Seattle: IASP Press, 2004, pp 3–18.

Prochaska JO, DiClemente CC. Towards a comprehensive, transtheoretical model of change: states of change and addictive behaviors. In: Miller WR, Heather N (Eds). *Applied Clinical Psychology,* 2nd ed. *Treating Behaviors.* New York: Plenum Press, 1998, pp 37–49.

Rainville P. Pain and emotions. In: Price DD, Bushnell MC (Eds). *Psychological Methods of Pain Control: Basic Science and Clinical Perspectives.* Progress in Pain Research and Management, Vol. 29. Seattle: IASP Press, 2004, pp 117–142.

Rainville P, Duncan GH, Price DD, Carrier B, Bushnell MC. Pain affect encoded in human anterior cingulate but not somatosensory cortex. *Science* 1997; 277:968–971.

Riley JL, Wade JB. Psychological and demographic factors that modulate the difference stages and dimensions of pain. In: Price DD, Bushnell MC (Eds). *Psychological Methods of Pain Control: Basic Science and Clinical Perspectives,* Progress in Pain Research and Management, Vol. 29. Seattle: IASP Press, 2004, pp 19–42.

Robinson JP. Evaluation of function and disability. In: Loeser JD, Butler SH, Chapman CR, Turk DC (Eds). *Bonica's Management of Pain.* Philadelphia: Lippincott Williams & Wilkins, 2001, pp 342–362.

Romano JM, Turner JA. Chronic pain and depression: does the evidence support a relationship? *Psychol Bull* 1985; 97:18–34.

Romano JM, Turner JA, Jensen MP, et al. Chronic pain patient-spouse behavioral interactions predict patient disability. *Pain* 1995; 63:353–360.

Romano JM, Jensen MP, Turner JA, Good AB, Hops H. Chronic pain patient-partner interactions: further support for a behavioral model of chronic pain. *Behav Ther* 2000; 31:415–440.

Rosenberger PH, Ickovics JR, Epel ES, D'Entremont D, Jokl P. Physical recovery in arthroscopic knee surgery: unique contributions of coping behaviors to clinical outcomes and stress reactivity. *Psychol Health* 2004; 19:307–320.

Rosenstiel AK, Keefe FJ. The use of coping strategies in chronic low back pain patients: relationship to patient characteristics and current adjustment. *Pain* 1983; 17:33–44.

Sanders SH. Operant conditioning with chronic pain: back to basics. In: Turk DC, Gatchel RJ (Eds). *Psychological Approaches to Pain Management: A Practitioner's Handbook.* New York: Guilford Press, 2002, pp 128–137.

Severeijns R, Vlaeyen JWS, van den Hout MA, Weber WEJ. Pain catastrophizing predicts pain intensity, disability, and psychological distress independent of the level of physical impairment. *Clin J Pain* 2001; 17:165–172.

Severeijns R, Vlaeyen JWS, van den Hout MA, Picavet HSJ. Pain catastrophizing is associated with health indices in musculoskeletal pain: a cross-sectional study in the Dutch community. *Health Psychol* 2004; 23:49–57.

Skinner EA, Edge K, Altman J, Sherwood H. Searching for the structure of coping: a review and critique of category systems for classifying ways of coping. *Psychol Bull* 2003; 129:216–269.

Smith SJA, Keefe FJ, Caldwell DS, Romano J, Baucom D. Gender differences in patient-spouse interactions: a sequential analysis of behavioral interactions in patients having osteoarthritic knee pain. *Pain* 2004; 112:183–187.

Spinhoven P, Ter Kuile M, Kole-Snijders AM, et al. Catastrophizing and internal pain control as mediators of outcome in the multidisciplinary treatment of chronic low back pain. *Eur J Pain* 2004; 8:211–219.

Steinhauser KE, Christakis NA, Clipp EC, et al. Factors considered important at the end of life by patients, family, physicians, and other care providers. *JAMA* 2000; 284:2476–2482.

Sufka KJ, Price DD. Gate control theory reconsidered. *Brain & Mind* 2002; 3:277–290.

Sullivan M. Exaggerated pain behavior: by what standard? *Clin J Pain* 2004; 20:433–439.

Sullivan MJ, Thorn B, Haythornthwaite JA, et al. Theoretical perspectives on the relation between catastrophizing and pain. *Clin J Pain* 2001; 17:52–64.

Symreng I, Fishman SM. Anxiety and pain. *Pain: Clin Updates* 2004; XII(7):1–6.

Syrjala KL, Chapko ME. Evidence for a biopsychosocial model of cancer treatment-related pain. *Pain* 1995; 61:69–79.

Tan G, Jensen MP, Robinson-Whelen S, Thornby JI, Monga T. Measuring control appraisals in chronic pain. *J Pain* 2002; 3:385–393.

Todd KH, Deaton C, D'Adamo AP, Goe L. Ethnicity and analgesic practice. *Ann Emerg Med* 2000; 35:11–16.

Turk DC, Flor H. Pain greater than pain behavior: the utility and limitations of the pain behavior construct. *Pain* 1987; 31:295.

Turk DC, Flor H. Chronic pain: a biobehavioral perspective. In: Gatchel RJ, Turk DC (Eds). *Psychosocial Factors in Pain: Clinical Perspectives.* New York: Guilford Press, 1999, pp 18–34.

Turk DC, Gatchel RJ. Psychosocial factors and pain: revolution and evolution. In: RJ Gatchel and DC Turk (Eds). *Psychosocial Factors in Pain.* New York: Guilford Press, 1999, pp 481–493.

Turk DC, Melzack R. *Handbook of Pain Assessment.* New York: Guilford Press, 2001.

Turk DC, Monarch ES. Biopsychosocial perspective on chronic pain. In: Turk DC, Gatchel RJ (Eds). *Psychological Approaches to Pain Management: A Practitioner's Handbook.* New York: Guilford Press, 2002, pp 3–29.

Turner JA, Aaron LA. Pain-related catastrophizing: what is it? *Clin J Pain* 2001; 17:65–71.

Turner JA, Romano JM. Psychological and psychosocial evaluation. In: Loeser JD, Butler SH, Chapman CR, Turk DC (Eds). *Bonica's Management of Pain.* Philadelphia: Lippincott Williams & Wilkins, 2001, pp 329–341.

Turner JA, Jensen MP, Romano JM. Do beliefs, coping, and catastrophizing independently predict functioning in patients with chronic pain? *Pain* 2000; 85:115–125.

Vlaeyen JWS, Linton SJ. Fear-avoidance and its consequences in chronic musculoskeletal pain: a state of the art. *Pain* 2000; 85:317–332.

von Baeyer CL, Spagrun LJ. Social development and pain in children. In: McGrath PJ, Finley GA (Eds). *Pediatric Pain: Biological and Social Context,* Progress in Pain Research and Management, Vol. 26. Seattle, IASP Press, 2003, pp. 81–98.

Ward SE, Goldberg N, Miller-McCauley V, et al. Patient-related barriers to management of cancer pain. *Pain* 1993; 52:319–324.

Weisberg JN, Keefe FJ. Personality, individual differences, and psychopathology in chronic pain. In: Gatchel RJ, Turk DC (Eds). *Psychosocial Factors in Pain: Critical Perspectives.* New York: Guilford Press, 1999, pp 56–73.

Williams AC. Assessing chronic pain and its impact. In: Dworkin RH, Breitbart WS (Eds). *Psychosocial Aspects of Pain: A Handbook for Health Care Providers,* Progress in Pain Research and Management, Vol. 27. Seattle: IASP Press, 2004, pp 97–116.

Williams DA. Evaluating acute pain. In: Dworkin RH, Breitbart WS (Eds). *Psychosocial Aspects of Pain: A Handbook for Health Care Providers,* Progress in Pain Research and Management, Vol. 27. Seattle: IASP Press, 2004, pp 79–96.

Wolfe F. Determinants of WOMAC function, pain and stiffness scores: evidence for the role of low back pain, symptom counts, fatigue and depression in osteoarthritis, rheumatoid arthritis and fibromyalgia. *Rheumatology* 1999; 38:355–361.

Core Curriculum for Professional Education in Pain, edited by J. Edmond Charlton, IASP Press, Seattle, © 2005.

12

Sex and Gender Issues in Pain

I.   Understand the differences in the terms "sex" and "gender" (Pardue et al. 2001).

   A.   Be aware of the biological (e.g. physical, anatomical, developmental) and chromosomal differences between males and females (human and nonhuman), which are typically referred to as "sex."

   B.   Be aware that "gender" refers to one's self-identity as being female or male, based on social and environmental as well as biological factors.

II. Understand the nature of sex differences in the epidemiology of pain in relation to age and reproductive history.

   A.   Know that in population-based surveys, women typically report more frequent and/or severe pain than men (Unruh 1996).

   B.   Know that women are at greater risk for several chronic painful disorders, including temporomandibular disorders, fibromyalgia, migraine headache, interstitial cystitis, joint pain, irritable bowel syndrome, complex regional pain syndrome, and trigeminal neuralgia (Unruh 1996; Jones and Nyberg 1997; LeResche 1999; Buckwalter and Lappin 2000; Dao and LeResche 2000). Be aware that these differences vary with age and are associated with endogenous or exogenous sex hormone changes, for example, in the case of migraine headaches (Silberstein 2001). Women are at greater risk for autoimmune disorders that have a pain component, such as rheumatoid arthritis, lupus, and scleroderma (Buckwalter and Lappin 2000).

   C.   Know that men are at greater risk for some pain disorders, including cluster headache and pancreatitis (Dodick et al. 2000; Lin et al. 2000).

   D.   Recognize that several pain conditions are unique to reproductive organs—either to women, including dysmenorrhea, vulvodynia, and labor pain, or to men, such as testicular pain and pain associated with prostatitis (Wesselmann and Reich 1996).

   E.   Know that some studies suggest greater procedural and postoperative pain among females than males (Froehlich et al. 1997; Averbuch and Katzper 2000; Taenzer et al. 2000), while other studies have reported no sex differences (Lander et al. 1990; Gear et al. 1996).

III. Understand sex differences in nociceptive responses and pain perception in both animal (acute and chronic) and human (acute) experimental pain models.

   A.   Know that nonhuman animal models reveal sex differences in nociceptive responses, but the results vary across pain assays. For example, females are more sensitive to electrical stimuli and to chemical provocations such as formalin (Aloisi et al. 1994, 1995; Mogil et al. 2000). Be aware that findings from studies of heat stimuli are less consistent, with more studies than not reporting no sex differences (Mogil et al. 2000).

   B.   Know that hormonal responses to nociceptive stimuli differ according to sex (Aloisi 1997).

   C.   Know that among humans, women report lower pain thresholds and tolerances than men, and that ratings of suprathreshold stimuli are often higher among women than men across a wide range of painful stimuli (Fillingim and Maixner 1995; Riley et al. 1998).

IV.   Understand differences in analgesic responses both within the same sex (e.g., during childbearing) and between sexes.

   A.   Know that endogenous analgesic responses can differ both quantitatively and qualitatively by sex (Bodnar et al. 1988; Mogil et al. 1993) and that there are female-specific endogenous analgesic systems, including pregnancy-induced analgesia (Gintzler and Liu 2000) and analgesia produced by vaginocervical stimulation (Komisaruk and Whipple 2000).

   B.   Be aware that nonhuman animal research, primarily in rodents, suggests greater opioid analgesia in males than females (Fillingim and Ness 2000; Kest et al. 2000). Limited research on non-opioid analgesics suggests that sex differences may also be present for these agents (Walker and Carmody 1998; Chiari et al. 1999).

   C.   Know that among humans, research suggests that sex differences can be measured between mu- and kappa-opioid agonists. For example, following oral surgery, females experienced either more robust or more prolonged analgesia than males using kappa- (or weak mu-) opioid analgesics (Miaskowski et al. 2000). Be aware that limited experimental research suggests that women show greater analgesic responses to potent mu-opioid agonists (Sarton et al. 2000; Zacny 2002).

   D.   Know that for nonsteroidal anti-inflammatory drugs, the variability in response may be gender-related such that females demonstrate less effect than males (Walker and Carmody 1998), although findings of no sex difference have also emerged (Averbuch and Katzper 2000).

V.   Understand biological and psychosocial contributions to sex differences in pain responses (Fillingim 2000).

   A.   Know that developmental factors influence the structural and functional sex differences in nervous system development (McEwen 2001). Be aware that brain function and activation during pain can differ between males and females (Paulson et al. 1998).

   B.   Know that sex hormone receptors can influence nociceptive activity through genomic and nongenomic or membrane effects (Aloisi 2000).

   C.   Know that sex differences in immune responses can contribute to sex differences in pain sensitivity (Da Silva 1999; Gregory et al. 2000).

   D.   Be aware of the normal biological differences between the sexes, e.g., weight and body mass composition, as they apply to pharmacokinetic differences as well as cyclical hormonal variations with age (Berkley and Holdcroft 1999).

   E.   Know that hormonal fluctuations associated with the estrous or menstrual cycle have been associated with pain and analgesia (Riley et al. 1999; Fillingim and Ness 2000). Exogenous hormones have also been related to clinical pain (LeResche et al. 1997; Wise et al. 2000; Musgrave et al. 2001) and to experimental pain sensitivity (Fillingim and Edwards 2001).

   F.   Know that genetic factors appear to determine some sex differences in pain and analgesia (Mogil 2000).

   G.   Know that multiple psychosocial variables may contribute to sex differences in clinical and experimental pain responses, including (but not limited to) anxiety (Edwards et al. 2000), abuse history (Spertus et al. 1999), coping (Affleck et al. 1999; Keefe et al. 2000), gender roles (Robinson et al. 2001), and family history (Fillingim et al. 2000).

VI.   Understand that the patient's sex may influence treatment seeking, delivery of treatment, and treatment effectiveness.

   A.   Know that women seek more pain-related health care than men (Unruh 1996; Barsky et al. 2001), and that women in the general population are more likely than men to use prescription narcotics (Eggen 1993; Simoni-Wastila 2000).

B.   Know that women are more likely than men to suffer an adverse effect after analgesia (Ciccone and Holdcroft 1999).

C.   Know that women and men presenting with pain complaints (e.g., ischemic cardiac pain or back pain) may be offered different diagnostic tests and/or treatments (Safran et al. 1997; Roger et al. 2000; Weisse et al. 2001).

D.   Be aware that some research suggests that rehabilitation and multidisciplinary pain treatment produces more robust clinical improvement in women than men (Jensen et al. 2001), while other findings indicate similar treatment gains for women and men (Mannion et al. 2001).

E.   Be aware that the determinants of treatment effectiveness may differ for women and men (Burns et al. 1998).

VII.   Understand the factors that may influence the outcome of pain experiments or therapies for men and women.

A.   Know that health care delivery occurs in a sociocultural context and that the characteristics of providers and patients and the setting in which health care is provided may influence women and men in different ways.

B.   Know that the attitude of the person matters and that within-sex variation in pain is greater than between-sex variation in pain.

C.   Know that time (e.g., daily circadian rhythms) and environmental factors (e.g., music, lighting) may influence women and men differently.

REFERENCES

Affleck G, Tennen H, Keefe FJ, et al. Everyday life with osteoarthritis or rheumatoid arthritis: independent effects of disease and gender on daily pain, mood, and coping. *Pain* 1999; 83:601–609.

Aloisi AM. Sex differences in pain-induced effects on the septo-hippocampal system. *Brain Res Brain Res Rev* 1997; 25:397–406.

Aloisi AM. Sensory effects of gonadal hormones. In: Fillingim RB (Ed). *Sex, Gender, and Pain,* Progress in Pain Research and Management, Vol. 17. IASP Press, Seattle, 2000, pp 7–24.

Aloisi AM, Albonetti ME, Carli G. Sex differences in the behavioural response to persistent pain in rats. *Neurosci Lett* 1994; 179:09–82.

Aloisi AM, Sacerdote P, Albonetti ME, Carli G. Sex-related effects on behaviour and beta-endorphin of different intensities of formalin pain in rats. *Brain Res* 1995; 699:242–249.

Averbuch M, Katzper M. A search for sex differences in response to analgesia. *Arch Intern Med* 2000; 160:3424–3428.

Barsky AJ, Peekna HM, Borus JF. Somatic symptom reporting in women and men. *J Gen Intern Med* 2001; 16:266–275.

Berkley KJ, Holdcroft A. Sex and gender differences in pain. In: Wall PD, Melzack R (Eds). *Textbook of Pain.* Edinburgh: Churchill-Livingstone, 1999, pp 951–965.

Bodnar RJ, Romero MT, Kramer E. Organismic variables and pain inhibition: roles of gender and aging. *Brain Res Bull* 1988; 21:947–953.

Buckwalter JA, Lappin DR. The disproportionate impact of chronic arthralgia and arthritis among women. *Clin Orthop* 2000; 87:159–168.

Burns JW, Johnson BJ, Devine J, Mahoney N, Pawl R. Anger management style and the prediction of treatment outcome among male and female chronic pain patients. *Behav Res Ther* 1998; 36:1051–1062.

Chiari A, Tobin JR, Pan HL, Hood DD, Eisenach JC. Sex differences in cholinergic analgesia I: a supplemental nicotinic mechanism in normal females. *Anesthesiology* 1999; 91:1447–1454.

Ciccone GK, Holdcroft A. Drugs and sex differences: a review of drugs relating to anaesthesia. *Br J Anaesth* 1999; 82:255–265.

Da Silva JA. Sex hormones and glucocorticoids: interactions with the immune system. *Ann Acad Sci NY* 1999; 876:102–117; discussion 117–118, 102–117.

Dao TT, LeResche L. Gender differences in pain. *J Orofac Pain* 2000; 14:169–184.

Dodick DW, Rozen TD, Goadsby PJ, Silberstein SD. Cluster headache. *Cephalalgia* 2000; 20:787–803.

Edwards RR, Augustson E, Fillingim RB. Sex-specific effects of pain-related anxiety on adjustment to chronic pain. *Clin J Pain* 2000; 16:46–53.

Eggen AE. The Tromso Study: frequency and predicting factors of analgesic drug use in a free-living population (12–56 years). *J Clin Epidemiol* 1993; 46:1297–1304.

Fillingim RB. *Sex, Gender, and Pain,* Progress in Pain and Research Management, Vol. 17. Seattle: IASP Press, 2000.

Fillingim RB, Edwards RR. The association of hormone replacement therapy with experimental pain responses in postmenopausal women. *Pain* 2001; 92:229–234.

Fillingim RB, Maixner W. Gender differences in the responses to noxious stimuli. *Pain Forum* 1995; 4:209–221.

Fillingim RB, Ness TJ. Sex-related hormonal influences on pain and analgesic responses. *Neurosci Biobehav Rev* 2000; 24:485–501.

Fillingim RB, Edwards RR, Powell T. Sex-dependent effects of reported familial pain history on clinical and experimental pain responses. *Pain* 2000; 86:87–94.

Froehlich F, Thorens J, Schwizer W, et al. Sedation and analgesia for colonoscopy: patient tolerance, pain, and cardiorespiratory parameters. *Gastrointest Endosc* 1997; 45:1–9.

Gear RW, Gordon NC, Heller PH, et al. Gender difference in analgesic response to the kappa-opioid pentazocine. *Neurosci Lett* 1996; 205:207–209.

Gintzler AR, Liu NJ. Ovarian sex steroids activate antinociceptive systems and reveal gender-specific mechanisms. In: Fillingim RB (Ed). *Sex, Gender, and Pain,* Progress in Pain Research and Management, Vol. 17. Seattle: IASP Press, 2000, pp 89–108.

Gregory MS, Duffner LA, Faunce DE, Kovacs EJ. Estrogen mediates the sex difference in post-burn immunosuppression. *J Endocrinol* 2000; 164:129–138.

Jensen IB, Bergstrom G, Ljungquist T, Bodin L, Nygren AL. A randomized controlled component analysis of a behavioral medicine rehabilitation program for chronic spinal pain: are the effects dependent on gender? *Pain* 2001; 91:65–78.

Jones CA, Nyberg L. Epidemiology of interstitial cystitis. *Urology* 1997; 49(Suppl):2–9.

Keefe FJ, Lefebvre JC, Egert JR, et al. The relationship of gender to pain, pain behavior, and disability in osteoarthritis patients: the role of catastrophizing. *Pain* 2000; 87:325–334.

Kest B, Sarton E, Dahan A. Gender differences in opioid-mediated analgesia: animal and human studies. *Anesthesiology* 2000; 93:539–547.

Komisaruk BR, Whipple B. How does vaginal stimulation produce pleasure, pain, and analgesia? In: Fillingim RB (Ed). *Sex, Gender, and Pain,* Progress in Pain Research and Management, Vol. 17. Seattle: IASP Press, 2000, pp 109–134.

Lander J, Fowler Kerry S, Hill A. Comparison of pain perceptions among males and females. *Can J Nurs Res* 1990; 22:39–49.

LeResche L. Gender considerations in the epidemiology of chronic pain. In: Crombie IK, Croft PR, Linton SJ, LeResche L, Von Korff M (Eds). *Epidemiology of Pain.* Seattle: IASP Press, 1999, pp 43–52.

LeResche L, Saunders K, Von Korff MR, Barlow W, Dworkin SF. Use of exogenous hormones and risk of temporomandibular disorder pain. *Pain* 1997; 69:153–160.

Lin Y, Tamakoshi A, Matsuno S, et al. Nationwide epidemiological survey of chronic pancreatitis in Japan. *J Gastroenterol* 2000; 35:136–141.

Mannion AF, Junge A, Taimela S, et al. Active therapy for chronic low back pain: part 3. Factors influencing self-rated disability and its change following therapy. *Spine* 2001; 26:920–929.

McEwen BS. Estrogen's effects on the brain: multiple sites and molecular mechanisms. *J Appl Physiol* 2001; 91:2785–2801.

Miaskowski C, Gear RW, Levine JD. Sex-related differences in analgesic responses. In: Fillingim RB (Ed). *Sex, Gender, and Pain,* Progress in Pain Research and Management, Vol. 17. Seattle: IASP Press, 2000, pp 209–230.

Mogil JS. Interactions between sex and genotype in the mediation and modulation of nociception in rodents. In: Fillingim RB (Ed). *Sex, Gender, and Pain,* Progress in Pain Research and Management, Vol. 17. Seattle: IASP Press, 2000, pp 25–40.

Mogil JS, Sternberg WF, Kest B, Marek P, Liebeskind JC. Sex differences in the antagonism of stress-induced analgesia: effects of gonadectomy and estrogen replacement. *Pain* 1993; 53:17–25.

Mogil JS, Chesler EJ, Wilson SG, Juraska JM, SternbergWF. Sex differences in thermal nociception and morphine antinociception in rodents depend on genotype. *Neurosci Biobehav Rev* 2000; 24:375–389.

Musgrave DS, Vogt MT, Nevitt MC, Cauley JA. Back problems among postmenopausal women taking estrogen replacement therapy. *Spine* 2001; 26:1606–1612.

Pardue ML, Wizemann TM, Wizemann TM, Pardue ML. *Exploring the Biological Contributions to Human Health: Does Sex Matter?* Washington, DC: National Academy Press, 2001.

Paulson PE, Minoshima S, Morrow TJ, Casey KL. Gender differences in pain perception and patterns of cerebral activation during noxious heat stimulation in humans. *Pain* 1998; 76:223–229.

Riley JL, Robinson ME, Wise EA, Myers CD, Fillingim RB. Sex differences in the perception of noxious experimental stimuli: a meta-analysis. *Pain* 1998; 74:181–187.

Riley JLI, Robinson ME, Wise EA, Price DD. A meta-analytic review of pain perception across the menstrual cycle. *Pain* 1999; 81:225–235.

Robinson ME, Riley JL III, Myers CD, et al. Gender role expectations of pain: relationship to sex differences in pain. *Pain* 2001; 2:251–257.

Roger VL, Farkouh ME, Weston SA, et al. Sex differences in evaluation and outcome of unstable angina. *JAMA* 2000; 283:646–652.

Safran DG, Rogers WH, Tarlov AR, McHorney CA, Ware JE Jr. Gender differences in medical treatment: the case of physician-prescribed activity restrictions. *Soc Sci Med* 1997; 45:711–722.

Sarton E, Olofsen E, Romberg R, et al. Sex differences in morphine analgesia: an experimental study in healthy volunteers. *Anesthesiology* 2000; 93:1245–1254.

Silberstein SD. Headache and female hormones: what you need to know. *Curr Opin Neurol* 2001; 14:323–333.

Simoni-Wastila L. The use of abusable prescription drugs: the role of gender. *J Womens Health Gend Based Med* 2000; 9:289–297.

Spertus IL, Burns J, Glenn B, Lofland K, McCracken L. Gender differences in associations between trauma history and adjustment among chronic pain patients. *Pain* 1999; 82:97–102.

Taenzer AH, Clark C, Curry CS. Gender affects report of pain and function after arthroscopic anterior cruciate ligament reconstruction. *Anesthesiology* 2000; 93:670–675.

Unruh AM. Gender variations in clinical pain experience. *Pain* 1996; 65:123–167.

Walker JS, Carmody JJ. Experimental pain in healthy human subjects: gender differences in nociception and in response to ibuprofen. *Anesth Analg* 1998; 86:1257–1262.

Weisse CS, Sorum PC, Sanders KN, Syat BL. Do gender and race affect decisions about pain management? *J Gen Intern Med* 2001; 16:211–217.

Wesselmann U, Reich SG. The dynias. *Semin Neurol* 1996; 16:63–74.

Wise EA, Riley JL III, Robinson ME. Clinical pain perception and hormone replacement therapy in post-menopausal females experiencing orofacial pain. *Clin J Pain* 2000; 16:121–126.

Zacny JP. Gender differences in opioid analgesia in human volunteers: cold pressor and mechanical pain (CPDD abstract). *NIDA Res Monogr* 2002; 182:22–23.

Part III
Treatment of Pain

Core Curriculum for Professional Education in Pain, edited by J. Edmond Charlton, IASP Press, Seattle, © 2005.

13

Opioids

I. Understand the classification of opioid compounds (Casey and Parfitt 1986; Gutstein and Akil 2001; Uppington 2002).

    A. Identify and differentiate the various subclasses and specific drugs that are used clinically and are agonists at the mu-opioid receptor:

        1. Alkaloids (including semisynthetic alkaloids) such as morphine, hydromorphone, oxymorphone, codeine, oxycodone, hydrocodone, dihydrocodeine, and heroin.

        2. Synthetic opioids, including phenylpiperidine derivatives (such as fentanyl, sufentanil, alfentanil, remifentanil, and meperidine [pethidine]), diphenylheptane derivatives (such as methadone and propoxyphene), and morphinan derivatives (such as levorphanol).

    B. Identify and differentiate those opioid drugs that are used clinically and are partial agonists at the mu receptor:

        1. Semisynthetic alkaloids, including buprenorphine.

        2. Synthetic opioids, including the morphinan dezocine.

        3. Tramadol (which also has non-opioid analgesic effects).

    C. Identify and differentiate those opioid drugs that are used clinically and are known as the mixed agonists-antagonists because they possess antagonist activity at the mu-opioid receptor and agonist activity at another opioid receptor subtype (e.g., the kappa receptor):

        1. Semisynthetic alkaloids, including nalbuphine.

        2. Synthetic opioids, including benzomorphan derivatives (such as pentazocine) and morphinan derivatives (such as butorphanol).

    D. Identify and differentiate those opioid drugs that are used clinically and are pure antagonists of the opioid receptor, including:

        1. Naloxone.

        2. Naltrexone.

    E. Identify and differentiate the major classes of the endogenous opioid peptides, and know the precursor molecules for each.

        1. The precursor proopiomelanocortin yields beta-endorphin.

        2. The precursor prodynorphin yields the dynorphin peptides.

        3. The precursor proenkephalin yields the enkephalin peptides.

II. Understand those aspects of basic opioid pharmacology that are relevant to the use of opioid drugs in clinical practice for acute, chronic, and cancer-related pain.

    A. Understand the core structure shared by all opioids and how structural modifications alter binding to opioid receptors and the resultant pharmacodynamic activities of the related compounds (Casey and Parfitt 1986; Pasternak 1993; Gutstein and Akil 2001).

    B. Understand the importance of physical properties of opioid drugs (Gutstein and Akil 2001).

        1. Understand how the lipid solubility and pKa of an opioid influences transport across biological membranes and affects its pharmacokinetics (Bernards 1999).

2. Understand the particular importance of lipid solubility in determining the pharmacodynamics following intraspinal and other routes of opioid administration (Carr and Cousins 1998; Gourlay 2002).

C. Understand the major findings related to opioid receptor pharmacology (Dickenson 1994; Kieffer and Gaveriaux-Ruff 2003; Cheng et al. 2004; Fields 2004).

1. The major types of opioid receptors: mu (MOR/OPRM), delta (DOR/OPRD) and kappa (KOR/OPRK), their subtypes, and the receptor selective actions that have been identified (Kieffer and Gaveriaux-Ruff 2003).
2. Localization of opioid receptors in relation to sites likely to be involved in analgesia, and the concept of state-dependent opioid control of pain (Stein et al. 2003; Fields 2004).
3. Cloning and molecular characterization of opioid receptors as members of the G-protein-receptor superfamily (Kieffer and Gaveriaux-Ruff 2003).
4. The localization of opioid receptors both inside and outside the nervous system and the implications of this localization for widespread involvement of opioid mechanisms in the modulation of mood, affect, learning, and memory acquisition and in the physiological functioning of many organ systems, including the cardiovascular, gastrointestinal, hormonal, and immune systems (Dickenson 1994; Gutstein and Akil 2001; Stein et al. 2003).
5. The intracellular events produced by binding of the opioid receptor, including activation of second messenger systems (e.g., G protein, protein kinase C), interaction with other receptors (e.g., *N* methyl D aspartate), electrophysiological outcomes (e.g., hyperpolarization due to opening of potassium channels or closing of calcium channels) (Dickenson 1994; Mayer et al. 1995; Kieffer and Gaveriaux-Ruff 2003; Eguchi 2004), and endocytosis (Finn and Whistler 2001).
6. Understand that other receptor types have been identified, such as opioid-receptor-like 1 receptor (ORL1; Zeilhofer et al. 2003).

D. Understand tolerance and physical dependence (Yaksh 1991; Mayer et al. 1999; Vanderah et al. 2001; Kieffer and Evans 2002).

1. Be able to define tolerance and physical dependence.
2. Recognize the multiple types of tolerance (e.g., associative or behavioral vs. non-associative or pharmacological) and that tolerance can develop to many opioid effects. Some effects such as constipation and miosis are more resistant to the development of tolerance.
3. Understand the multiple mechanisms that may be responsible for opioid tolerance or physical dependence (Akil et al. 1997).
4. Understand opioid-induced hyperalgesia and its relevance in clinical pain management and tolerance (Ballantyne and Mao 2003).

E. Recognize that the mechanisms that produce tolerance are not the only factors that can reduce opioid efficacy and that the following pathological processes, which have the same result, may be more important clinically (Dickenson 1994; Portenoy 1994, 2002; Mayer et al. 1999; Gourlay 2002; Desmeules et al. 2004):

1. Increased nociception due to progression of a tissue damaging lesion.
2. Sensitization of central nervous system neurons, rendering them less responsive to opioid mechanisms.
3. Transmission of nociceptive information along afferent pathways that are usually non-nociceptive and are less subject to modulation by opioid mechanisms.
4. Pharmacokinetic processes, such as the production of active metabolites that may have antianalgesic effects or pharmacokinetic interaction (induction of liver enzymes like CYP 3A4 with decreased methadone concentrations).

III. Know those aspects of clinical opioid pharmacology that are relevant to the use of opioid drugs in patient care (Lipman and Gauthier 1997; Gutstein and Akil 2001; Gourlay 2002; Uppington 2002).

A. Be able to define the terms efficacy, maximal efficacy, relative efficacy, responsiveness, potency (for acute and chronic opioid administration), and relative potency (Portenoy 1994).

B. Understand the differences in clinical effects among pure opioid agonists, partial agonists, mixed agonists-antagonists, and antagonists.

   1. Recognize that the existence of a ceiling effect for analgesia limits the utility of the partial agonist and mixed agonist-antagonist drugs for the management of chronic pain.

   2. Understand that the mixed agonist-antagonist opioids are more likely to cause psychotomimetic effects than are the pure agonist opioids.

   3. Understand that the partial agonists and mixed agonist-antagonist drugs have a ceiling effect for respiratory depression, in contrast to the pure agonist opioids.

   4. Understand that abstinence can be precipitated when a partial agonist or mixed agonist-antagonist is administered to a patient who is physically dependent on a pure agonist drug.

C. Understand the various factors that results in the great individual variability in opioid response in terms of pharmacokinetics and pharmacodynamics. This pronounced variability, combined with changes in responsiveness over time, mandates individualization of opioid doses based on a continuing process of assessment (analgesia and adverse effects) and dose titration (Bandolier Web Site; Ballantyne and Mao 2003; Kalso et al. 2004). There is a requirement to regularly reassess the dose to optimize the analgesic response and minimize adverse effects.

D. Be aware of the varied routes of administration by which opioids can be delivered and the benefits and limitations of each route (Bruera and Neumann 1999; Gourlay 2001, 2002).

   1. Systemic administration:

      a. Oral.
      b. Sublingual.
      c. Buccal.
      d. Rectal.
      e. Transdermal (and the emerging area of iontophoretic transdermal drug delivery).
      f. Subcutaneous, via intermittent injection or continuous infusion.
      g. Intramuscular, via intermittent injection.
      h. Intravenous, via intermittent injection or continuous infusion.
      i. Pulmonary.
      j. Nasal.

   2. Cerebrospinal administration:

      a. Spinal epidural, via intermittent injection or continuous infusion.
      b. Spinal intrathecal, via intermittent injection or continuous infusion.
      c. Intraventricular.

   3. Peripheral:

      a. Local/topical for inflammatory conditions such as mucositis, skin ulcerations, or arthritis (Stein et al. 2003).

E. Understand the clinical factors that influence the decision to use specific routes of administration in the management of acute and chronic pain (Carr and Cousins 1998; Gourlay 2001, 2002; Macintyre and Ready 2001; Uppington 2002; ANZCA 2005).

   1. Be aware of the efficacy and utility of noninvasive routes, particularly the oral route, when treating chronic pain.

   2. Be aware that the need for rapid onset of analgesia may justify the parenteral route.

   3. Understand that infusions can eliminate bolus effects (peak concentration toxicity or pain recurrence at the end of the dosing interval).

4. Understand that patient controlled analgesia can provide appropriate patients an effective means to continually adjust treatment to meet analgesic needs.
5. Recognize that intraspinal administration (epidural or subarachnoid) may be able to reduce the opioid adverse effects associated with systemic opioid administration.
6. Understand that slow transdermal systems are not suitable for opioid titration.

F. Understand that equianalgesic dose tables are derived from relative potency data and recognize the need to adjust doses when changing drugs or routes of administration (Bruera et al. 1996; Pereira et al. 2001). Understand the important interindividual differences in the relative equianalgesic dose conversions and the need to used different conversion ratios when switching to another opioid when the patient has already been on a high opioid dose for some time.

G. Understand major pharmacokinetic and pharmacodynamic considerations for each opioid drug and for each formulation and route of administration used clinically.

1. Know important pharmacokinetic information for each drug (Gourlay 1998, 2002; Gutstein and Akil 2001; Andersen et al. 2003).

   a. Elimination half life.
   b. Whether active metabolites exist, and their contribution to the analgesic response and/or adverse event profile; for example, meperidine [pethidine] (with its toxic metabolite, normeperidine [norpethidine]) and morphine (with its active opioid metabolite, morphine-6-glucuronide).
   c. Influence of patient characteristics, including age (changes associated with very young age and old age) and major organ dysfunction (changes associated with disease of the kidneys or liver) and the impact of concomitantly administered drugs on these pharmacokinetic parameters. There may be other conditions such as sleep apnea that render the patient more sensitive to opioids.

2. Know relevant pharmacokinetic and pharmacodynamic information for each formulation and route of administration (Carr and Cousins 1998; Gourlay 1998, 2001, 2002).

   a. Bioavailability.
   b. Time-action profile for a single dose, including time of onset, time to peak effect, and duration of effect.
   c. Time-action profile for repeated doses and infusions, including time of onset and time to approach steady state.

3. Understand that individual variation in metabolic processes may be genetically determined and the impact on the efficacy and/or toxicity of opioid drugs (Poulsen et al. 1996; Eckhardt al, 1998; Desmeules et al. 2004).

   a. Genetic variability in the activity of the cytochrome P450 2D6 enzyme influences the endogenous conversion of codeine to morphine and oxycodone to oxymorphone and the impact this variability has on pharmacodynamics in terms of analgesia and side effects.
   b. Understand the extensive role of cytochrome P450 3A4 in the metabolism of opioids (e.g., methadone) and a multitude of other drugs that can be administered concomitantly (Gourlay 2002).

      i. That levels of this enzyme can be induced by concomitantly administered drugs, resulting in reduced blood opioid concentrations, and the impact this might have on the pharmacodynamic response.
      ii. That blood opioid concentrations can be significantly increased by the co-administration of other drugs that are also metabolized via cytochrome P450 3A4 (competitive inhibition); the concomitantly administered drugs are not necessarily analgesic drugs.

2. Understand that variability in the glucuronidation of morphine influences the ratio of active glucuronidated metabolites to the parent compound (Faura et al. 1998).

a. Understand the difference in glucuronide ratios in neonates compared to older children and adults.

b. Understand the impact of renal impairment on metabolite ratios.

c. Understand the routes of administration that bypass hepatic first pass metabolism (i.v., i.m., transdermal, rectal, local, epidural, and intrathecal) have lower metabolite production compared to oral, buccal, and sublingual.

d. Understand that duration of morphine therapy does not influence morphine glucuronidation ratios (Andersen et al. 2004).

H. Understand the potential for additive analgesic effects but not adverse effects that can occur with the combination of opioids and other drugs.

1. Systemic opioids combined with nonopioid analgesics or adjuvant analgesics (such as ketamine; Bell et al. 2003).

2. Intraspinal opioids combined with local anesthetics and/or alpha-2-adrenergic agonists (Walker et al. 2002).

I. Recognize that specific clinical guidelines have been recommended for different patient populations and that the techniques needed for optimal therapy differ for the following conditions:

1. Postoperative and procedure-related acute pain (Macintyre and Ready 2001; Mitra and Sinatra 2004; ANZCA 2005).

2. Cancer-related pain (Hanks et al. 2001; American Pain Society 2005).

3. Chronic nonmalignant pain (Kalso et al. 2003; Pain Society 2004).

4. Chronic or recurrent pain due to medical illness such as sickle cell anemia (Jacobson et al. 1997), headache (Bach 1999).

J. Understand the potential adverse effects and toxicities of opioid drugs (Carr and Cousins et al. 1998; Bruera and Neumann 1999; Gutstein and Akil 2001; Gibson 2003; Kalso et al. 2004).

1. Know the clinical presentation and management strategies for common adverse effects, including constipation, nausea, somnolence, mental clouding, and urinary retention.

2. Know that respiratory depression is rare during chronic opioid use.

3. Know that tolerance develops to the psychomotor effects of opioids.

4. Be aware that adverse effects and toxicity may be more likely with specific patient characteristics such as advanced age, major organ dysfunction (e.g., renal disease, chronic encephalopathy, chronic obstructive pulmonary disease, sleep apnea), and with concurrent centrally acting drugs (e.g., benzodiazepines).

5. Be aware that chronic opioid prescription may reduce hormonal levels (notably testosterone), which may effect libido, particularly in men (Roberts et al. 2002; Ballantyne and Mao 2003).

K. Understand the use of naloxone to treat acute opioid overdose (Manfredi et al. 1996; Wanger et al. 1998).

1. Know the risks associated with naloxone administration to patients receiving chronic opioid therapy, including abstinence and recurrent pain, and understand the value of careful titration using a dilute solution of naloxone.

2. Be aware that naloxone should only be given to patients receiving chronic opioid therapy to reverse respiratory depression or impending respiratory depression.

3. Know that naloxone has a short half-life and that repeated injections or an infusion are usually needed to effectively treat opioid overdose.

L. Understand that the risk of abstinence mandates dose tapering after a few days of frequent dosing with an opioid drug, and be aware of the techniques used to discontinue these drugs safely, including the rate of the taper, substitution withdrawal with a long half-life opioid, and the use of clonidine to prevent abstinence (Gowing et al. 2003; Umbricht et al. 2003).

M. Know the definitions of addiction (i.e., loss of control over drug use, compulsive use, and continued use despite harm), physical dependence (withdrawal syndrome that can be produced by abrupt cessation, rapid dose reduction, decreasing blood level of the drug, and/or administration of an antagonist), psychological dependence (dependence on opioid drugs for their psychic effects), and tolerance (state of adaptation in which exposure to a drug induces changes that result in a diminution of one or more of the drug's effects over time); understand the implications of the therapeutic use of a potential drug of abuse (Portenoy 1994; Savage 2002, Savage et al. 2003). (See also Section I for guidelines.)

1. Understand the need to monitor the patient for the appearance of aberrant drug-related behavior during chronic therapy.
2. Be aware of the various diagnoses that may account for aberrant drug-related behavior and understand the assessment that is needed to accurately characterize the patient's response.
3. Be aware of the approaches to the management of the patient who exhibits aberrant drug-related behavior during long-term opioid treatment of chronic pain.

REFERENCES

Akil H, Meng F, Devine DP, Watson SJ. Molecular and neuroanatomical properties of the endogenous opioid system: implications for treatment of opiate addiction. *Semin Neurosci* 1997; 9:70–83.

American Pain Society, *Principles of Analgesic Use in the Treatment of Acute and Chronic Cancer Pain,* 5th ed. Skokie, IL: American Pain Society, 2005.

Andersen G, Christrup L, Sjogren P. Relationships among morphine metabolism, pain and side-effects during long term treatment: an update. *J Pain Symptom Manage* 2003; 25:74–91.

Andersen G, Sjogren P, Hansen SH, et al. Pharmacological consequences of long-term morphine treatment in patients with cancer and chronic non-malignant pain. *Eur J Pain* 2004; 8:263–271.

ANZCA. *Acute Pain Management: Scientific Evidence.* The Australian and New Zealand College of Anaesthetists, 2005. Available at: www.anzca.edu.au/publications/acutepain.htm. Accessed 24 July, 2005.

Bach FW. Opioids in headache. In: Kalso E, McQuay HJ, Wiesenfeld-Hallin Z (Eds). *Opioid Sensitivity of Chronic Noncancer Pain.* Seattle: IASP Press, 1999, pp 367–370.

Ballantyne JC, Mao J. Opioid therapy for chronic pain. *N Engl J Med* 2003; 349:1943–1953.

Bandolier Website. Available at: www.jr2.ox.ac.uk/bandolier/. Accessed 24 July, 2005.

Bell RF, Eccleston C, Kalso E. Ketamine as adjuvant to opioids for cancer pain. A qualitative systematic review. *J Pain Symptom Manage* 2003; 26:867–875.

Bernards CM. Clinical implications of physiochemical properties of opioids. In: Stein C (Ed). *Opioids in Pain Control: Basic and Clinical Aspects.* Cambridge: Cambridge University Press, 1999, pp 166–187.

Bruera E, Neumann CM. Opioid toxicities-assessment and management. In: Max M (Ed). *Pain 1999: An Updated Review.* Seattle: IASP Press, 1999, pp 443–457.

Bruera E, Pereira J, Watanabe S, et al. Opioid rotation in patients with cancer pain. A retrospective comparison of dose ratios between methadone, hydromorphone, and morphine. *Cancer* 1996; 78:852–857.

Carr DB, Cousins MJ. Spinal route of analgesia: opioids and future options. In: Cousins MJ, Bridenbaugh PO (Eds). *Neural Blockade in Clinical Anaesthesia and the Management of Pain,* 3rd ed. Philadelphia: Lippincott-Raven, 1998, pp 915–983.

Casey AF, Parfitt RT. *Opioid Analgesics: Chemistry and Receptors.* New York: Plenum Press, 1986.

Cheng W-J, Porreca F, Woods JH. *The Delta Receptor.* New York: Marcel Dekker, 2004.

Desmeules JA, Piguet V, Ehret GB, et al. Pharmacogenetics, pharmacokinetics, and analgesia. In: Mogil JS (Ed). *The Genetics of Pain,* Progress in Pain Research and Management, Vol. 28. Seattle: IASP Press, 2004, pp 211–237.

Dickenson AH. Where and how do opioids act? In: Gebhart GF, Hammond DL, Jensen TS (Eds). *Proceedings of the 7th World Congress on Pain,* Progress in Pain Research and Management, Vol. 2. Seattle: IASP Press, 1994, pp 525–552.

Eckhardt K, Li S, Ammon S, et al. Same incidence of adverse drug events after codeine administration irrespective of the genetically determined differences in morphine formation. *Pain* 1998; 76:27–33.

Eguchi M. Recent advances in selective opioid receptor agonists and antagonists. *Med Res Rev* 2004; 24:182–212.

Faura CC, Collins SL, Moore AM, et al. Systematic review of factors affecting the ratios of morphine and its major metabolites. *Pain* 1998; 74:43–53.

Fields H. State-dependent opioid control of pain. *Nat Rev Neurosci* 2004; 5:565–575.

Finn AK, Whistler JL. Endocytosis of the mu-opioid receptor reduces tolerance and a cellular hallmark of opiate withdrawal. *Neuron* 2001; 32:829–839.

Gibson SJ. Pain and aging: the pain experience over the adult lifespan. In: Dostrovsky JO, Carr DB, Koltzenburg M (Eds). *Proceedings of the 10th World Congress on Pain,* Progress in Pain Research and Management, Vol. 24. Seattle: IASP Press, 2003, pp 767–790.

Gourlay GK. Sustained relief of chronic pain: pharmacokinetics of SR morphine. *Clin Pharmacokin* 1998; 35:173–190.

Gourlay GK. Treatment of cancer pain with transdermal fentanyl. *Lancet Oncol* 2001; 2:165–172.

Gourlay GK. Clinical pharmacology of opioids in the treatment of pain. In: Giamberardino MA (Ed). *Pain 2002: An Updated Review.* Seattle: IASP Press, 2002, pp 381–394.

Gowing L, Farrell M, Ali R, et al. Alpha-2 adrenergic agonists for the management of opioid withdrawal. *Cochrane Database Syst Rev* 2004;4:CD002024.

Gutstein HB, Akil H. Opioid analgesics. In: Hardman JG, Limbird LE, Gilman AG (Eds). *The Pharmacological Basis of Therapeutics,* 10th ed. New York: McGraw-Hill, 2001, pp 569–619.

Hanks GW, de Conno F, Cherney N, et al. Morphine and alternative opioids in cancer pain: the EAPC recommendations. *Br J Cancer* 2001; 84:587–593.

Jacobson SJ, Kopecky EA, Joshi P, Babul N. Randomised trial of oral morphine for painful episodes of sickle-cell disease in children. *Lancet* 1997; 350:1358–1361.

Kalso E, Allan L, Dellemijn PLI, et al. Recommendation for using opioids in chronic non-cancer pain. *Eur J Pain* 2003; 7:381–386.

Kalso E, Edwards J, Moore RA, et al. Opioids in chronic non-cancer pain: systematic review of efficacy and safety. *Pain* 2004; 112:372–380.

Kieffer BL, Evans CJ. Opioid tolerance—in search of the Holy Grail. *Cell* 2002; 108:587–590.

Kieffer BL, Gaveriaux-Ruff C. Exploring the opioid system by gene knockout. *Prog Neurobiol* 2002; 66:285–306.

Lipman AG, Gauthier ME. Pharmacology of opioid drugs: basic principles. In: Portenoy RK, Bruera E (Eds). *Topics in Palliative Care,* Vol 1. New York: Oxford University Press, 1997, pp 137–161.

Manfredi PL, Ribeiro S, Chandler SW, Payne R. Inappropriate use of naloxone in cancer patients with pain. *J Pain Symptom Manage* 1996; 11:131–134.

Mayer DJ, Mao J, Price DD. The development of morphine tolerance and dependence is associated with translocation of protein kinase C. *Pain* 1995; 61:365–374.

Mayer DJ, Mao J, Holt J, et al. Cellular mechanisms of neuropathic pain, morphine tolerance, and their interactions. *Proc Natl Acad Sci USA* 1999; 96:7731–7736.

Macintyre PE, Ready LB. *Acute Pain Management: A Practical Guide,* 2nd ed. London: WB Saunders, 2001.

Mitra S, Sinatra RS. Perioperative management of acute pain in the opioid-dependent patient. *Anesthesiology* 2004; 101:212–217.

Pain Society. Recommendations for the appropriate use of opioids for persistent non-cancer pain. A consensus statement prepared on behalf of the Pain Society, the Royal College of Anaesthetists, the Royal College of General Practitioners and the Royal College of Psychiatrists. March 2004. Available at: www.britishpainsociety.org/pdf/opioids_doc_2004.pdf. Accessed 24 July, 2005.

Pereira J, Lawlor P, Vigano A, et al. Equianalgesic dose ratios for opioids: a critical review and proposals for long-term dosing. *J Pain Symptom Manage* 2001; 22:672–687.

Poulsen L, Brosen K, Arendt-Nielsen L, et al. Codeine and morphine in the extensive and poor metabolizers of sparteine: pharmacokinetic, analgesic effects and side-effect. *Eur J Clin Pharmacol* 1996; 51:289–295.

Portenoy RK. Opioid tolerance and responsiveness: research findings and clinical observations. In: Gebhart GF, Hammond DL, Jensen TS (Eds). *Proceedings of the 7th World Congress on Pain,* Progress in Pain Research and Management, Vol. 2. Seattle: IASP Press, 1994, pp 595–619.

Portenoy RK. Opioid and adjuvant analgesics. In: Max M (Ed). *Pain 1999: An Updated Review—Refresher Course Syllabus.* Seattle: IASP Press, 1999, pp 3–18.

Portenoy RK. Clinical strategies for the management of cancer pain poorly responsive to systemic opioid therapy. In: Giamberardino MA (Ed). *Pain 2002: An Updated Review—Refresher Course Syllabus.* Seattle: IASP Press, 2002, pp 19–27.

Roberts LJ, Finch P, Pullan PT, et al. Sex hormones suppression by intrathecal opioids: a prospective study. *Clin J Pain* 2002; 18:144–148.

Savage SR. Assessment for addiction in pain-treatment settings. *Clin J Pain* 2002; (Suppl 4)18:S28–38.

Savage SR, Joranson DE, Covington EC, et al. Definitions related to the medical use of opioids: evolution towards universal agreement. *J Pain Symptom Manage* 2003; 26:655–667.

Stein C, Schäfer M, Machelska H. Attacking pain at its source: new perspectives on opioids. *Nat Med* 2003; 9:1003–1008.

Umbricht A, Hoover DR, Tucker MJ, et al. Opioid detoxification with buprenorphine, clonidine, or methadone in hospitalized heroin-dependent patients with HIV infection. *Drug Alcohol Depend* 2003; 69:263–272.

Uppington J. Opioids. In: Ballantyne J, Fishman SM, Abdi S (Eds). *The Massachusetts General Hospital Handbook of Pain Management,* 2nd ed. Philadelphia: Lippincott Williams & Wilkins, 2002, pp 103–123.

Vanderah TW, Ossipov MH, Lai J, et al. Mechanisms of opioid-induced pain and antinociceptive tolerance: descending facilitation and spinal dynorphin. *Pain* 2001; 92:5–9.

Walker SM, Goundas LC, Cousins MJ, et al. Combination spinal analgesic chemotherapy: a systematic review. *Anesth Analg* 2002; 95:674–715.

Wanger K, Brough L, Macmillan I, et al. Intravenous vs subcutaneous naloxone for out-of-hospital management of presumed opioid overdose. *Acad Emerg Med* 1998; 5:293–299.

Yaksh TL. Tolerance: factors involved in changes in the dose-effect relationship with chronic drug exposure. In: Basbaum AI, Besson J-M (Eds). *Towards a New Pharmacotherapy of Pain.* New York: John Wiley & Sons, 1991, pp 157–180.

Zeilhofer HU, Reinscheid RK, Okuda-Ashitaka E. Nociceptin, nocistatin, and pain. In: Dostrovsky JO, Carr DB, Koltzenburg M (Eds). *Proceedings of the 10th World Congress on Pain, Progress in Pain Research and Management*, Vol. 24. Seattle: IASP Press, 2003, pp 469–480.

Core Curriculum for Professional Education in Pain, edited by J. Edmond Charlton, IASP Press, Seattle, © 2005.

14

Antipyretic Analgesics: Nonsteroidals, Acetaminophen, and Phenazone Derivatives

I.   Pharmacodynamics (Paulus 1985; Taiwo and Levine 1988; Kantor 1989; Handwerker 1991; McCormack and Brune 1991; Brune et al. 1992; Malmberg and Yaksh 1992; Williams 1993; Dray 1994; Laneuville et al. 1994; McCormack 1994; Neugebauer et al. 1994; Vane et al. 1994; Freston 1999; Tramer et al. 2000; Brune and Neubert 2001; Brune 2002)

A.   Know the following about nonsteroidal anti-inflammatory drugs (NSAIDs):

1.   All nonselective NSAIDs or their active metabolites are acids. These acids accumulate in inflamed tissue, the gastrointestinal (GI) tract, the kidney, and the bone marrow.
2.   NSAIDs inhibit cyclooxygenases (COX-1 and COX-2), which produce prostaglandins from arachidonic acid.
3.   There are two cyclooxygenase enzymes (COX-1, COX-2) with overlapping location of expression. They are both constitutive and inducible, but to differing degrees. Both COX-1 and COX-2 isoforms are involved in inflammation and in renal and GI functions.
4.   Some are more COX-2 selective than others and have been deemed COX-2 inhibitors.
5.   Prostaglandins sensitize nociceptors to the actions of other mediators of pain (histamine, bradykinin, and hydrogen ions) in the periphery and facilitate pain-related neuronal activities in the spinal cord.
6.   NSAIDs reduce leukocyte invasion in inflamed tissue.
7.   NSAIDs enhance the production of leukotrienes from arachidonic acid.
8.   Leukotrienes are mediators of pseudoallergic and allergic reactions.
9.   There is little difference in analgesia with nonselective and COX-2-selective drugs.
10. Dose-response and side-effect curves are not superimposable.

B.   Know the characteristics of nonacidic antipyretic analgesics, i.e., acetaminophen, phenazone, propyphenazone, and dipyrone (active metabolites of 4-methylaminophenazone and others):

1.   They are weak bases or neutral substances.
2.   They penetrate easily into the central nervous system (CNS) and reach equally high concentrations throughout the body.
3.   They are weak inhibitors of cyclooxygenases.
4.   They enhance leukotriene production.
5.   They exert their main actions in the CNS (inhibition of pain and fever); the mediators involved are not fully defined.
6.   Dipyrone has some antispasmodic action.
7.   The selective COX-2 inhibitors are non-acidic.

II. Pharmacokinetics

A.   Be aware of the following properties of NSAIDs:

1.   Absorption usually begins in the stomach (aspirin, hydrolyzed, and unhydrolyzed); all others are absorbed in the small intestine.
2.   For some, parenteral administration is available.
3.   Onset of action depends on the speed of absorption.

4. They are mostly unchanged at elimination, usually after conjugation reactions (salicylic acid, diflunisal, ketoprofen, indomethacin) or by conjugation after oxidation (diclofenac, ibuprofen, piroxicam, and most others).
5. They show different elimination half-lives: a short half-life (1–6 hours) for diclofenac, flurbiprofen, ibuprofen, and ketoprofen; intermediate half-life (about 12–24 hours) for naproxen, diflunisal, and nabumetone (active metabolite); long half-life (days) for piroxicam, phenylbutazone, tenoxicam, and oxaprozin.
6. Elimination is slowed in the elderly.
7. They have interactions with other acids in plasma protein binding and tubular excretion.
8. COX-2 inhibitors usually have intermediate to long half-lives.
9. There are sustained- or extended-release forms of short-half-life NSAIDS.

B. Be aware of the following properties of acetaminophen and phenazone derivatives:

1. They are absorbed in the small intestine (acetaminophen, dipyrone).
2. Parenteral administration is possible.
3. They are metabolized in the liver; half-life is 2 hours for acetaminophen, 5–25 hours for phenazone, and 2–10 hours for propyphenazone and dipyrone.
4. Elimination occurs by renal excretion of the metabolites.
5. Elimination is slowed in liver disease and in the elderly.

III. Know the side effects and drug interactions for these drugs (Brune and Lanz 1985; Paulus 1985; Murray and Brater 1993; Figueras et al. 1994; Langman et al. 1994; Komhoff 1997; Feinstein 2000; Fitzgerald et al. 2001; Crofford 2002; McQuay and Moore 2003; Wright 2002):

A. NSAIDs (COX-2-selective, nonselective)

1. GI tract: irritations (10%), bleeding ulcerations, perforations (1 per 10,000); serious side effects are least prominent with ibuprofen, most prominent with azapropazone and piroxicam. COX-2-selective drugs may have fewer GI side effects, but more data are needed.
2. Kidney damage: occasional (little difference between nonselective and COX-2 selective); risk of nephropathy from combination analgesics (non-phenacetin) is still unresolved.
3. Liver damage: occasional, particularly seen with aspirin (in children) and diclofenac (in adults); most likely with lipid-soluble and enterohepatic cycling drugs.
4. Bone marrow damage: aplastic anemia (most prominent with phenylbutazone).
5. Pseudoallergic reactions (10%, particularly in asthmatics, patients with neurodermatitis, and children with nasal polyposis and related conditions); sulfa allergy question (celecoxib).
6. Hypotension.
7. Occasional severe allergic reactions (Steven's Johnson syndrome, Lyell syndrome, shock).
8. Aspirin: inhibition of platelet aggregation for days; cofactor in Reye's syndrome in children.
9. Ketorolac: inhibition (for days) of platelet aggregation.
10. There is accumulating evidence of an increased risk of the use of COX-2 inhibitors in cardiovascular disease. Caution is advised if use of these agents is contemplated.

B. Acetaminophen, phenazone, and derivatives

1. Acetaminophen.

    a. Permanent liver damage with overdosage or chronic high dose in susceptible populations (alcoholics).
    b. Long-term effects in patients abusing combinations (analgesic nephropathy, urinary tract tumors).

2. Phenazone and derivatives.

    a. Allergic skin reactions (frequent) and pseudoallergic reactions (rare severe skin reactions).
    b. Risk of agranulocytosis low but real (1 per 100,000 weekly treatment periods for dipyrone).
    c. Shock cases occasional, as with NSAIDs.

IV. Know the major indications for use of these drugs (Kantor 1989; McCormack and Brune 1991; Brune et al. 1992; Levy et al. 1995; Sinatra 2002):

    A. NSAIDs (nonselective, COX-2 selective)

        1. Chronic intensive inflammatory pain, e.g., rheumatoid arthritis (diclofenac, indomethacin, piroxicam).

        2. Phasic intensive inflammatory pain, as in osteoarthrosis (diclofenac, ibuprofen, ketoprofen; short half-life).

        3. Acute post-traumatic or postoperative pain (diclofenac, flurbiprofen, ibuprofen, ketoprofen; short half-life).

        4. Headache (ibuprofen, ketoprofen, naproxen).

        5. Dysmenorrhea.

        6. COX-2-selective drugs are used in all these conditions, but data are unclear on the risk-benefit ratio except during the perioperative period (minimal platelet effect) and with a history of GI bleeding. Caution should be exercised in their use.

        7. Preemptive analgesia, multimodal analgesia: use COX-2-selective or nonselective drugs?

    B. Acetaminophen

        1. Some forms of headache.

        2. Fever (e.g., in children).

REFERENCES

Bennett A, Tavares IA. COX-2 inhibitors compared and contrasted. *Exp Opin Pharmacother* 2002; 2(11):1859–1876.

Berger RG, Intelligent use of NSAIDs—where do we stand? *Exp Opin Pharmacother* 2001; 2(1):19–30.

Brune K. Next generation of everyday analgesics. *Am J Ther* 2002; 9:215–223.

Brune K, Lanz R. Pharmacokinetics of nonsteroidal anti-inflammatory drugs. In: Bonta IL, Bray MA, Pamham MJ (Eds). *Handbook of Inflammation*. Amsterdam: Elsevier Science, 1985, pp 413–449.

Brune K, Neubert A. Pharmacokinetic and pharmacodynamic aspects of the ideal COX-2 inhibitor: a pharmacologist's perspective. *Clin Exp Rheumatol* 2001; 19(Suppl 25):S51–S57.

Brune K, Geisslinger G, Menzel-Soglowek S. Pure enantiomers of 2-arylpropionic acids: tools in pain research and improved drugs in rheumatology. *J Clin Pharmacol* 1992; 32:944–952.

Crofford LJ. Specific Cyclooxygenase-2 inhibitors: what have we learned since they came into widespread use? *Curr Opin Rheumatol* 2002; 13:225–230.

Dray A. Tasting the inflammatory soup: the role of peripheral neurons. *Pain Rev* 1994; 1:153–171.

Figueras A, Capell D, Castel JM, Laporte JR. Spontaneous reporting of adverse drug reactions to nonsteroidal anti-inflammatory drugs. *Eur J Clin Pharmacol* 1994; 47:297–303.

Fitzgerald GA, Patrono C. The coxibs, selective inhibitors of cyclooxygenase-2. *N Engl J Med* 2001; 345(6):433–442.

Freston JW. Rationalizing cyclooxygenase (COX) inhibition for maximal efficacy and minimal adverse events. *Am J Med* 1999; 107(6A):S78–S89.

Handwerker HO. What peripheral mechanisms contribute nociceptive transmission and hyperalgesia? In: Basbaum AL, Besson JL (Eds). *Towards a New Pharmacotherapy of Drugs of Pain*. Chichester: John Wiley & Sons, 1991, pp 5–19.

Kantor TG. Concepts in pain control. *Semin Arthritis Rheum* 1989; 18:94–99.

Komhoff M, Grone H-J, Klein T, Setberth HW, Nusing RM. Localization of cyclooxygenase-1 and -2 in adult and fetal human kidney: implication for renal function. *Am J Physiol* 1997; 272:F460–468.

Laneuville O, Breuer DK, Dewitt DL, et al. Differential inhibition of human prostaglandin endoperoxide H synthases-1 and -2 by nonsteroidal anti-inflammatory drugs. *J Pharmacol Exp Ther* 1994; 271:927–934.

Langman MJS, Weil J, Wainwright P, et al. Risks of bleeding peptic ulcer associated with individual nonsteroidal anti-inflammatory drugs. *Lancet* 1994; 343:1075–1078.

Levy M, Zylber-Katz E, Rosenkranz B. Clinical pharmacokinetics of dipyrone and its metabolites. *Clin Pharmacokinet* 1995; 28:216–234.

Malmberg AB, Yaksh TL. Antinociceptive actions of spinal nonsteroidal anti-inflammatory agents on the formalin test in the rat. *J Exp Ther* 1992; 263:136–146.

McCormack K. Nonsteroidal anti-inflammatory drugs and spinal nociceptive processing. *Pain* 1994; 59:9–44.

McCormack K, Brune K. Dissociation between antinociceptive and inflammatory drugs. *Drugs* 1991; 41:533–545.

McQuay HJ, Moore RA. Side effects of COX-2 inhibitors and other NSAIDs. In: Dostrovsky JO, Carr DB, Koltzenburg M (Eds). *Proceedings of the 10th World Congress on Pain, Progress in Pain Research and Management,* Vol. 24. Seattle: IASP Press, 2003, pp 499–510.

Murray MD, Brater DC. Renal toxicity of the nonsteroidal anti-inflammatory drugs. *Annu Rev Pharmacol Toxicol* 1993; 32:435–465.

Neugebauer V, Schaible HG, He X, et al. Electrophysiological evidence for a spinal antinociceptive action of dipyrone. *Agents Actions* 1994; 41:62–70.

Paulus HE. FDA arthritis advisory committee meeting: postmarketing surveillance of nonsteroidal anti-inflammatory drugs. *Arthritis Rheum* 1985; 28:1168–1169.

Sinatra R. Role of COX-2 inhibitors in evolution of acute pain management. *J Pain Symptom Manage* 2002; 24:S18–S27.

Taiwo YO, Levine JD. Prostaglandins inhibit endogenous pain control mechanisms by blocking transmission at spinal noradrenergic synapses. *J Neurosci* 1988: 8:1346–1349.

Tramer MR, Moore RA, Reynolds JM, McQuay HJ. Quantitative estimation of rare adverse events which follow a biological progression: a new model applied to chronic NSAID use. *Pain* 2000; 85:139–182.

Vane JR, Mitchell JA, Appleton I, et al. Inducible isoforms of cyclooxygenase and nitric-oxide synthase in inflammation. *Proc Natl Acad Sci USA* 1994; 91:2046–2050.

Williams KM, Breit S, Day RO. Biochemical actions and clinical pharmacology of anti-inflammatory drugs. *Advances Drug Res* 1993; 24:121–152.

Wright JM. The double-edged sword of COX-2 selective NSAIDs. *CMAJ* 2002; 167(10):1131–1137.

Core Curriculum for Professional Education in Pain, edited by J. Edmond Charlton, IASP Press, Seattle, © 2005.

15

Antidepressants and Anticonvulsants

I.   Antidepressants (Magni 1991; Onghena and van Houdenhove 1992; Carette et al. 1994; Max 1994; McQuay et al. 1996; Sindrup and Jensen 1999; Kunz et al. 2000; Semenchuk et al. 2001; Sindrup 2003; Sindrup et al. 2003).

A.   Know the indications for the use of antidepressants.

1.   Be aware of those pain conditions for which support for the use of these drugs derives from controlled studies (e.g., migraine prophylaxis, tension headache, postherpetic neuralgia, diabetic and other painful polyneuropathies, postmastectomy pain syndrome, poststroke pain).

2.   Be aware of indications supported by empirical evidence (cancer pain with a neuropathic component).

3.   Be aware that antidepressants have an analgesic effect independent from their antidepressant effect, i.e., antidepressants are useful in pain patients both with depressed and normal mood.

B.   Know the specific drugs used for the treatment of pain.

1.   Know the different classes of antidepressants used in pain treatment (tricyclic antidepressants, serotonin and norepinephrine reuptake inhibitors, selective serotonin reuptake inhibitors).

2.   Know the major pharmacological differences between commonly used antidepressant drugs.

3.   Know which tricyclic antidepressants have analgesic efficacy proven by controlled trials (amitriptyline, desipramine, nortriptyline, imipramine, clomipramine, and maprotiline).

4.   Know the usefulness of serotonin norepinephrine reuptake inhibitors in painful polyneuropathy (venlafaxine) or in patients with different peripheral neuropathic pains (bupropion), and of some selective serotonin reuptake inhibitors (paroxetine and citalopram) in painful diabetic polyneuropathy.

5.   Know the major hypotheses to explain the efficacy of antidepressants in pain treatment.

C.   Know the principles of dosing antidepressants in the treatment of pain.

1.   Know the usual dosage range of different antidepressants in pain treatment.

2.   Know the difference between the antidepressant and analgesic dosage range for tricyclic antidepressants.

3.   When available, understand the value of drug blood levels in assessing optimum dose, potential toxicity, and compliance with therapy.

4.   Know that blood levels of tricyclic antidepressants vary greatly in patients taking identical doses.

5.   Be able to choose an appropriate endpoint for dosing, recognizing its empiric nature, e.g., intolerable side effects or drug blood levels in the toxic range.

6.   Understand the potential value in switching from one drug to another in the case of therapeutic failure.

7.   Know demographic, metabolic, or disease-related factors that may affect drug selection or dosage titration (e.g., age; cardiac, renal, or hepatic disease)

8.   Know important drug interactions with antidepressants (e.g., two drugs with serotonergic effect should not be combined due to the risk of serotonergic syndrome)

D.   Know the contraindications for different antidepressants (e.g., cardiac conduction disturbances, cardiac decompensation, recent myocardial infarction, and epilepsy for tricyclic antidepressants).

E. Know the common side effects of the antidepressant drugs used in the treatment of pain (e.g., sedation, dry mouth, memory impairment, urinary retention, orthostatic hypotension, and cardiac conduction abnormalities with tricyclic antidepressants).

II. Anticonvulsant drugs (McQuay et al. 1995; Backonja et al. 1998; Rowbotham et al. 1998; Sindrup and Jensen 1999)

A. Know the indications for the use of anticonvulsant drugs.

1. Know those syndromes for which the use of these drugs is supported by controlled studies (e.g., trigeminal neuralgia, painful diabetic neuropathy, postherpetic neuralgia, and central poststroke pain).
2. Know the other neuropathic pain syndromes in which these drugs are used, often with little hard evidence (including chronic postoperative pain, sciatica, peripheral nerve damage, and spinal cord injury).

B. Know the relative efficacy and adverse effects of the variety of available anticonvulsants, to include carbamazepine, phenytoin, valproate, clonazepam, gabapentin, lamotrigine, pregabalin, and other ion channel blockers.

C. Know the appropriate dosing regimen for each anticonvulsant used as an analgesic.

1. Understand the similarity between dosing for analgesic purposes and anticonvulsant dosing.
2. Have titration schedules in mind for the drugs, understanding the importance of low initial dosing and gradual upward titration to reduce adverse effects.
3. Understand the arguments for and against therapeutic drug monitoring (TDM) for anticonvulsants (value of blood levels in monitoring patient compliance, levels associated with effective analgesia, potential explanations for therapeutic failure versus cost or unavailability of TDM).

D. Know the potential toxicities of these drugs and how to advise the patient and other health care professionals what they should expect and how to deal with it.

REFERENCES

Backonja M, Beydoun A, Edwards KR, et al. Gabapentin for the symptomatic treatment of painful neuropathy in patients with diabetes mellitus. *JAMA* 1998; 280(21):1831–1836.

Carette S, Bell MJ, Reynolds WJ, et al. Comparison of amitriptyline, cyclobenzaprine, and placebo in the treatment of fibromyalgia. *Arthritis Rheum* 1994; 37:32–40.

Kunz NR, Goli V, Entsuah R. Venlafaxine extended release in the treatment of pain associated with diabetic neuropathy. *Neurology* 2000; (Suppl 3)54:A441.

Magni G. The use of antidepressants in the treatment of chronic pain. *Drugs* 1991; 42:730–748.

Max MB. Antidepressants as analgesics. In: Fields HL, Liebeskind JC (Eds). *Pharmacological Approaches to the Treatment of Chronic Pain: New Concepts and Critical Issues,* Progress in Pain Research and Management, Vol. 1, Seattle: IASP Press, 1994, pp 229–246.

McQuay H, Carroll D, Jadad AR, Wiffen P, Moore A. Anticonvulsant drugs for management of pain: a systematic review. *BMJ* 1995; 311(7012):1047–1052.

McQuay HJ, Tramèr M, Nye BA, et al. A systematic review of antidepressants in neuropathic pain. *Pain* 1996; 68:217–227.

Onghena P, van Houdenhove B. Antidepressant-induced analgesia in chronic non-malignant pain: a meta-analysis of 39 placebo-controlled studies. *Pain* 1992; 49:205–220.

Rowbotham M, Harden N, Stacey B, et al. Gabapentin for the treatment of postherpetic neuralgia. *JAMA* 1998; 280(21):1837–1842.

Semenchuk MR, Sherman S, Davis B. Double-blind, randomized trial of bupropion SR for the treatment of neuropathic pain. *Neurology* 2001; 57:1583–1588.

Sindrup SH. Antidepressants in chronic pain. In: Jensen TS, Wilson PR, Rice ASC (Eds). *Clinical Pain Management: Chronic Pain.* London: Arnold, 2003, pp 239–249.

Sindrup SH, Jensen TS. Efficacy of pharmacological treatments of neuropathic pain: an update and effect related to mechanism of drug action. *Pain* 1999; 83:389–400.

Sindrup SH, Bach FW, Madsen C, Jensen TS. Venlafaxine versus imipramine in painful polyneuropathy. A randomized, controlled trial. *Neurology* 2003; 60:1284–1289.

Core Curriculum for Professional Education in Pain, edited by J. Edmond Charlton, IASP Press, Seattle, © 2005.

16

Miscellaneous Agents

I.   Neuroleptic drugs (Beaver et al. 1966; Patt et al. 1994)

    A.   Know the indications for using neuroleptic drugs as adjuvant analgesics.

        1.   Know that methotrimeprazine is the only neuroleptic with analgesic potential supported by controlled studies.

        2.   Know the anecdotal evidence for using neuroleptic drugs in neuropathic pain.

        3.   Understand their potential value in treating patients with coexisting symptoms, such as nausea or anxiety.

        4.   Be aware of the lack of a theoretical basis for analgesic effects of neuroleptic drugs, and that the evidence for their efficiency is controversial at best.

    B.   Be aware of the potential toxicities of the neuroleptic drugs.

        1.   Know the potential for long-term, refractory movement disorders (for example, tardive dyskinesia) and consider this risk in the long-term administration of these drugs.

        2.   Be aware of the short-term, reversible toxicity, including other movement disorders (e.g., dystonic reactions), sedation, orthostatic hypotension, and the neuroleptic malignant syndrome.

        3.   Be aware that combining neuroleptics with tricyclic antidepressants may produce additive toxicity because of overlapping side effects.

II. Antihistamines (Stambaugh and Lance 1983; Rumore and Schlicting 1986)

    A.   Be aware of the literature supporting the use of antihistamines, specifically hydroxyzine, orphenadrine, and diphenhydramine, as analgesics.

    B.   Recognize the limited role played by these drugs in clinical pain management.

    C.   Understand the potential use of certain antihistamines as anxiolytics or antiemetics.

III. Analeptic drugs (Rozans et al. 2002; Bruera et al. 1987)

    A.   Be aware of the literature supporting the analgesic potential of analeptic drugs.

    B.   Understand the reasons for the limited role played by these drugs in the management of nonmalignant pain (e.g., tolerance on long-term administration, potential for precipitating psychosis, sleep disturbance, and cardiac toxicity).

    C.   Understand the potential value of these drugs in the treatment of cancer pain with coexisting opioid-induced sedation.

IV. Corticosteroids (Devor et al. 1985; Bruera et al. 1985; Watkins and Maier 2002)

    A.   Understand the literature supporting the use of corticosteroids in certain pain states.

        1.   Know the role of these drugs in the management of pain and other symptoms related to cancer (controlled studies in pain and nausea, anecdotal reports in lassitude, anorexia, and others).

        2.   Be aware of the laboratory evidence supporting the use of steroids in reducing both the magnitude and effects of nerve injury.

3. Understand the importance of immunological activation of the central nervous system during chronic pain syndromes and the potential for modification of this response by corticosteroids.

B. Understand the reasons for the limited role played by these drugs in the management of nonmalignant pain syndromes and their substantial potential for toxicity with short- or long-term use.

V. Muscle relaxants and antispasticity drugs (Dellemijn and Fields 1994 ; Arrezzo 2002; Dodick 2003; van Tulder et al. 2003; Raj 2003; Gobel 2004)

A. Know the potential indications for muscle relaxants as a short-term treatment for muscle spasm from a variety of causes.

B. Know the specific drugs used as systemic muscle relaxants and antispasticity agents.

1. Be aware of the pharmacology of specific drugs such as dantrolene, baclofen, and orphenadrine.
2. Understand the potential for using these drugs in combination.

C. Know the data supporting the use of muscle relaxant drugs for common musculoskeletal pain syndromes.

1. Be aware of the paucity of controlled studies.
2. Be aware of the lack of evidence of long-term benefit.
3. Understand that drug selection is empirical.

D. Know the appropriate dosing regimens and toxicity associated with these drugs.

E. Know the clinical pharmacology of botulinum toxin.

1. Be aware of the peripheral anti-spasticity effects and central analgesic effects of botulinum toxin.
2. Be aware of the different subtypes of botulinum toxin.
3. Be aware of the evidence supporting the use of botulinum toxin in headache of various etiologies, musculoskeletal pain syndromes, and the pain of neurological disease.
4. Be aware of the dosing regimens and potential side effects of botulinum toxin.

VI. NMDA antagonists (Mercadante et al. 2000; Hocking and Cousins 2003)

A. Understand the theoretical basis for the use of NMDA antagonist drugs in chronic pain states.

B. Be aware of the clinical pharmacology of ketamine.

1. Be aware of the use of ketamine in refractory neuropathic pain.
2. Be aware of the use of ketamine in opioid resistance/tolerance.
3. Be aware of the spectrum of side-effects associated with the use of ketamine (e.g., dysphoria, hallucinations, psychosis) and appropriate management strategies.
4. Be aware of appropriate oral and parenteral dosing regimens for ketamine.

VII. Local anesthetics and membrane-stabilizing drugs (Lindstrom and Lindblom 1987; Dejgard et al. 1988; Chabal et al. 1989; Rowbotham et al. 1991 ; Galer et al. 1993; Strichartz 1995)

A. Be aware of the evidence demonstrating the efficacy of certain antiarrhythmic drugs (e.g., mexiletine, tocainide) in neuropathic pain.

B. Know the rationale for the use of these drugs in neuropathic pain.

1. Understand that they block voltage-dependent sodium channels in a manner similar to some anticonvulsants (e.g., carbamazepine and lamotrigine).
2. Be familiar with the evidence from human and animal studies demonstrating sodium channel accumulation in damage to peripheral nerves and reduction in spontaneous and evoked activity in animal neuroma models.

C. Know the dosing regimens for these agents.

D. Be aware of the possibility for serious or irreversible toxicity with these agents (e.g., blood dyscrasias, malignant cardiac arrhythmias in susceptible patients).

VIII. Sympatholytic drugs (Verdugo and Ochoa 1994; Verdugo, Campero and Ochoa 1994; Jadad et al. 1995).

A. Know the rationale for the use of sympatholytic drugs in the management of sympathetically maintained pain.

B. Be aware of the limited and contradictory evidence for the use of these drugs in clinical pain management.

IX. Miscellaneous adjuvant analgesics (Fromm et al. 1984; Khan et al. 1999; Devers and Galer 2000; Robbins 2000; Campbell et al. 2001; Mason et al. 2004; Silberstein 2004).

A. Know that baclofen is effective in trigeminal neuralgia and is often used for other neuropathic lancinating pain.

B. Understand the difficulty in interpreting evidence relating to the use of cannabinoids as analgesics.

1. Be aware of the evidence indicating that cannabinoids have analgesic activity but that this activity is compromised by significant side effects.
2. Understand that the scientific debate relating to therapeutic use of cannabinoids is generally subservient to the concurrent political debate.

C. Know that drugs modifying serotonergic pathways (pizotifen, methysergide, and triptan drugs) are of proven efficacy for migraine headache.

D. Understand the basis for the analgesic effects of alpha-2 adrenergic agents (clonidine, tizanidine, dexmedetomidine) together with the use of these agents via the oral, parenteral, and neuroaxial routes.

E. Be aware of the evidence from controlled studies for the use of topical agents in neuropathic pain syndromes such as diabetic neuropathy and postherpetic neuralgia.

1. Be aware of the use of lidocaine patch technology in relieving the symptoms of localized neuropathic pain.
2. Be aware of the use of capsaicin in both low- and high-potency preparations in the management of neuropathic, musculoskeletal, and arthritic pain.

REFERENCES

Arezzo JC. Possible mechanisms for the effects of botulinum toxin on pain. *Clin J Pain* 2002; 18(6 Suppl):S125–132.

Beaver WT, Wallenstein SL, Houde RW, Rogers A. A comparison of the analgesic effects of methotrimeprazine and morphine in patients with cancer. *Clin Pharmacol Ther* 1966; (7):436–446.

Bruera E, Roca E, Cedaro L, Cararro S, Chacon R. Action of oral methylprednisolone in terminal cancer patients: a prospective, randomised, double-blind controlled study. *Cancer Treat Rep* 1985; (69):751–754.

Bruera E, Chadwick S, Brenneis C, Hanson J, MacDonald RN. Methylphenidate associated with narcotics for the treatment of cancer pain. *Cancer Treat Rep* 1987; (71):67–70.

Campbell FA, Tramer MR, Carroll D, et al. Are cannabinoids an effective and safe treatment option in the management of pain? A qualitative systematic review. *BMJ* 2001; 323(7303):13–16.

Chabal C, Russell LC, Burchiel KJ. The effect of intravenous lidocaine, tocainide and mexiletine on spontaneously active fibres originating in rat sciatic neuromas. *Pain* 1989; (38):333–338.

Dejgard A, Petersen P, Kastrup J., Mexiletine for treatment of chronic painful diabetic neuropathy. *Lancet* 1988;1(8575–8576):9–11.

Dellemijn PL, Fields HL. Do benzodiazepines have a role in chronic pain management? *Pain* 1994; 57:137–152.

Devers A, Galer BS. Topical lidocaine patch relieves a variety of neuropathic pain conditions: an open-label study. *Clin J Pain* 2000; 16(3):205–208.

Devor M, Govrin-Lippmann R, Raber P. Corticosteroids suppress ectopic neural discharge originating in experimental neuromas. *Pain* 1985; 22:127–137.

Dodick DW. Botulinum neurotoxin for the treatment of migraine and other primary headache disorders: from bench to bedside. *Headache* 2003; 43(Suppl 1):S25–33.

Fromm GH, Terence CF, Chatta AS. Baclofen in the treatment of trigeminal neuralgia. *Ann Neurol* 1984; (15):240–247.

Galer BS, Miller KV, Rowbotham MC. Response to intravenous lidocaine infusion differs based on clinical diagnosis and site of nervous system injury. *Neurology* 1993; (43):1233–1235.

Gobel H. Botulinum toxin in migraine prophylaxis. *J Neurol* 2004; 251(Suppl 1):8–11.

Hocking G, Cousins MJ. Ketamine in chronic pain management: an evidence-based review. *Anesth Analg* 2003; 97(6):1730–1739.

Jadad AR, Carroll D, Glynn CJ, McQuay HJ. Intravenous regional sympathetic blockade for pain relief in reflex sympathetic dystrophy: a systematic review and a randomized, double-blind crossover study. *J Pain Symptom Manage* 1995; 10(1):13–20.

Khan ZP, Ferguson CN, Jones RM. Alpha-2 and imidazoline receptor agonists: their pharmacology and therapeutic role. *Anaesthesia* 1999; 54(2):146–165.

Lindstrom P, Lindblom U. The analgesic effect of tocainide in trigeminal neuralgia. *Pain* 1987; 28:45–50.

Mason L, Moore RA, Derry S, Edwards JE, McQuay HJ. Systematic review of topical capsaicin for the treatment of chronic pain. *BMJ* 2004; 328(7446):991.

Mercadante S, Arcuri E, Tirelli W, Casuccio A. Analgesic effect of intravenous ketamine in cancer patients on morphine therapy: a randomized, controlled, double-blind, crossover, double-dose study. *J Pain Symptom Manage* 2000; 20(4):246–252.

Patt RB, Proper G, Reddy S. The neuroleptics as adjuvant analgesics. *J Pain Symptom Manage* 1994;9(7):446–453.

Raj PP. Botulinum toxin therapy in pain management. *Anesthesiol Clin N Am* 2003; 21(4):715–731.

Robbins W. Clinical applications of capsaicinoids. *Clin J Pain* 2000; 16(2 Suppl):S86–89.

Rowbotham MC, Reisner-Keller LA, Fields HL. Both intravenous lidocaine and morphine reduce the pain of postherpetic neuralgia. *Neurology* 1991; 41(7):1024–1028.

Rozans M, Dreisbach A, Lertora JJ, Kahn MJ. Palliative uses of methylphenidate in patients with cancer: a review. *J Clin Oncol* 2002; 20(1):335–339.

Rumore MM, Schlichting DA. Clinical efficacy of antihistamines as analgesics. *Pain* 1986; 25:7–22.

Silberstein SD. Migraine. *Lancet* 2004; 363(9406):381–391.

Stambaugh JE, Lance C. Analgesic efficacy and pharmacokinetic evaluation of meperidine and hydroxyzine, alone and in combination. *Cancer Invest* 1983; (Suppl 1):111–117.

Strichartz G. Protracted relief of experimental neuropathic pain by systemic local anesthetics: how, where, and when. *Anesthesiology* 1995; 83(4):654–655.

van Tulder MW, Touray T, Furlan AD, Solway S, Bouter LM. Cochrane Back Review Group. Muscle relaxants for nonspecific low back pain: a systematic review within the framework of the Cochrane Collaboration. *Spine* 2003; 28(17):1978–1992.

Verdugo RJ, Ochoa JL. 'Sympathetically maintained pain.' I. Phentolamine block questions the concept. *Neurology* 1994; 44(6):1003–1010.

Verdugo RJ, Campero M, Ochoa JL. Phentolamine sympathetic block in painful polyneuropathies. II. Further questioning of the concept of 'sympathetically maintained pain'. *Neurology* 1994; 44(6):1010–1014.

Watkins L, Maier SF. Beyond neurons: evidence that immune and glial cells contribute to pathological pain states. *Physiol Rev* 2002; 82(4):981–1011.

Core Curriculum for Professional Education in Pain, edited by J. Edmond Charlton, IASP Press, Seattle, © 2005.

17

Psychological Treatments (Cognitive-Behavioral and Behavioral Interventions)

I.   For the following intervention strategies, understand the evidence base, theoretical rationale, assessment procedures, indications, specific details of the treatment approach, and efficacy (Flor et al. 1992; Keefe et al. 1992; Turk and Melzack 1992; NIH Technology Assessment Panel 1996; Compas et al. 1998; Holroyd et al. 1998, 2001; Morley et al. 1999; Guzman et al. 2001; Turner and Romano 2001; Turk and Monarch 2002).

   A.   Understand relaxation strategies: progressive muscle relaxation, autogenic training, guided imagery, cue controlling and other strategies (Bernstein et al. 2000; Turner and Romano 2001).

   B.   Know the cognitive-behavioral treatments of pain: cognitive therapy, cognitive restructuring, problem solving, and communication skills training (Keefe et al. 1996a; Turk and Okifuji 1999; Turner and Romano 2001).

   C.   Be familiar with the techniques of operant therapy, e.g., contingency management for pain behavior and well behavior, reinforcement, stimulus and response generalization, quotas and goal setting, and medication management (Fordyce 1976; Keefe and Lefebvre 1994; Fordyce 2001; Flor et al. 2002; Sanders 2002).

   D.   Be familiar with the use of graded exposure in vivo to reduce the effects of pain-related anxiety or fears of pain and disability (McCracken et al. 1992; Vlaeyen et al. 2001, 2002).

   E.   Be familiar with the use of biofeedback in pain management, e.g., using electromyographic (EMG) and temperature feedback (Flor and Birbaumer 1993; Jessup and Gallegos 1994; Schwartz 1995; Arena and Blanchard 2002).

   F.   Understand the potential for and methods available to produce hypnoanalgesia and other hypnotic effects (Spanos et al. 1994; Syrjala and Abrams 2002).

   G.   Be familiar with psychological strategies for preparing patients for painful medical procedures and implantation of neuroaugmentative devices including spinal cord stimulators and drug delivery systems (Williams 1999).

   H.   Be familiar with the potential benefits of stress management via private emotional disclosure (including expressive writing) among patients with rheumatoid arthritis and other stress-exacerbated pain conditions (Kelley et al. 1997; Smyth et al. 1999).

   I.   Be familiar with the integration of psychological therapies with rehabilitation therapies, e.g., physical therapy, occupational therapy, and vocational rehabilitation (Feuerstein and Zastowny 1996).

   J.   Be aware of group therapy and how to assess patients for the likely efficacy of group therapy approaches (Keefe et al. 1996a; Keel et al. 1998).

   K.   Be aware of cognitive-behavioral interventions used to treat pain in children and adolescents (McGrath and Hillier 1996).

   L.   Understand the behavioral interventions used to improve sleep in patients with persistent pain (stimulus control, sleep hygiene, cognitive-behavioral therapy) (Morin et al. 1993, 1994).

M. Understand strategies used to involve spouses, caregivers, and significant others in behavioral and cognitive-behavioral pain management interventions (e.g., Keefe et al. 1996b).

N. Be familiar with behavioral and motivational strategies for enhancing patient adherence and preventing relapse (Keefe and Van Horn 1993; Myers and Midence 1998; Martin et al. 2000; Turner and Romano 2001; Kerns et al. 2002).

O. Be familiar with the behavioral interventions used in primary care settings to prevent chronic pain (Linton and Bradley 1996).

P. Be familiar with the use of early intervention techniques for helping patients cope with chronically painful diseases such as rheumatoid arthritis (e.g., Sharpe et al. 2001).

Q. Be familiar with relapse prevention training and methods for enhancing maintenance and generalization of therapeutic improvements (McGrath and Manion 1990; Turk and Rudy 1991; Keefe and Van Horn 1993).

II. Have a basic understanding of the medical/physiological aspects of the pain problem, e.g., disease severity, prognosis, common medical and surgical treatments. Recognize behavioral components and the importance of the social context of all biological interventions (motivational factors, relationship factors, suggestion, trust, and adherence) (Turk and Rudy 1991). Be able to recognize the psychological effects of biological interventions, e.g., effects and side effects of medications that can compromise functioning or impair psychological test performance.

III. Be aware of the need to treat comorbid psychological problems that may accompany pain (DeGood and Dane 1996).

IV. Recognize the application of various cognitive and behavioral strategies to specific pain syndromes such as temporomandibular disorder pain, neck and back pain, fibromyalgia, arthritis pain, burn pain, and postoperative pain (Kendall 1983; Keefe et al. 1990a,b; Dworkin et al. 1994; Linton and Ryberg 2001; Williams et al. 2002).

V. Be familiar with how the various separate approaches can be integrated including different cognitive-behavioral treatments and combined behavioral and drug treatments (Flor and Birbaumer 1991; Holroyd et al. 2001; Turk 2001; Polatin and Gajraj 2002), and be aware of the economic benefits of integrating cognitive-behavioral and drug treatments (Conrad and Deyo 1994; McCarberg 2000; Gatchel 2001).

VI. Be familiar with the transtheoretical model of behavioral change and with motivational interviewing techniques used to address patients at different stages of change (Kerns et al. 1997; Keefe et al. 2000; Dijkstra et al. 2001).

VII. Recognize common process factors in cognitive-behavioral and self-management interventions including rapport, engendering hope and positive expectations, developing a therapeutic alliance, communication strategies, support, and suggestion (Lorig and Holman 1993).

VIII. Be familiar with placebo effects and nonspecific effects on treatment outcome (Turner et al. 1994; Turner 2001).

IX. Understand the racial, ethnic, and cultural factors to consider in the psychological treatment of pain (Edwards et al. 2001).

X. Know the role of clinical decision-making in matching interventions to patients' needs (Turk 1990; Rudy et al. 1992; Turk and Okifuji 2001).

REFERENCES

Arena JG, Blanchard EB. Biofeedback for chronic pain disorders: a primer. In: Turk DC, Gatchel RJ (Eds). *Psychological Approaches to Pain Management: A Practitioner's Handbook*. New York: Guilford Press, 2002, pp 159–186.

Bernstein DA, Borkovec TD, Hazlett-Stevens H. New directions in progressive relaxation training. Westport, CT: Praeger, 2000, p 171.

Compas BE, Haaga DA, Keefe FJ, Leitenberg H, Williams DA. Sampling of empirically supported treatments from health psychology: smoking, chronic pain, cancer, and bulimia nervosa. *J Consult Clin Psychol* 1998; 66:89–112.

Conrad DA, Deyo RA. Economic decision analysis in the diagnosis and treatment of low back pain: a methodologic primer. *Spine* 1994; 19:2101S–2106S.

DeGood DE, Dane JR. The psychologist as a pain consultant in outpatient, inpatient, and work settings. In: Gatchel RJ, Turk DC (Eds). *Psychological Approaches to Pain Management: A Practitioner's Handbook*. New York: Guilford Press, 1996, pp 403–437.

Dijkstra A, Vlaeyen JW, Rijnen H, et al. Readiness to adopt the self-management approach to cope with chronic pain in fibromyalgia patients. *Pain* 2001; 90:37–45.

Dworkin SF, Turner JA, Wilson L, et al. Brief group cognitive-behavioral intervention for temporomandibular disorders. *Pain* 1994; 59:175–187.

Edwards RR, Doleys DM, Fillingim RB, Lowery D. Ethnic differences in pain tolerance: clinical implications in a chronic pain population. *Psychosom Med* 2001; 63:316–323.

Feuerstein M, Zastowny TR. Occupational rehabilitation: multidisciplinary management of work-related musculoskeletal pain and disability. In: Gatchel R, Turk DC (Eds). *Psychological Approaches to Pain Management: A Practitioner's Handbook*. New York: Guilford Press, 1996, pp 403–437.

Flor H, Birbaumer N. Comprehensive assessment and treatment of chronic back pain patients without physical disabilities. In: Bond MR, Charlton JE, Woolf CJ (Eds). *Proceedings of the VIth World Congress on Pain*, Progress in Pain Research Management, Vol. 4. Amsterdam: Elsevier, 1991, pp 229–234.

Flor H, Birbaumer N. Comparison of EMG biofeedback, cognitive behavior therapy, and conservative medical treatment for chronic musculoskeletal pain. *J Consult Clin Psychol* 1993; 61:653–658.

Flor H, Fydrich T, Turk DC. Efficacy of multi disciplinary pain treatment centers: a meta analytic review. *Pain* 1992; 49:221–230.

Flor H, Knost B, Birbaumer N. The role of operant conditioning in chronic pain: an experimental investigation. *Pain* 2002; 95:111–118.

Fordyce WE. *Behavioral Methods for Chronic Pain and Illness*. St. Louis: CV Mosby, 1976, 113–126.

Fordyce WE. Operant or contingency therapies. In: Loeser JD (Ed). *Bonica's Management of Pain*. Philadelphia: Lippincott Williams and Wilkins, 2001, pp 1745–1750.

Gatchel RJ. A biopsychosocial overview of pretreatment screening of patients with pain. *Clin J Pain* 2001; 17:192–199.

Guzman J, Esmail R, Karjalainen K, et al. Multidisciplinary rehabilitation for chronic low back pain: systematic review. *BMJ* 2001; 322:511–516.

Holroyd KA, Holm JE, Hursey KG, et al. Recurrent vascular headache: home based behavioral treatment versus abortive pharmacological treatment. *J Consult Clin Psychol* 1988; 56:218–223.

Holroyd KA, O'Donnell FJ, Stenland M, et al. Management of chronic tension-type headache with tricyclic antidepressant medication, stress management therapy, and their combination: a randomized controlled trial. *JAMA* 2001; 285:2208–2215.

Jessup BA, Gallegos X. Relaxation and biofeedback. In: Wall PD, Melzack R (Eds). *Textbook of Pain,* 3rd ed. Edinburgh: Churchill Livingstone, 1994, pp 1321–1336.

Keefe FJ, Lefebvre JC. Behaviour therapy. In: Wall PD, Melzack R (Eds). *Textbook of Pain,* 3rd ed. Edinburgh: Churchill Livingstone, 1994, pp 1367–1380.

Keefe FJ, Van Horn Y. Cognitive-behavioral treatment of rheumatoid arthritis pain: understanding and enhancing maintenance of treatment gains. *Arthritis Care Res* 1993, 6:213–222.

Keefe FJ, Caldwell DS, Williams DA, et al. Pain coping skills training in the management of osteoarthritic knee pain: a comparative study. *Behav Ther* 1990a, 21:49–62.

Keefe FJ, Caldwell DS, Williams DA, et al. Pain coping skills training in the management of osteoarthritic knee pain: follow-up results. *Behav Ther* 1990b; 21:435–448.

Keefe FJ, Dunsmore J, Burnett R. Behavioral and cognitive-behavioral approaches to chronic pain: recent advances and future directions. *J Consult Clin Psychol* 1992; 60:528–536.

Keefe FJ, Beaupre PM, Gil KM. Group therapy for patients with chronic pain. In: Turk DC, Gatchel RJ (Eds). *Psychological Approaches to Pain Management: A Practitioner's Handbook*. New York: Guilford Press, 1996a.

Keefe FJ, Caldwell DS, Baucom D, et al. Spouse-assisted coping skills training in the management of osteoarthritis knee pain. *Arthritis Care Res* 1996b; 9:279–291.

Keefe FJ, Lefebvre JC, Kerns RD, et al. Understanding the adoption of arthritis self-management: stages of change profiles among arthritis patients. *Pain* 2000, 87:303–314.

Keel PJ, Bodokey C, Gerhard U, Muller W. Comparison of integrated group therapy and group relaxation training for fibromyalgia. *Clin J Pain* 1998; 63:232–238.

Kelley JE, Lumley MA, Leisen JCC. Health effects of emotional disclosure in rheumatoid arthritis patients. *Health Psychol* 1997; 16:331–340.

Kendall PC. Stressful medical procedures: cognitive behavioral strategies for stress management and prevention. In: Meichenbaum DH, Jaremko ME (Eds). *Stress Reduction and Prevention*. New York: Plenum, 1983, pp 159–190.

Kerns RD, Rosenburg R, Jamison R, et al. Readiness to adopt a self-management approach to chronic pain: the Pain Stages of Change Questionnaire. *Pain* 1997; 72:227–234.

Kerns RD, Otis JD, Wise EA. Treating families of chronic pain patients: applications of a cognitive-behavioral transactional model. In: Turk DC, Gatchel RJ (Eds). *Psychological Approaches to Pain Management: A Practitioner's Handbook*. New York: Guilford Press, 2002, pp 256–275.

Linton SJ, Bradley LA. Strategies for the prevention of chronic pain. In: Gatchel RJ, Turk DC (Eds). *Psychological Approaches to Pain Management: A Practitioner's Handbook*. New York: Guilford Press, 1996, pp 438–457.

Linton SJ, Ryberg M. A cognitive-behavioral group intervention as prevention for persistent neck and back pain in a non-patient population: a randomized controlled trial. *Pain* 2001; 90:83–90.

Lorig K, Holman H. Arthritis self-management studies: a twelve-year review. *Arthritis Rheum* 1993; 20:17–28.

Martin KA, Bowen DJ, Dunbar-Jacob J, Perri MG. Who will adhere? Key issues in the study and prediction of adherence in randomized controlled trials. *Control Clin Trials* 2000; 21:195S–199S.

McCarberg B. Cost effectiveness of chronic pain programs. *Am Pain Soc Bull* 2000; 10:12–14.

McCracken LM, Zayfert C, Gross RT. The Pain Anxiety Symptoms Scale: development and validation of a scale to measure fear of pain. *Pain* 1992; 50:67–73.

McGrath PA, Hillier LM. Controlling children's pain. In: Gatchel RJ, Turk DC (Eds). *Psychological Approaches to Pain Management: A Practitioner's Handbook.* New York: Guilford Press, 1996, pp 331–370.

McGrath PJ, Manion IG. Prevention of pain problems. In: Craig KD, Weiss SM (Eds). *Health Enhancement, Disease Prevention and Early Intervention: Biobehavioral Perspectives.* New York: Springer, 1990, pp 269–286.

Morin CM, Kowatch RA, Barry T, Walton E. Cognitive-behavior therapy for late-life insomnia. *J Consult Clin Psychol* 1993; 61:137–146.

Morin CM, Culbert JP, Schwartz SM. Nonpharmacological interventions for insomnia: a meta-analysis of treatment efficacy. *Am J Psychiatry* 1994; 151:1172–1180.

Morley S, Eccleston C, Williams AC de C. Systematic review and meta-analysis of randomized controlled trials of cognitive behaviour therapy for chronic pain in adults, excluding headache. *Pain* 1999; 80:1–13.

Myers LB, Midence K (Eds). *Adherence to Treatment in Medical Conditions.* London: Harwood Academic, 1998.

NIH Technology Assessment Panel on Integration of Behavioral and Relaxation Approaches into the Treatment of Chronic Pain and Insomnia. Integration of behavioral and relaxation approaches into the treatment of chronic pain and insomnia. *JAMA* 1996; 276:313–318.

Polatin PB, Gajraj NM. Integration of pharmacotherapy with psychological treatment of chronic pain. In: Turk DC, Gatchel RJ (Eds). *Psychological Approaches to Pain Management: A Practitioner's Handbook.* New York: Guilford Press, 2002, pp 276–298.

Rudy TE, Turk DC, Kubinski JA, Zaki HS. Differential treatment responses of TMD patients as a function of psychological characteristics. *Pain* 1992; 61:103–112.

Sanders SH. Operant conditioning with chronic pain: back to basics. In: Turk DC, Gatchel RJ (Eds). *Psychological Approaches to Pain Management: A Practitioner's Handbook.* New York: Guilford Press, 2002, pp 128–137.

Schwartz MS. *Biofeedback: A Practitioner's Guide,* 2nd ed. New York: Guilford Press, 1995.

Sharpe L, Sensky T, Timberlake N, Ryan B. A blind, randomized controlled trail of cognitive-behavioural intervention for patients with recent onset rheumatoid arthritis: preventing psychological and physical disability. *Pain* 2001: 89:275–283.

Smyth JM, Stone AA, Hurewitz A, Kaell A. Effects of writing about stressful experiences on symptom reduction in patients with asthma or rheumatoid arthritis. *JAMA* 1999; 281:1304–1309.

Spanos NP, Carmanico SJ, Ellis JA. Hypnotic analgesia. In: Wall PD, Melzack R (Eds). *Textbook of Pain,* 3rd ed. Edinburgh: Churchill Livingstone, 1994, pp 1349–1366.

Syrjala KL, Abrams JR. Hypnosis and imagery in the treatment of pain In: Turk DC, Gatchel RJ (Eds). *Psychological Approaches to Pain Management: A Practitioner's Handbook.* New York: Guilford Press, 2002, pp 187–209.

Turk DC. Customizing treatment for chronic pain patients: who, what, and why. *Clin J Pain* 1990; 6:255–270.

Turk DC. Combining somatic and psychosocial treatment for chronic pain patients: perhaps 1 + 1 does = 3. *Clin J Pain* 2001; 17:281–283.

Turk DC, Melzack R. The measurement of pain and the assessment of people experiencing pain. In: Turk DC, Melzack R (Eds). *Handbook of Pain Assessment.* New York: Guilford Press, 1992, pp 3–12.

Turk DC, Monarch ES. Biopsychosocial perspective on chronic pain. In: Turk DC, Gatchel RJ (Eds). *Psychological Approaches to Pain Management: A Practitioner's Handbook.* New York: Guilford Press, 2002, pp 1–29.

Turk DC, Okifuji AD. A cognitive behavioral approach to pain management. In: Wall PD, Melzack R (Eds). *Textbook of Pain.* London: Churchill Livingstone, 1999, pp 1431–1444.

Turk DC, Okifuji A. Matching treatment to assessment of patients with chronic pain. In: Turk DC, Melzack R (Eds). *Handbook of Pain Assessment,* 2nd ed. New York: Guilford, 2001, pp 400–414.

Turk DC, Rudy TE. Neglected topics in the treatment of chronic pain patients: relapse, noncompliance and adherence enhancement. *Pain* 1991; 44:5–28.

Turner JA. Nonspecific treatment effects. In: Loeser JD (Ed). *Bonica's Management of Pain,* 3rd ed. Philadelphia: Lippincott Williams and Wilkins, 2001, pp 1649–1656.

Turner JA, Romano JM. Cognitive-behavioral therapy for chronic pain. In: Loeser JD (Ed). *Bonica's Management of Pain,* 3rd ed. Philadelphia: Lippincott Williams and Wilkins, 2001, pp 1751–1758.

Turner JA, Deyo RA, Loeser JD, et al. The importance of placebo effects in pain treatment and research. *JAMA* 1994; 271:1609–1614.

Vlaeyen JWS, de Jong J, Geilen M, Heuts PHT G, van Breukelen G. Graded exposure in vivo in the treatment of pain-related fear: a replicated single-case experimental design in four patients with chronic low back pain. *Behav Res Ther* 2001; 39:151–166.

Vlaeyen JWS, de Jong JR, Sieben JM, Crombez G. Graded exposure in vivo for pain-related fear. In: Gatchel R, Turk DC (Eds). *Psychological Approaches to Pain Management.* New York: Guilford Press, 2002.

Williams DA. Acute pain (including painful medical procedures). In: Gatchel RJ, Turk DC (Eds). *Psychosocial Factors in Pain.* New York: Guilford Publications, 1999.

Williams DA, Cary M, Groner KH, et al. Improving physical functional status in patients with fibromyalgia: a brief cognitive-behavioral intervention. *J Rheumatol* 2002; 29.

Core Curriculum for Professional Education in Pain, edited by J. Edmond Charlton, IASP Press, Seattle, © 2005.

18

Psychiatric Evaluation and Treatment

I. General principles

    A. Be aware that chronic pain is associated with a large number of psychiatric and psychological comorbidities including depression, anxiety, drug dependence, somatoform disorders, and bipolar disorder (Fishbain et al. 1998)

    B. Know that patients with diffuse complaints and widespread pain are at greater risk of psychiatric disorder and functional impairment than are patients with specific and/or localized complaints.

    C. Be able to make a diagnosis of major depression and dysthymic disorder and to distinguish these forms of mental disorder from the depressive symptoms that often accompany chronic pain.

    D. Be able to diagnose other psychiatric disorders that might present with pain as a symptom (such as a panic disorder presenting with nonorganic chest pain, post-traumatic stress disorder, or the rare presentation of psychotic disorders with delusional pain) as well as psychiatric disorders that might be comorbid with pain (e.g., obsessive-compulsive disorder).

    E. Be alert to the possibility of comorbid alcohol or nonalcohol substance abuse disorders that might increase pain disability or impede response to rehabilitation. The diagnosis must be based on a clinical examination, including a detailed mental state evaluation, and not solely on questionnaire methods (Goli and Fozdar 2002).

II. Drug treatment

    A. Know the indications for the use of antidepressants for both mood and anxiety disorders (Goli and Fozdar 2002).

    B. Understand the indications, contraindications, efficacy, use, drug interactions, and side effects of classical and newer or alternative antidepressants for treating comorbid mood or anxiety disorders in patients with pain. This would include the use of first-generation agents (e.g., tricyclics, including nortriptyline and desipramine, and monoamine oxidase inhibitors, including phenelzine), as well as selective serotonin reuptake inhibitors (SSRIs, e.g., fluoxetine and paroxetine), serotonergic-noradrenergic reuptake inhibitors (e.g., venlafaxine and mirtazapine), and noradrenergic-dopaminergic reuptake inhibitors (e.g., bupropion).

    C. Understand the use of other antidepressant/mood-stabilizing agents (e.g., lithium, valproate, and carbamazepine). Because mood disorders are often treatment resistant, use of augmentation and combination strategies should be understood.

    D. Be familiar with the use and roles of antidepressants and anxiolytics (e.g., benzodiazepines) to treat generalized anxiety disorder, panic disorder, social phobias, and obsessive-compulsive disorder.

    E. Be aware of the pharmacotherapy of psychotic disorders with first-generation and atypical neuroleptics (Breitbart 1998). Delirium can complicate the clinical picture of patients with pain due to diseases associated with pain and their therapy, as well as being a complication of opioid therapy, and thus it is important to be aware of the use of typical and atypical neuroleptics for delirium.

    F. Understand the efficacy of psychopharmacological agents as analgesics, and their application for specific conditions.

G. Be aware that antidepressants do have an analgesic effect outside of their antidepressant effect (Fishbain 2000a) and that the SSRI antidepressants may have a greater analgesic effect than the non-SSRIs (Fishbain 2000b).

H. Be aware of the limitations of antidepressant medications and that data demonstrating their efficacy is strong only for selected neuropathic pain syndromes (e.g., Max et al. 1992), migraine and tension headache syndromes, and perhaps atypical facial pain (e.g., see Magni 1991; Onghena and Van Houdenhove 1992), although evidence is developing that chronic low back pain may be responsive (e.g., Atkinson et al. 1999).

I. Recognize that there is little evidence that antidepressants are effective for nonspecific or mixed pain states, and that their role as analgesics in rheumatoid disorders and fibromyalgia is not yet clear.

J. Understand the potential differential efficacy of noradrenergic antidepressants, compared to serotonergic antidepressants (Max et al. 1992), as well as the possibility that there may be concentration-response effects (Sindrup et al. 1985, 1991).

K. Recognize that the evidence is very limited on the efficacy of mood stabilizers, benzodiazepines, and neuroleptics (except methotrimeprazine) as analgesics (e.g., Atkinson et al. 1994).

L. Be aware of the use of anticonvulsants as an aid to analgesia (e.g., olanzapine, gabapentin, and tiagabine) (Covington 1998; Khojainova et al. 2002).

III. Psychotherapy

A. Be aware of the different forms of psychotherapy for depression including supportive, cognitive, behavioral, marital and family, interpretative, and group therapy (Pilowsky and Barrow 1990; Flor et al. 1992).

B. Understand that, of these forms of psychotherapy used in pain management, the evidence base is strongest for cognitive-behavioral treatment (Williams et al. 2002).

C. Be aware that psychotherapeutic intervention (specifically cognitive-behavioral treatment) may offer significant benefits to patients with painful illnesses such as rheumatoid arthritis (Sharpe et al. 2001), osteoarthritis (Keefe et al. 1990), or sickle cell disease (Gil et al. 1996).

IV. Anxiety

A. Be able to discriminate anxiety conditions (e.g., panic disorder or post-traumatic stress disorder) that may augment pain and suffering in patients with chronic pain (Sharp and Harvey 2001).

B. Understand the application of the different forms of psychotherapy for anxiety disorders, for example, supportive, cognitive, behavioral, marital and family, interpretative, and group therapy (Keefe et al. 1992). Note that high anxiety is associated with heightened pain and may disrupt the use of self control strategies in coping with pain (McCracken et al. 1993; Biedermann and Schefft 1994).

C. Be aware that the SSRI antidepressants are now utilized in treating a wide range of anxiety syndromes.

V. Anger

A. Be aware that anger is an emotion that is frequently seen in chronic pain patients (Fernandez and Turk 1995) and that anger intensity relates to perceived pain interference (Kerns et al. 1994).

B. Be aware that anger may be a specific affective component of pain along with fear and sadness (Fernandez and Milburn 1994) and may be an important concomitant of the depression seen in chronic pain (Wade et al. 1990).

C. Be aware that patients with persistent pain may be at risk for violent behaviors (Fishbain et al. 2000b). Those patients demonstrating significant anger should be evaluated for potential violent behaviors. The presence of anger in a chronic pain patient should alert the pain physician to a syndrome that may be treatable by psychopharmacology or cognitive-behavioral therapy.

VI. Opioids

    A. Be familiar with the use of opioids for chronic noncancer pain in which there is objective nociceptive pathology that is related to and consistent with the pain syndrome.

    B. Understand the difference among the concepts of addiction, tolerance and dependence.

    C. Be familiar with the controversy over opioid medication in patients who have a history of substance abuse or do not have a demonstrable nociceptive source of pain (Ciccone et al. 2000; Robinson et al. 2001; Reid et al. 2002).

    D. Understand substance-abuse-related issues including withdrawal symptoms. Be familiar with detoxification for the chronic pain patient (Chabal et al. 1992; Fishbain et al. 1992a; Sees and Clark 1992; Jamison et al. 1994) and be aware of the protocols for opioid and sedative detoxification (Fishbain et al. 1992b, 1993).

    E. Understand the characteristics, different properties, and use of full agonist opioid agents, partial agonists, and mixed agonist-antagonist opioid drugs.

    F. Understand the use of adjunctive agents to enhance opioid therapy and be aware of evidence that aspirin, acetaminophen, and selected nonsteroidal anti-inflammatory drugs augment analgesia at a given dose of opioid, whereas neuroleptics, hydroxyzine, benzodiazepines, and antidepressants do not.

    G. Be aware of the importance of patient instruction and education regarding use of opioids, in order to minimize sense of stigmatization, lessen fears of addiction, and set the stage for appropriate use.

    H. Understand the potential application of opioid treatment contracts to help guide expectations around the use of opioids, particularly when there are concerns about diversion of opioids.

    I. Understand the medical-legal documentation relevant to patient instruction, selection, and follow-up of patients on opioid therapy.

VII. Somatization

    A. Be aware that some patients with persistent pain may demonstrate somatic complaints or pain out of proportion to the alleged organic findings, indicating that they may be suffering from a conversion disorder or hypochondriasis (Fishbain 2000a).

    B. In treating patients with somatoform disorders, including hypochondriasis, understand the importance of:

        1. Developing a therapeutic relationship with the patient
        2. Shifting the emphasis of intervention away from symptom alleviation and toward functional restoration
        3. Avoiding reliance on invasive diagnostic or surgical interventions. Understand the application of the other techniques recommended for patients with somatization disorder and hypochondriasis, including cognitive, behavioral, marital, and family therapy (Smith et al. 1986; Tunks and Merskey 1990; Merskey 1994).

VIII. The interview

    A. Know the value of interviewing a spouse or other relatives and evaluating information about the case obtained from a relative.

    B. Be aware that interviewing a spouse or significant other can be useful in corroborating premorbid behavior, mood, personality, and functional status (Kerns et al. 2002).

    C. Understand that discussions leading up to an appreciation by all parties of the implications of pain, and of other social or interpersonal problems exacerbated or ameliorated by chronic pain, are often of value in pain management (Kerns et al. 2002).

    D. Understand that training both patient and spouse in pain control skills may be beneficial (Keefe et al. 1996).

IX.   Beliefs and strategies

    A.   Understand the importance of coping strategies for the control of pain and the current status of this area of pain treatment research (Lester and Keefe 1997).

    B.   Understand that coping strategies may differ among individuals and may be affected by age and gender (Elton et al. 1994; Keefe et al. 2000).

    C.   Understand the important contribution that catastrophizing and fear-avoidance beliefs make to pain and disability (Sullivan et al. 2001; Vlaeyen et al. 2002).

    D.   Understand the importance of prior experiences with pain and illness in influencing how persons cope with pain. Be aware that persons who have suffered abuse may be at risk for chronic pain (Alexander et al. 1998).

    E.   Understand that in seeking medical care, chronic pain patients may have treatment goals that differ widely from those of the treating professional (Hazard et al. 1993; Leeman et al. 2000); a patient's satisfaction with care will be determined by whether his or her goals for treatment are met (Hazard et al. 1993).

    F.   Be familiar with the role of iatrogenic factors (inappropriate or excessive investigation or the use of spurious diagnosis) in contributing to chronic pain.

    G.   Be familiar with the importance of instructing the patient in risks associated with invasive medical procedures and passive modalities when performed on patients with unrealistic expectations.

    H.   Understand how to negotiate a balance of treatment goals (e.g., pain relief vs. functional improvement). Recognize the role of economic and social disincentives to rehabilitation, such as financial compensation (Rohling et al. 1995) or spousal relationships (Romano et al. 1992).

    I.   Be aware of the impact that current or future litigation may have on disability and pain (Main and Spanswick 1995).

X.   Sleep

    A.   Be aware that many chronic pain patients complain of sleep disturbance (Menefee et al. 2000). Be familiar with the variety of sleep disorders experienced by persons having chronic pain.

    B.   Recognize that sleep laboratory analyses show that patients with persistent pain sleep less than do insomniacs and demonstrate nocturnal myoclonus and alpha intrusions (Atkinson et al. 1988a,b) and that patients with high pain intensities report significantly less sleep (Atkinson et al. 1988a).

    C.   Be aware that these chronic sleep disturbances are better treated with sedating antidepressants (e.g. amitriptyline, doxepin, trazodone, nefazodone, or mirtazapine) than with benzodiazepines or other sedatives (Menefee et al. 2000).

    D.   Be familiar with treatments available to treat sleep disorders including behavioral instruction on proper sleep "hygiene" (observing scheduled sleep times and avoiding caffeine-containing compounds) and antidepressants in low dose (e.g. trazodone, doxepin, or mirtazapine) (Morin et al. 1994; NIH Technology Assessment Panel 1996).

XI.   Vocation and personality

    A.   Know the value of evaluation of the patient's past work level and educational attainment and be able to refer patients for appropriate psychological testing for both intellectual capacity and vocational preference.

    B.   Be able to identify patients for whom vocational guidance, further education, and retraining may lead to rehabilitation (Schade et al. 1999; Feuerstein et al. 2001).

C. Be able to advise on the effects of chronic pain upon personality, to provide insight and support for the patient, to interpret the situation to the family and other relatives and interested persons, and to advise on cognitive-behavioral treatments.

D. Be able to introduce suitable cognitive and behavioral pain management measures or recognize when it is appropriate to refer for the patient for special evaluation and therapy (Turk and Okifuji 2001; Turner and Romano 2001).

E. Know that personality disorders are common in chronic pain patients (Gatchel et al. 1996; Weisberg 2000).

F. Be aware of the role of personality in the patient's premorbid and current presentation.

G. Know that there does not appear to be strong empirical support for the notion of a "pain-prone personality" (Turk and Solovay 1984; Gatchel 1991).

H. Recognize that individuals without a history of personality disorders may appear personality disordered due to the exacerbation of premorbid personality characteristics resulting from pain and subsequent stressors (Weisberg and Keefe 1997).

I. Be aware that patients with chronic pain are at greater risk for suicidal behaviors and suicide completion and that those in greater pain may be at greatest risk (Fishbain 1999).

REFERENCES

Alexander RW, Bradley LA, Alarcon GS, et al. Sexual and physical abuse in women with fibromyalgia: association with outpatient health care utilization and pain medication usage. *Arthritis Care Res* 1998; 11:102–115.

Atkinson JH, Slater MA, Grant I, Patterson TL, Garfin SR. Depressed mood in chronic low back pain: relationship with stressful life events. *Pain* 1988a; 35:47–55.

Atkinson JH, Ancoli Isra el S, Slater MA, Garfin SR, Gitlin JC. Subjective sleep disturbance in chronic back pain. *Clin J Pain* 1988b; 4:225–232.

Atkinson JH, Slater MA, Doctor JA, Klapow J. Psychopharmacologic agents in the treatment of pain syndromes. In: Tollison CD, Satterthwaite JR, Tollison JW (Eds). *Handbook of Pain Management,* 2nd ed. Baltimore: Williams & Wilkins, 1994, pp 181–214.

Atkinson JH, Slater MA, Wahlgren DR, et al. Effects of noradrenergic and serotonergic antidepressants on chronic low back pain intensity. *Pain* 1999; 83:137–145.

Biedermann JJ, Schefft BK. Behavioral, physiological, and self evaluative effects of anxiety on the self control of pain. *Behav Modif* 1994; 18:89–105.

Breitbart W. Psychotropic adjuvant analgesics for pain in cancer and AIDS. *Psychooncology* 1998; 7:333–345.

Chabal C, Jacobson L, Chaney EF, Mariano AJ. Narcotics for chronic pain, yes or no? A useless dichotomy. *APS J* 1992; 1:376–381.

Ciccone DS, Just N, Bandilla EB, et al. Psychological correlates of opioid use in patients with chronic nonmalignant pain: a preliminary test of the downhill spiral hypothesis. *J Pain Symptom Manage* 2000; 20:180–192.

Covington EC. Anticonvulsants for neuropathic pain and detoxification. *Cleve Clin J Med* 1998; 65(Suppl 1):SI21–29.

Elton NH, Magdi MH, Treasure J, Treasure H. Coping with chronic pain: some patients suffer more. *Br J Psychiatry* 1994; 165:802–807.

Fernandez E, Milburn TW. Sensory and affective predictors of overall pain and emotions associated with affective pain. *Clin J Pain* 1994; 10:3–9.

Fernandez E, Turk DA. The scope and significance of anger in the experience of chronic pain. *Pain* 1995; 61:165–175.

Feuerstein M, Berkowitz SM, Haufler AJ, Lopez MS, Huang GD. Working with low back pain: workplace and individual psychosocial determinants of limited duty and lost time. *Am J Ind Med* 2001; 40:627–638.

Fishbain DA. The association of chronic pain and suicide. *Semin Clin Neuropsychiatry* 1999; 4(3):221–227.

Fishbain DA. *The Somatizing Disorders: Diagnostic and Treatment Approaches for Pain Medicine in Practical Pain Management,* 3rd ed. In: Tollison D (Ed). Lippincott & Williams & Wilkins, 2000a, pp 580–594.

Fishbain DA. Evidence-based data on pain relief with antidepressants. *Ann Med* 2000b; 32(5):305–316.

Fishbain DA, Rosomoff HL, Rosomofff RS. Drug abuse, dependence, and addiction in chronic pain patients. *Clin J Pain* 1992a; 8:77–85.

Fishbain DA, Rosomoff HL, Rosomoff RS. Detoxification of nonopiate drugs in the chronic pain setting and clonidine opiate detoxification. *Clin J Pain* 1992b; 8:191–203.

Fishbain DA, Rosomoff HL, Cutler R, Rosomoff RS. Opiate detoxification protocols. *Ann Clin Psychiatry* 1993; 5:53–65.

Fishbain DA, Cutler RB, Rosomoff HL, Rosomoff RS. Comorbidity between psychiatric disorders and chronic pain. *Curr Rev Pain* 1998; 2(1):1–10.

Fishbain DA, Cutler RB, Rosomoff HL, Rosomoff RS. Evidence-based data from animal and human experimental studies on pain relief with antidepressants. *Pain Med* 2000a; 1(4):310–316.

Fishbain DA, Cutler RB, Rosomoff HL, Rosomoff RS. Risk for violent behavior in patients with chronic pain: evaluation and management in the pain facility setting: a review and case reports. *Pain Med* 2000b; 1(2):140–155.

Flor H, Fydrich T, Turk DC. Efficacy of multi disciplinary pain treatment centers: a meta analytic review. *Pain* 1992; 49:221–230.

Gatchel RJ. Early developments of physical and mental deconditioning in painful spinal disorders. In: Mayer TG, Mooney V, Gatchel RJ (Eds). *Contemporary Conservative Care for Painful Spinal Disorders.* Philadelphia: Lea & Febiger, 1991, pp 278–289.

Gatchel RJ, Garofalo JP, Ellis E, Holt C. Major psychological disorders in acute and chronic TMD: an initial examination. *J Am Dent Assoc* 1996; 127:1365–1374.

Gil KM, Wilson JJ, Edens JL, et al. Effects of cognitive coping skills training on coping strategies and experimental pain sensitivity in African American adults with sickle cell disease. *Health Psychol* 1996; 15:3–10.

Goli V, Fozdar M. Chronic pain and depression. *Econ Neurosci* 2002; 4:40–47.

Hazard RG, Haugh LD, Green PA, Jones PL. Chronic low back pain: the relationship between patient satisfaction and pain, impairment, and disability outcomes. *Spine* 1993; 19:881–887.

Jamison RN, Anderson KO, Peeters Asdourian C, Ferrante FM. Survey of opioid use in chronic nonmalignant pain patients. *Reg Anesth* 1994; 19:225–230.

Keefe FJ, Caldwell DS, Williams DA, et al. Pain coping skills training in the management of osteoarthritic knee pain: a comparative study. *Behav Ther* 1990; 21:49–62.

Keefe FJ, Dunsmore J, Burnett R. Behavioral and cognitive-behavioral approaches to chronic pain: recent advances and future directions. *J Consult Clin Psychol* 1992; 60:528–536

Keefe FJ, Caldwell DS, Baucom D, et al. Spouse-assisted coping skills training in the management of osteoarthritis knee pain. *Arthritis Care Res* 1996; 9:279–291.

Keefe FJ, Lefebvre JC, Egert J, et al. The relationship of gender to pain, pain behavior, and disability in osteoarthritis patients: the role of catastrophizing. *Pain* 2000; 87:325–334.

Kerns RD, Rosenberg R, Jacon MC. Anger expression and chronic pain. *J Behav Med* 1994; 17:57–62.

Kerns RD, Otis JD, Wise EA. Treating families of chronic pain patients: applications of a cognitive-behavioral transactional model. In: Turk DC, Gatchel RJ (Eds). *Psychological Approaches to Pain Management: A Practitioners Handbook.* New York: Guilford, 2002, pp 256–275.

Khojainova N, Santiago-Palma J, Kornick C, Breitbart W, Gonzales GR. Olanzapine in the management of cancer pain. *J Pain Symptom Manage* 2002; 23:346–350.

Leeman G, Polatin P, Gatchel R, et al. Managing secondary gain in patients with pain associated disability. *J Workers Comp* 2000; 9:25–43.

Lester N, Keefe FJ. Coping with chronic pain. In: Baum A, McManus C, Newman S, Weinman J, West R (Eds). *Cambridge Handbook of Psychology, Health and Medicine.* Cambridge: Cambridge University Press, 1997.

Magni G. The use of antidepressants in the treatment of chronic pain: a review of the current evidence. *Drugs* 1991; 42:730–748.

Main CJ, Spanswick CC. 'Functional overlay' and illness behaviour in chronic pain: distress or malingering? Conceptual difficulties in medico-legal assessment of personal injury claims. *J Psychosom Res* 1995; 39:737–753.

Max MB, Lynch SA, Muir J, et al. Effects of desipramine, amitriptyline, and fluoxetine on pain in diabetic neuropathy. *N Engl J Med* 1992; 326:1250–1256.

McCracken LM, Gross RT. Does anxiety affect coping with chronic pain? *Clin J Pain* 1993; 9:253–259.

McCracken LM, Gross RT, Sorg PJ, Edmands TA. Prediction of pain in patients with chronic low back pain: effects of inaccurate prediction and pain related anxiety. *Behav Res Ther* 1993; 31:647–652.

Menefee LA, Cohen JM, Anderson WR, et al. Sleep disturbance in chronic pain: a comprehensive review of the literature. *Pain Med* 2000; 1:156–172.

Merskey H. Pain and psychological medicine. In: Wall PD, Melzack R (Eds). *Textbook of Pain,* 3rd ed. Edinburgh: Churchill Livingstone, 1994, pp 903–920.

Morin CM, Culbert JP, Schwartz SM. Non-pharmacological interventions for insomnia: a meta-analysis of treatment efficacy. *Am J Psychiatry* 1994; 151:1172–1180.

NIH Technology Assessment Panel. Integration of behavioral and relaxation approaches into the treatment of chronic pain and insomnia. NIH Technology Assessment Panel on Integration of Behavioral and Relaxation Approaches into the Treatment of Chronic Pain and Insomnia. *JAMA* 1996; 276:313–318.

Onghena P, Van Houdenhove B. Antidepressant-induced analgesia in chronic non-malignant pain: a meta-analysis of 39 placebo-controlled studies. *Pain* 1992; 49:205–220.

Pilowsky I, Barrow CG. A controlled study of psychotherapy and amitriptyline used individually and in combination in the treatment of chronic intractable (psychogenic) pain. *Pain* 1990; 40:3–19.

Reid MC, Engles-Horton LL, Weber MB, et al. Use of opioid medications for chronic noncancer pain syndromes in primary care. *J Gen Intern Med* 2002; 17(3):173–179.

Robinson R, Gatchel P, Polatin P, et al. Screening for problematic prescription opioid use. *Clin J Pain* 2001; 17:191–228.

Rohling ML, Binder LM, Langhinrichsen-Rohling J. Money matters: a meta-analytic review of the association between financial compensation and the experience and treatment of chronic pain. *Health Psychol* 1995; 14:537–547.

Romano JM, Turner JA, Friedman LS, et al. Sequential analysis of chronic pain behaviors and spouse responses. *J Consult Clin Psychol* 1992; 60:777–782.

Schade V, Semmer N, Main CJ, Hora J, Boos N. The impact of clinical, morphological, psychosocial and work-related factors on the outcome of lumbar discectomy. *Pain* 1999; 80:239–249.

Sees KL, Clark HW. Opioid use in the treatment of chronic pain: assessment of addiction. *J Pain Symptom Manage* 1992; 8:257–264.

Sharp TJ, Harvey AG. Chronic pain and posttraumatic stress disorder: mutual maintenance? *Clin Psychol Rev* 2001; 21(6):857–877.

Sharpe L, Sensky T, Timberlake N, Ryan B. A blind, randomized controlled trail of cognitive-behavioural intervention for patients with recent onset rheumatoid arthritis: preventing psychological and physical disability. *Pain* 2001: 89:275–283.

Sindrup SH, Gram LF, Skjold T, Froland A, Beck-Nielsen H. Concentration-response relationship in imipramine treatment of diabetic neuropathy symptoms. *Clin Pharmacol Ther* 1985; 47:387–394.

Sindrup SH, Grodum E, Gram LF, Beck-Nielsen H. Concentration-response relationship in paroxetine treatment of diabetic neuropathy symptoms: a patient-blinded dose escalation study. *Ther Drug Monit* 1991; 13:408–414.

Smith GR, Monson RA, Ray DC. Psychiatric consultation in somatization disorder: a randomized controlled study. *N Engl J Med* 1986; 314:1407–1413.

Sullivan MJL, Thorn B, Haythornthwaite J, et al. Theoretical perspectives on the relation between catastrophizing and pain. *J Clin Pain* 2001; 17:52–64.

Tunks E, Merskey H. Psychotherapy of pain. In: Bonica JJ (Ed). *The Management of Pain,* 2nd ed. Philadelphia: Lea and Febiger, 1990.

Turk DC, Okifuji A. Matching treatment to assessment of patients with chronic pain. In: Turk DC, Melzack R (Eds). *Handbook of Pain Assessment,* 2nd ed. United Kingdom: Elsevier Science, 2001, pp 400–414.

Turk DC, Solovay P. Chronic pain as a variant of depressive disease: a critical reappraisal. *J Nerv Ment Dis* 1984; 172:398–404.

Turner JA, Romano JM. Cognitive-behavioral therapy for chronic pain. In: Loeser JD (Ed). *Bonica's Management of Pain.* Baltimore: Lippincott Williams and Wilkins, 2001, pp 1751–1758.

Vlaeyen JWS, de Jong JR, Sieben JM, Crombez G. Graded exposure in vivo for pain-related fear. In: Gatchel R, Turk DC (Eds). *Psychological Approaches to Pain Management.* New York: Guilford, 2002.

Wade JB, Price DD, Hamer RM, Schwartz SM. An emotional component analysis of chronic pain. *Pain* 1990; 40:303–310.

Weisberg JN. Studies investigating the prevalence of personality disorders in patients with chronic pain. In: Gatchel RJ, Weisberg JN (Eds). *Personality Characteristics of Patients with Pain.* Washington, DC: American Psychological Association, 2000, pp 221–239.

Weisberg JN, Keefe FJ. Personality disorders in the chronic pain population: basic concepts, empirical findings, and clinical implications. *Pain Forum* 1997; 6(1):1–9.

Williams DA, Cary MA, Groner KH, et al. Improving physical functional status in patients with fibromyalgia: a brief cognitive behavioral intervention. *J Rheumatol* 2002; 29:1280–1286.

Core Curriculum for Professional Education in Pain, edited by J. Edmond Charlton, IASP Press, Seattle, © 2005.

19

Stimulation-Produced Analgesia

I. Know different peripheral stimulation techniques used to produce analgesia (Pan et al. 2000; White et al. 2001).

   A. Transcutaneous electrical nerve stimulation (TENS) (Kalra et al. 2001).

   B. Acupuncture-like TENS (Melzack and Wall 1984; Gadsby and Flowerdew 2000).

   C. Acupuncture, dry needle (Karakurum et al. 2001), or electroacupuncture (Ulett et al. 1998).

   D. Vibration (Lundeberg et al. 1987), acupressure (Kurland 1976; Weaver 1985).

II. Understand the postulated mechanisms of peripheral stimulation-induced analgesia.

   A. Segmental

      1. Low-intensity, high-frequency electrical stimulation selectively activates large-diameter, low-threshold A-beta afferent fibers, to produce segmental inhibition of dorsal horn neurons, thus reducing nociceptive afferent evoked responses (Levin and Hui-Chan 1993).
      2. Know about the inhibitory interneurons in the substantia gelatinosa and the chemical mediators, including gamma-butyric amino acid (GABA) (Chakrabarti et al. 1988), glycine, etc.
      3. Know the historical contribution of the spinal gate control theory in pain perception and modulation (Melzack and Wall 1965).

   B. Extrasegmental

      1. Stimulation of small-diameter, higher-threshold A-beta, A-delta (and part of C) fibers activates descending inhibitory pathway, and also inhibits the descending facilitatory pathway from the brain stem, to suppress the excitability of the dorsal horn neurons (Liu et al. 1986; Takeshige et al. 1992).
      2. Know about the synaptic pharmacology of descending inhibition and facilitation systems, the on/off cells in the medulla, and diffuse noxious inhibitory controls (Takeshige et al. 1992; Kalra et al. 2001).
      3. Know about the endogenous opioid peptides and anti-opioid peptides in pain control (Chen and Han 1992; Sluka et al. 1999; Cutler 2001; Han 2001; Kalra et al. 2001).

   C. Cortical

      1. Know that high-level cognitive/emotional inputs initiate poorly understand mechanisms at different levels of the neuraxis to control nociceptive sensory processing (Hennig et al. 2000).
      2. Know that this is likely to contribute to the efficacy of suggestion, placebo, and many folk medicine therapies.
      3. Know about the use of brain-imaging techniques to study the contribution of higher nervous activities in pain control (Wu et al. 1999).

   D. Peripheral

      1. Limited evidence suggests that peripheral stimulation alters blood flow and peripheral chemicals (Cramp et al. 2002).

III.   Be aware of the parameters of stimulation (Gopalkrishnan and Sluka 2000)

  A.   Conventional TENS (Carroll et al. 2001)

    1.   High frequency (50–100 Hz), low intensity (paresthesia, not painful), small pulse width (50–200 μs).
    2.   Electrode localization: cover the painful region.
    3.   Duration: about 30 minutes.

  B.   Acupuncture-like TENS (Levin and Hui-Chan 1993; Gadsby and Flowerdew 2000)

    1.   Low frequency (2–4 Hz), higher intensity (to tolerance threshold), longer pulse width (100–400 μs).
    2.   Alternating low (2–4 Hz) and high (50–100 Hz) frequency, each lasting for 3 seconds (Hamza et al. 1999a, b).
    3.   Electrode localization: usually at traditional Chinese acupuncture points, or trigger points, but one can also use it at the painful region.
    4.   Duration: about 30 minutes.

  C.   Acupuncture, dry needling, or electroacupuncture

    1.   For dry needling, the needle is manipulated by rotation and multiple insertion (Gunn et al. 1980; McMillan et al. 1997).
    2.   For electroacupuncture, the needle shafts are connected to an electrical stimulator.
    3.   Localization: traditional Chinese acupuncture points, or trigger points.
    4.   Duration: variable.

  D.   Vibration (Guieu et al. 1991)

    1.   Electro-mechanical, high-frequency (100–200 Hz) and low-intensity (strong but not painful).
    2.   Localization: over the painful area.
    3.   Duration: usually 30 minutes, shorter than 45 minutes (Hamza et al. 1999a, b).

IV.   Be familiar with the clinical applications of neuroaugmentative therapies.

  A.   Conventional TENS or vibration

    1.   TENS reduces pain in different acute and chronic pain conditions including low back pain (Marchand et al. 1993; Brosseau et al. 2002), deafferentation pain, causalgia (Meyer and Fields 1972), pain during delivery (Allaire 2001; Gentz 2001), acute orofacial pain (Hansson and Ekblom 1983), acute and chronic arthritic pain (Roche et al. 1984; Hardware and Lacey 2002).
    2.   The analgesic effect of TENS is generally not sufficient to manage for intense acute pain such as in dental surgery but can reduce anesthetic requirement during surgery (Bourke et al. 1984).
    3.   Similar results are reported for vibration analgesia (Lundeberg 1984; Ter Riet et al. 1990; Guieu et al. 1991).
    4.   Even if analgesic effects of TENS are generally reported as brief and fading over time, some long-term benefits are reported, for some patients (Junnila 1987a,b; Johnson et al. 1991; Thomas et al. 1999).

  B.   Acupuncture-like TENS or hyperstimulation

    1.   As for TENS, hyperstimulation has been successfully used for different chronic and acute pain conditions (Wang et al. 1997), but its painful character may limit patients' acceptance (Marwick 1997).
    2.   The diffuse quality of hyperstimulation may be useful in some pain conditions where the stimulation can not be applied to the painful site.

C.   Acupuncture

1.   As for TENS and vibration, several studies report good results with acupuncture for different pain conditions. However, a meta-analysis of the literature reveals highly contradictory results. Most clinical trials are poorly designed. Efficacy is still debatable (Xi et al. 1992; Thomas and Lundberg 1994; Ernst et al. 2002).

2.   The neurobiological rationale for this type of treatment has been explored extensively (Han 1989; Ulett et al. 1998), but much work remains to be done.

V.   Efficacy

A.   Know that the results of treatment are variable in clinical and experimental studies. Be aware that no clear criteria have been identified to decide whether a patient will benefit from neuroaugmentative treatment (Halbert et al. 2002).

B.   Understand that the analgesic effect of TENS may be potentiated by repetitive use and that the efficacy of treatment may improve over time (Johnson et al. 1991; Marchand et al. 1993).

C.   Know that even if the suggestibility and predisposition of the patients are important contributors, TENS and vibration are better than placebo in some studies, but failures are common. Be aware of the difficulty in designing placebo treatments to compare with neuroaugmentative therapy (Marchand 1993; Marchand et al. 1993; Sanchez 1998; Shen 2001; Vickers 2001; Ernst et al. 2002).

D.   Be aware of the relatively short duration of the effects, and the possibility of development of tolerance over time (Han 2001).

REFERENCES

Allaire AD. Complementary and alternative medicine in the labor and delivery suite. *Clin Obstet Gynecol* 2001; 44:681–691.

Bourke DL, Smith BA, Erickson J, Gwartz B, Lessard L. TENS reduces halothane requirements during hand surgery. *Anesthesiology* 1984; 61:769–772.

Brosseau L, Milne S, Robinson V, et al. Efficacy of the transcutaneous electrical nerve stimulation for the treatment of chronic low back pain: a meta-analysis. *Spine* 2002; 27:596–603.

Carroll D, Moore RA, McQuay HJ, et al. Transcutaneous electrical nerve stimulation (TENS) for chronic pain. *Cochrane Database Syst Rev* 2001; CD003222.

Chakrabarti S, Ganguly A, Poddar MK. Possible involvement of the GABAergic system in dopaminergic-cholinergic interactions in electroacupuncture-induced analgesia. *Methods Find Exp Clin Pharmacol* 1988; 10:545–549.

Chen XH, Han JS. All three types of opioid receptors in the spinal cord are important for 2/15 Hz electroacupuncture analgesia. *Eur J Pharmacol* 1992; 211:203–210.

Cramp FL, McCullough GR, Lowe AS, Walsh DM. Transcutaneous electric nerve stimulation: the effect of intensity on local and distal cutaneous blood flow and skin temperature in healthy subjects. *Arch Phys Med Rehabil* 2002; 83:5–9.

Cutler D. Acupuncture and opioids. *Trends Pharmacol Sci* 2001; 22:400–401.

Ernst E, White AR, Wider B. Acupuncture for back pain: meta-analysis of randomised controlled trials and an update with data from the most recent studies. *Schmerz* 2002; 16:129–139.

Gadsby JG, Flowerdew MW. Transcutaneous electrical nerve stimulation and acupuncture-like transcutaneous electrical nerve stimulation for chronic low back pain. *Cochrane Database Syst Rev* 2000; CD000210.

Gentz BA. Alternative therapies for the management of pain in labor and delivery. *Clin Obstet Gynecol* 2001; 44:704–732.

Gopalkrishnan P, Sluka KA. Effect of varying frequency, intensity, and pulse duration of transcutaneous electrical nerve stimulation on primary hyperalgesia in inflamed rats. *Arch Phys Med Rehabil* 2000; 81:984–990.

Guieu R, Tardy-Gervet MF, Roll JP. Analgesic effects of vibration and transcutaneous electrical nerve stimulation applied separately and simultaneously to patients with chronic pain. *Can J Neurol Sci* 1991; 18:113–119.

Gunn CC, Milbrandt WE, Little AS, Mason KE. Dry needling of muscle motor points for chronic low-back pain: a randomized clinical trial with long-term follow-up. *Spine* 1980; 5:279–291.

Halbert J, Crotty M, Cameron ID. Evidence for the optimal management of acute and chronic phantom pain: a systematic review. *Clin J Pain* 2002; 18:84–92.

Hamza MA, Ghoname ES, White PF, et al. Effect of the duration of electrical stimulation on the analgesic response in patients wtih low back pain. *Anesthesiology* 1999a; 91:1622–1627.

Hamza MA, White PF, Ahmed HE, Ghoname EA. Effect of the frequency of transcutaneous electrical nerve stimulation on the postoperative opioid analgesic requirement and recovery profile. *Anesthesiology* 1999b; 91:1232–1238.

Han JS. Opioid and anti-opioid peptides: a model of Yin-Yang balance in acupuncture mechanisms of pain modulation. In: Stux G, Hammerschlag R (Eds). *Clinical Acupuncture, Scientific Basis.* Berlin: Springer, 2001, pp 51–68.

Han JS. Central neurotransmitters and acupuncture analgesia. In: Pomerranz B, Stux G (Eds). *Scientific Bases of Acupuncture.* Springer-Verlag, 1989, pp 7–34.

Hansson P, Ekblom A. Transcutaneous electrical nerve stimulation (TENS) as compared to placebo TENS for the relief of acute orofacial pain. *Pain* 1983; 15:157–165.

Hardware B, Lacey A. Acupuncture and other alternative therapies in rheumatoid arthritis. *Prof Nurse* 2002; 17:437–439.

Hennig J, Lacour M, Hui KK, et al. Acupuncture modulates the limbic system and subcortical gray structures of the human brain: evidence from fMRI studies in normal subjects. *Hum Brain Mapp* 2000; 9:13–25.

Johnson MI, Ashton CH, Thompson JW. An in-depth study of long-term users of transcutaneous electrical nerve stimulation (TENS): implications for clinical use of TENS. *Pain* 1991; 44:221–229.

Junnila SY. Long-term treatment of chronic pain with acupuncture. Part I. *Acupunct Electrother Res* 1987a; 12:23–36.

Junnila SY. Long-term treatment of chronic pain with acupuncture. Part II. *Acupunct Electrother Res* 1987b; 12:125–138.

Kalra A, Urban MO, Sluka KA. Blockade of opioid receptors in rostral ventral medulla prevents antihyperalgesia produced by transcutaneous electrical nerve stimulation (TENS). *J Pharmacol Exp Ther* 2001; 298:257–263.

Karakurum B, Karaalin O, Coskun O, et al. The 'dry-needle technique': intramuscular stimulation in tension-type headache. *Cephalalgia* 2001; 21:813–817.

Kurland HD. Treatment of headache pain with auto-acupressure. *Dis Nerv Syst* 1976; 37:127–129.

Levin MF, Hui-Chan CW. Conventional and acupuncture-like transcutaneous electrical nerve stimulation excite similar afferent fibers. *Arch Phys Med Rehabil* 1993; 74:54–60.

Liu X, Zhu B, Zhang SX. Relationship between electroacupuncture analgesia and descending pain inhibitory mechanism of nucleus raphe magnus. *Pain* 1986; 24:383–396.

Lundeberg T, Hode L, Zhou J. A comparative study of the pain-relieving effect of laser treatment and acupuncture. *Acta Physiol Scand* 1987; 131:161–162.

Lundeberg T. Vibratory stimulation for the alleviation of pain. *Am J Chin Med* 1984; 12:60–70.

Marchand S, Charest J, Li J, et al. Is TENS purely a placebo effect? A controlled study on chronic low back pain. *Pain* 1993; 54:99–106.

Marwick C. Acceptance of some acupuncture applications. *JAMA* 1997; 278:1725–1727.

McMillan AS, Nolan A, Kelly PJ. The efficacy of dry needling and procaine in the treatment of myofascial pain in the jaw muscles. *J Orofac Pain* 1997; 11:307–314.

Melzack R, Wall PD. Pain mechanisms: a new theory. *Science* 1965; 150:971–979.

Melzack R, Wall PD. Acupuncture and transcutaneous electrical nerve stimulation. *Postgrad Med J* 1984; 60:893–896.

Meyer GA, Fields HL. Causalgia treated by selective large fibre stimulation of peripheral nerve. *Brain* 1972; 95:163–168.

Pan CX, Morrison RS, Ness J, Fugh-Berman A, Leipzig RM. Complementary and alternative medicine in the management of pain, dyspnea, and nausea and vomiting near the end of life: a systematic review. *J Pain Symptom Manage* 2000; 20:374–387.

Roche PA, Gijsbers K, Belch JJ, Forbes CD. Modification of induced ischaemic pain by transcutaneous electrical nerve stimulation. *Pain* 1984; 20:45–52.

Sanchez AM. Does the choice of placebo determine the results of clinical studies on acupuncture? *Forsch Komplementarmed* 1998; 5(Suppl S1):8–11.

Shen J. Research on the neurophysiological mechanisms of acupuncture: review of selected studies and methodological issues. *J Altern Complement Med* 2001; 7(Suppl 1): S121–S127.

Sluka KA, Deacon M, Stibal A, Strissel S, Terpstra A. Spinal blockade of opioid receptors prevents the analgesia produced by TENS in arthritic rats. *J Pharmacol Exp Ther* 1999; 289:840–846.

Takeshige C, Sato T, Mera T, Hisamitsu T, Fang J. Descending pain inhibitory system involved in acupuncture analgesia. *Brain Res Bull* 1992; 29:617–634.

Ter Riet G, Kleijnen J, Knipschild P. Acupuncture and chronic pain: a criteria-based meta-analysis. *J Clin Epidemiol* 1990; 43:1191–1199.

Thomas KJ, Fitter M, Brazier J, et al. Longer-term clinical and economic benefits of offering acupuncture to patients with chronic low back pain assessed as suitable for primary care management. *Complement Ther Med* 1999; 7:91–100.

Thomas M, Lundberg T. Importance of modes of acupuncture in the treatment of chronic nociceptive low back pain. *Acta Anaesthesiol Scand* 1994; 38:63–69.

Ulett GA, Han S, Han JS. Electroacupuncture: mechanisms and clinical application. *Biol Psychiatry* 1998; 44:129–138.

Vickers A. Acupuncture for treatment for chronic neck pain: reanalysis of data suggests that effect is not a placebo effect. *BMJ* 2001; 323:1306–1307.

Wang B, Tang J, White PF, et al. Effect of the intensity of transcutaneous acupoint electrical stimulation on the postoperative analgesic requirement. *Anesth Analg* 1997; 85:406–413.

Weaver MT. Acupressure: an overview of theory and application. *Nurse Pract* 1985; 10:38–9, 42.

White PF, Li S, Chiu JW. Electroanalgesia: its role in acute and chronic pain management. *Anesth Analg* 2001; 92:505–513.

Wu MT, Hsieh JC, Xiong J, et al. Central nervous pathway for acupuncture stimulation: localization of processing with functional MR imaging of the brain—preliminary experience. *Radiology* 1999; 212:133–141.

Xi D, Han J, Zhang Z, Sun Z. Acupuncture treatment of rheumatoid arthritis and exploration of acupuncture manipulations. *J Tradit Chin Med* 1992; 12:35–40.

Core Curriculum for Professional Education in Pain, edited by J. Edmond Charlton, IASP Press, Seattle, © 2005.

20

Interventional Pain Management Including Nerve Blocks and Lesioning

I.   Know the anatomy of critical peripheral and central nervous system (CNS) regions as it relates to analgesic nerve blocks (Cousins and Bromage 1988; Hogan 1991; Abram and Boas 1992; Brockway and Chambers 2003; Waldman and Winnie 1996).

A. Spine

1. Bony vertebral column
2. Spinal cord, meninges, nerve roots, dorsal root ganglion

B. Peripheral nervous system

1. Brachial, femoral, and sacral plexuses
2. Cranial nerves
3. Peripheral nerves of spinal origin: emphasis on nerves that are commonly involved in entrapment neuropathies, e.g., lateral femoral cutaneous, occipital, ulnar, median

C. Autonomic nervous system

1. Sympathetic efferent system

a. Cells or origin in spinal cord
b. Rami communicantes
c. Sympathetic chain
d. Postganglionics

2. Visceral (sympathetic) afferent system

a. Innervation of visceral structures
b. Sympathetic chain afferents from somatic structures

II. Be familiar with the general principles of the pharmacology and use of drugs used for nerve blocks.

A. Local anesthetics (Covino 1988; Charlton 2003)

1. Neural blocking mechanisms
2. Be aware of systemic effects:

a. CNS toxic effects
b. Nonconvulsant effects (e.g., analgesia)
c. Cardiotoxic effects

3. Pharmacokinetics (Tucker and Mather 1988)

a. Peripheral nerve block
b. Subarachnoid block
c. Epidural block

B. Know the pharmacology of opioids as they relate to regional analgesia (Cousins et al. 1988a; Dickinson 1991; McQuay 1991; Ready 2001).

1. Receptor types and function

2. Spinal and brain effects
3. Pharmacokinetics of spinal intrathecal and epidural application

C. Know commonly used neurolytic agents (Myers and Katz 1988; Jain and Gupta 1996).

1. Alcohol, phenol, botulinus toxin (Arnon 2001)
2. Pathological (neurotoxic) effects

   a. Blood vessels
   b. Spinal cord

3. Know the complications of neurolytic therapy (Butler and Charlton 2001).

   a. Denervation dysesthesia
   b. Peripheral neuralgia

D. Know about the use of locally injected corticosteroids (Rowlingson 1994).

1. Effect on nerve roots, peripheral nerves
2. Systemic effects
3. Pharmacokinetics of soluble, "depo" preparations

III. Know how nerve blocks are used for diagnostic purposes and pain control (Buckley 2001). All practitioners should understand the clinical indications, risks, and complications associated with the use of nerve blocks. All practitioners, including those outside of the field of anesthesiology, should be aware of the treatment of problems that may arise during the performance of these procedures. The patient should have a clear understanding of the reason(s) for the procedure and the likely benefit to be derived. Where there is no evidence base to indicate likely benefit, the patient should be made aware of this.

A. Myofascial trigger point injection (Travell 1993)

B. Common peripheral blocks (Buckley 2001)

1. Occipital
2. Lateral femoral cutaneous
3. Intercostal

C. Sympathetic blocks (Abram and Boas 1992; Abram and Haddox 1992)

1. Lumbar sympathetic
2. Stellate ganglion

D. Epidural steroid injections (National Health and Medical Research Council 1994)

E. Celiac plexus block and hypogastric plexus block (Waldman and Winnie 1996)

F. Intraspinal opioids

1. Techniques of catheter placement: intrathecal, epidural (Waldman and Winnie 1996)
2. Administration techniques

   a. Bolus
   b. External infusion
   c. Subcutaneous post
   d. Implantable infusion pump

G. Intrathecal and epidural neurolytic blocks (Cousins et al. 1988b)

H. Phenol motor point block (Halpern and Meelhuysen 1966)

I. Cryoneurolysis (Saberski 1996)

J. Radiofrequency lesions (Kline 1996)

IV.   Know how to recognize and treat the side effects and complications of nerve blocks (Abram and Hogan 1992; Murphy and O'Keefe 1992).

    A.   Spinal and epidural blocks

    B.   Paravertebral somatic and sympathetic blocks

    C.   Peripheral nerve blocks

    D.   Muscle, joint, and bursa injections

    E.   Continuous infusion therapy

REFERENCES

Abram SE, Boas RA. Sympathetic and visceral nerve blocks. In: Benumot JL (Ed). *Procedures in Anesthesia and Intensive Care.* Philadelphia: Lippincott, 1992, pp 787–806.

Abram SE, Haddox JD. Chronic pain management. In: Barash PG, Cullen BF, Stoelting RK (Eds). *Clinical Anesthesia,* 2nd ed. Philadelphia: Lippincott, 1992, pp 1579–1607.

Abram SE, Hogan QH. Complications of peripheral nerve blocks. In: Saidman L, Benumof J. (Eds). *Anesthesia and Perioperative Complications.* St. Louis: Mosby, 1992, pp 52–76.

Arnon SS, Schechter R, Inglesby TV, et al. Working Group on Civilian Biodefense. Botulinum toxin as a biological weapon: medical and public health management. *JAMA* 2001; 285(8):1059–1070.

Butler SH, Charlton JE. Neurolytic blockade and hypophysectomy. In: Loeser JD (Ed). *Bonica's Management of Pain,* 3rd ed. Lippincott, Williams & Wilkins, 2001, pp 1967–2006.

Brockway M, Chambers WA. Anatomy and physiology of the vertebral canal. In: Wildsmith JAW, Armitage EN, McClure JH (Eds). *Principles and Practice of Regional Anesthesia,* 3rd ed. Edinburgh: Churchill Livingstone, 2003, p 111–124.

Charlton JE. Managing the block. In: Wildsmith JAW, Armitage EN, McClure JH (Eds). *Principles and Practice of Regional Anesthesia,* 3rd ed. Edinburgh: Churchill Livingstone, 2003, pp 91–109.

Cousins MJ, Bromage PR. Epidural neural blockade. In: Cousins MJ, Bridenbaugh PO (Eds). *Neural Blockade,* 2nd ed. Philadelphia: Lippincott, 1988, pp 253–360.

Cousins MJ, Cherry DA, Gourlay GK. Acute and chronic pain: use of spinal opioids. In: Cousins MJ, Bridenbaugh PO (Eds). *Neural Blockade in Clinical Anesthesia and Management of Pain,* 2nd ed. Philadelphia: Lippincott, 1988, pp 955–1029.

Cousins MJ, Dwyer B, Gibb D. Chronic pain and neurolytic blockade. In: Cousins MJ, Bridenbaugh PO (Eds). *Neural Blockade in Clinical Anesthesia and Management of Pain,* 2nd ed. Philadelphia: Lippincott, 1988, pp 1053–1084.

Covino BC. Clinical pharmacology of local anesthetic agents. In: Cousins MJ, Bridenbaugh PO (Eds). *Neural Blockade in Clinical Anesthesia and Management of Pain,* 2nd ed. Philadelphia: Lippincott, 1988, pp 111–144.

Dickinson AH. Mechanism of the analgesic actions of opiates and opioids. *Br Med Bull* 1991; 47:690–702.

Halpern D, Meelhuysen FE. Phenol motor point block in the management of muscular hypertonia. *Arch Phys Med Rehabil* 1966; 47:659–664.

Hogan QH. Lumbar epidural anatomy. *Anesthesiology* 1991; 75:767–775.

Jain S, Gupta R. Neurolytic agents in clinical practice. In: Waldman SR, Winnie AP (Eds). *Interventional Pain Management.* Saunders, 1996, pp 167–171.

Kline MR. Radiofrequency techniques in clinical practice. In: Waldman SR, Winnie AP (Eds). *Interventional Pain Management.* Saunders, 1996, pp 185–217.

Loeser JD (Ed). *Bonica's Management of Pain,* 3rd ed. Philadelphia: Lippincott Williams & Wilkins, 2001.

McQuay HJ. Opioid clinical pharmacology and routes of administration. *Br Med Bull* 1991; 47:703–717.

Murphy TM, O'Keefe D. Complications of spinal, epidural, and caudal anesthesia. In: Benumof JL, Saidman LJ (Eds). *Anesthesia and Perioperative Complications.* Chicago: Mosby Year Book, 1992, pp 38–51.

Myers RR, Katz J. Neuropathology of neurolytic and semidestructive agents. In: Cousins MJ, Bridenbaugh PO (Eds). *Neural Blockade,* 2nd ed. Philadelphia: Lippincott, 1988, pp 1031–1052.

National Health and Medical Research Council. Epidural use of steroids in the management of back pain. Canberra: National Health and Medical Research Council, 1994, p 13.

Ready LB. Regional analgesia with intraspinal opioids. In: Loeser JD (Ed). *Bonica's Management of Pain,* 3rd ed. Lippincott, Williams & Wilkins, 2001, pp 1953–1966.

Saberski LR. Cryoneurolysis in clinical practice. In: Waldman SR, Winnie AP (Eds). *Interventional Pain Management.* Saunders, 1996, pp 172–184.

Scott DB. *Techniques of Regional Anaesthesia.* Norwalk: Appleton and Lange, 1989.

Travell JA, Simons DG. *Myofascial Pain and Dysfunction: The Trigger Point Manual,* Vol. 1. Baltimore: Williams & Wilkins, 1983.

Tucker JA, Mather LE. Properties, absorption and distribution of local anesthetic agents. In: Cousins MJ, Bridenbaugh PO (Eds). *Neural Blockade,* 2nd ed. Philadelphia: Lippincott, 1988, pp 47–110.

Waldman SR, Patt RB. In: Waldman SR, Winnie AP (Eds). *Interventional Pain Management.* Saunders, 1996, pp 360–374.

Waldman SR, Winnie AP (Eds). *Interventional Pain Management.* Saunders, 1996.

Core Curriculum for Professional Education in Pain, edited by J. Edmond Charlton, IASP Press, Seattle, © 2005.

21

Surgical Pain Management

I.   General principles (White and Sweet 1969; Willis 1985; Tasker 1987; Gybels and Sweet 1989; North and Levy 1996; Loeser 2000; Burchiel 2002)

   A.   Know the general health issues that are relevant to successful surgical procedures.

   B.   Know the importance of the following in evaluating a patient for surgery:

      1.   Disease causing pain
      2.   Life expectancy
      3.   Adequate trial of nonsurgical management, including physical, pharmacological, and psychological strategies
      4.   Cancer versus noncancer pain, including the role of cancer in neural injury pain
      5.   Pain due to injury to the nervous system
      6.   Role of nerve blocks in patient evaluation
      7.   Identification and assessment of psychological and environmental factors influencing pain behavior
      8.   Patient's, family's, and referring physician's expectations of surgical treatment

II.   Specific procedures: indications, techniques, and outcomes

   A.   General (Tasker 1994b; Gybels and Sweet 1989; Burchiel 2002)

      1.   Be aware of the complications of ablative surgery to relieve pain and of the likelihood of pain recurrence.
      2.   Be aware of the advantages and disadvantages of percutaneous and open surgical approaches ablative surgery and stereotactic radiosurgery.
      3.   Be aware of the need for outcomes-based evidence.

   B.   Peripheral neurectomy (White and Sweet 1969; Aids to the Examination 1986; Tasker 1987; Gybels and Sweet 1989; Loeser et al. 1990; Loeser 1994; Devor and Seltzer 1999)

      1.   Know the utility of peripheral neurectomy in pain management.
      2.   Be aware of proposed mechanisms for pain caused by injury to the nervous system including iatrogenic injuries, and the role of neuromas.
      3.   Know the utility of nerve relocation surgery.
      4.   Understand the unique features of tic douloureux which usually affects the trigeminal but very rarely the VIIth and IXth cranial nerves.

   C.   Sympathectomy (Gybels and Sweet 1989; Tasker and Lougheed 1990; Bennett 1994; Hardy and Bay 1995)

      1.   Know the indications for sympathectomy for pain relief.

         a.   Pain of vascular origin
         b.   Visceral pain

      2.   Know how to evaluate a patient by tests of sympathetic function and by use of local or regional anesthesia.
      3.   Be aware of CRPS types I and II and diagnostic issues.

4. Know available techniques and outcome data.
5. Know how to evaluate the adequacy of a sympathectomy for pain relief.

D. Spinal dorsal rhizotomy including ganglionectomy (Gybels and Sweet 1989, Taub et al. 1995; Taha 2002)

1. Know the indications:

   a. Cancer pain.
   b. Neuropathic pain syndromes.

2. Be aware of the various techniques, open and percutaneous.
3. Know how to interpret the results of nerve blocks in planning spinal dorsal rhizotomy.
4. Know the expected outcomes.

E. Anterolateral cordotomy spinothalamic tractotomy (White and Sweet 1969; Willis 1985; Sweet and Poletti 1994; Tasker 1995)

1. Indications: cancer pain
2. Know the available techniques: open and percutaneous, CT guided, X-ray guided.
3. Understand their relative outcomes with respect to:

   a. Pain recurrence
   b. Complications
   c. The pathophysiology of respiratory difficulties

F. Dorsal root entry zone (DREZ) procedures, spinal and medullary (Nashold et al. 1995)

1. Know the indications:

   a. Plexus avulsion injuries
   b. Postherpetic neuralgia
   c. Spinal cord and cauda equina injuries
   d. Other neuropathic pains

2. Be aware of the techniques of Nashold and Sindou.
3. Know the outcomes data.

G. Commissural myelotomy (Gybels and Sweet 1989; Nauta et al. 2002)

1. Know that the major indication is midline cancer pain in the pelvic area.
2. Be aware of the techniques:
   a. Open
   b. Percutaneous
   c. Cervical or lumbar spinal cord segments
3. Recognize that pain relief may not be restricted to the region of hypalgesia or the somatotopy of the area lesioned.

H. Facet rhizolysis (Bogduk 1988; North et al. 1994)

1. Know the indications.
2. Understand the innervation of the facet joints.
3. Know how to evaluate diagnostic nerve blocks.
4. Be aware of the different techniques under local and general anesthesia with and without physiological localization.
5. Be aware of outcomes data.

I. Operations on the cranial nerve roots (Sweet 1990; Burchiel 1999)

1. Know the indications for:
    a. Tic douloureux (V, rarely IX–X)

        i.   Understand how to diagnose tic.
        ii. Know the techniques available for tic:

             (a) Percutaneous radiofrequency (RF) rhizolysis
             (b) Percutaneous glycerol injection
             (c) Microcompression
             (d) Microvascular decompression
             (e) Open V rhizotomy in posterior fossa
             (f) Open IX–X rhizotomy
             (g) Stereotactic radiosurgery

    b. Cancer (rarely): percutaneous RF rhizolysis

2. Be aware of the expected outcomes and recurrence rates.

J. Destructive procedures on the brain and brainstem (Willis 1985; Gybels and Sweet 1989; Jannetta et al. 1990; Bouckoms 1994; Jeanmonod et al. 1994; Sweet and Poletti 1994; Ballantine et al. 1995; Young 2000)

1. Appreciate that the stereotactic approach is probably the chief technique by which such procedures are accomplished.
2. Understand the basic principles of stereotaxis: use of frames, imaging, computer assistance, physiology, and RF lesion-making.
3. Know that cancer pain has been the major indication for these procedures.
4. Be aware of the procedures currently in use:

    a. Stereotactic mesencephalic tractotomy
    b. Stereotactic medial thalamotomy
    c. Stereotactic central lateral thalamotomy
    d. Stereotactic cingulumotomy

5. Be aware of use of stereotactic radiosurgery to make stereotactic lesions in brain and cranial nerve roots.
6. Be aware of anecdotal nature of the outcome data.

K. Neurostimulation techniques (Willis 1985; Levy et al. 1987; Young and Rinaldi 1994; Gybels and Nuttin 2000; Meyerson and Linderoth 2000)

1. Be aware of:

    a. The historical development of neurostimulation techniques
    b. The general principles of stimulation techniques:

        i.   Safety principles in the use of chronic stimulation
        ii.   The role of test stimulation
        iii. Follow-up and management of the patient with an implanted stimulator
        iv   Troubleshooting when stimulation fails
        v.   Be aware of the proposed pathophysiological principles thought to be at work in chronic stimulation for the relief of pain

2. Peripheral nerve stimulation

    a. Know the indications: neuropathic pain
    b. Techniques and equipment available
    c. Outcomes data

3. Spinal cord stimulation

    a. Know the indications.

        i.   Neuropathic pain

        ii. Pain of degenerative disc disease and failed back surgery syndrome

            (a) Leg pain

            (b) Low back pain

    b. Know the cord stimulation sites for treating pain in different parts of the body.

    c. Recognize the need to produce paresthesia in the region of pain.

    d. Techniques:

        i.   Open with insertion of plate-type electrodes.

        ii. Percutaneous: be aware of the different electrode arrays available and their proposed indications.

        iii. Be aware of the two basic methods of chronic stimulation: radiofrequency-coupled and totally implantable and programmable.

4. Deep brain stimulation (DBS)

    a. Be aware that there are two basic DBS techniques, paresthesiae-producing and medial stimulation.

    b. Be aware of the suggested rationale for each.

    c. Know the indications.

        i.   Neuropathic pain

        ii. Failed back surgery syndrome

        iii. Cancer and other nociceptive pain

    d. Be aware of the equipment available (similar to that for spinal cord stimulation).

    e. Be aware of outcomes data and difficulties of outcome assessment.

5. Cortical stimulation (Tsubokawa al. 1991; Mertens et al. 1999)

    a. Techniques and complications

    b. Indications

    c. Outcomes

L. Epidural spinal and intrathecal opioid administration (Cousins and Mather 1984; Garber and Hassenbusch 2002; Gybels and Sweet 1989; Lenzi et al. 1995)

1. Know the indications:

    a. Cancer pain

    b. Noncancer pain

2. Understand the physiological basis (Chapter 5).

3. Know how to use test-dosing.

4. Be aware of techniques, routes, and complications.

    a. Intraspinal:

        i.   Epidural

        ii. Intrathecal

    b. Intraventricular

    c. Implanted pumps and external pumps

5. Understand the determination of dosage of opiate and its continued administration, the management of the equipment, and how to troubleshoot problems.

6. Be aware of other drugs that can be utilized in addition to opiates.

7. Understand outcomes data.

REFERENCES

Aids to the Examination of the Peripheral Nervous System. London: Bailliere Tindall, 986.

Burchiel KD (Ed). Trigeminal neuralgia. *Tech Neurosurg* 1999; 5:199–266.

Burchiel KJ. *Surgical Management of Pain.* New York: Thieme, 2002.

Cousins MJ, Mather LE. Intrathecal and epidural administration of opioids. *Anesthesiology* 1984; 61:276–310.

Devor M, Seltzer Z. Pathophysiology of damaged nerves in relation to chronic pain. In: Wall PD, Melzack R (Eds). *Textbook of Pain,* 4th ed. Edinburgh: Churchill Livingstone, 1999, pp 129–165.

Garber JD, Hassenbusch SJ. Innovative intrathecal analgesics. In: Burchiel KJ (Eds). *Surgical Management of Pain.* New York: Thieme, 2002, pp 948–957.

Gybels JM, Nuttin BJ. Peripheral nerve stimulation. In: Loeser JD (Ed). *Bonica's Management of Pain,* 3rd ed. Philadelphia: Lippincott, 2000, pp 1851–1855.

Gybels JM, Sweet WH. *Neurosurgical Treatment of Persistent Pain.* Basel: Karger, 1989.

Hardy RW, Bay JW. Surgery of the sympathetic nervous system. In: Schmidek HH, Sweet WH (Eds). *Operative Neurosurgical Techniques,* 3rd ed. Philadelphia: Saunders, 1995, pp 1637–1646.

Jeanmonod D, Magnin M, Morel A. A thalamic concept of neurogenic pain. In: Gebhart GF, Hammond DL, Jensen TS (Eds). *Proceedings of the 7th World Congress on Pain,* Progress in Pain Research and Management, Vol. 2. Seattle: IASP Press, 1994, pp 767–788.

Lenzi A, Galli G, Marini G. Intraventricular morphine in the treatment of pain secondary to cancer. In: Schmidek HH, Sweet WH (Eds). *Operative Neurosurgical Techniques,* 3rd ed. Philadelphia: Saunders, 1995, pp 1431–1441.

Levy RM, Lamb S, Adams JE. Treatment of chronic pain by deep brain stimulation: long term follow-up and review of literature. *Neurosurgery* 1987; 21:885–893.

Loeser JD. Ablative neurosurgical operations-introduction. In: Loeser JD (Ed). *Bonica's Management of Pain,* 3rd ed. Philadelphia: Lippincott, 2000, pp 2007–2010.

Loeser JD, Sweet WH, Ten JW Jr, Van Loveren H, Bonica JJ. Neurosurgical operations involving peripheral nerves. In: Bonica JJ (Ed). *The Management of Pain,* 2nd ed. Philadelphia: Lea & Febiger, 1990, pp 2044–2067.

Mertens P, Nuti C, Sindou M, et al. Precentral cortex stimulation for the treatment of central neuropathic pain. *Stereotact Funct Neurosurg* 1999; 73:122–125.

Meyerson BA, Linderoth B. Spinal cord stimulation. In: Loeser JD (Ed). *Bonica's Management of Pain,* 3rd ed. Philadelphia: Lippincott, 2000, pp 1856–1876.

Nashold JRB, Nashold BS Jr. Microsurgical DREZotomy in treatment of deafferentation pain. In: Schmidek HH, Sweet WH (Eds). *Operative Neurosurgical Techniques,* 3rd ed. Philadelphia: Saunders, 1995, pp 1623–1636.

Nauta HJW, Westlund KN, Willis WD. Midline myelotomy. In: Burchiel KJ (Ed). *Surgical Management of Pain.* New York: Thieme, 2000, pp 714–731.

North RB, Levy RM. *Neurosurgical Management of Pain.* New York: Springer-Verlag, 1996.

North RB, Han M, Zahurak M, Kidd DH. Radiofrequency lumbar facet denervation: analysis of prognostic factors. *Pain* 1994; 57:77–83.

Sindou M, Mertens P, Garcia-Larrea L. Surgical procedures for neuropathic pain. *Neurosurg Q* 2001; 11:45–46.

Sindou MP. Dorsal root entry zone lesions. In: Burchiel KJ (Ed). *Surgical Management of Pain.* New-York: Thieme, 2002, pp 701–703.

Sindou MP. Microsurgical DREZotomy. In: Schmidek HH, Sweet WH (Eds). *Operative Neurosurgical Techniques.* Philadelphia: Saunders, 2000, pp 2445–2459.

Sweet WH, Poletti CE. Operations in the brain stem and spinal canal, with an appendix on open cordotomy. In: Wall PD, Melzack R (Eds). *Textbook of Pain,* 3rd ed. Edinburgh: Churchill Livingstone, 1994, pp 1113–1135.

Sweet WH. Treatment of trigeminal neuralgia by percutaneous rhizotomy. In: Youmans JR (Ed). *Neurological Surgery: A Comprehensive Reference Guide to the Diagnosis and Management of Neurosurgical Problems,* 3rd ed. Philadelphia: Saunders, 1990, pp 3888–3921.

Taha JM. Dorsal root ganglionectomy and dorsal rhizotomy. In: Burchiel KJ (Ed). *Surgical Management of Pain.* New York: Thieme, 2002, pp 677–687.

Tasker RR, Lougheed WM. Neurosurgical techniques of sympathetic interruption. In: Stanton-Hicks M (Ed). *Pain and the Sympathetic Nervous System.* Boston: Kluwer, 1990, pp 165–190.

Tasker RR. Percutaneous cordotomy. In: Schmidek HH, Sweet WH (Eds). *Operative Neurosurgical Techniques,* 3rd ed. Philadelphia: Saunders, 1995, pp 1595–1611.

Tasker RR. The recurrence of pain after neurosurgical procedures. *Qual Life Res* 1994b; 3(Suppl 1):543–549.

Taub A, Robinson F, Taub E. Dorsal root ganglionectomy for intractable monoradicular sciatica. In: Schmidek HH, Sweet WH (Eds). *Operative Neurosurgical Techniques,* 3rd ed. Philadelphia: Saunders, 1995, pp 1585–1593.

Tsubokawa T, Katayama Y, Tamamoto T, Hirayama T, Koyama S. Chronic motor cortex stimulation for the treatment of central pain. *Acta Neurochir* 1991; (Suppl 52):137–139.

White JC, Sweet WH. *Pain and the Neurosurgeon.* Springfield: Charles C. Thomas, 1969.

Willis WD. The pain system: the neural basis of nociceptive transmission. In: Gildenberg PL (Ed). *The Mammalian Nervous System, Pain and Headache,* Vol. 8. Basel: Karger, 1985.

Young RF. Ablative brain operations for chronic pain. In: Loeser JD (Ed). *Bonica's Management of Pain,* 3rd ed. Philadelphia: Lippincott, 2000, pp 2048–2065.

Core Curriculum for Professional Education in Pain, edited by J. Edmond Charlton, IASP Press, Seattle, © 2005.

22

Physical Medicine and Rehabilitation

I. Temperature modalities

   A. Heat

      1. Understand that heat therapies and electrotherapies are usually administered in conjunction with other treatments (e.g., exercise, manual therapy).

      2. Know that heat and cold are both useful in reducing pain and spasm of musculoskeletal and neurological pathologies (Lehmann and deLateur 1999; Cameron 2003).

      3. Be aware of evidence that superficial heating of skin produces muscle relaxation due to decreased gamma-fiber activity and results in decreased spindle excitability, thus decreasing pain and spasm (Lehmann and deLateur 1999).

   B. Cold

      1. Know that cold reduces pain, bleeding, and swelling due to vasodilatation, which helps in healing and hematoma resolution and is an effective first-aid treatment post-injury when combined with rest, compression, and elevation (Dandy and Edwards 1999; Lehmann and deLateur 1999; Linchitz and Sorrell 2003).

      2. Know that ethyl chloride spray and ice massage are counterirritants that have been used in the treatment of myofascial pain (Travell and Simons 1998).

      3. Know that heat and cold can raise pain threshold significantly; ice therapy is more effective than heat (Lehmann and deLateur 1999; Cameron 2003).

   C. Practical use

      1. Know that heat is contraindicated in acute rheumatoid arthritis and in acute trauma, as it may increase bleeding tendency and edema (Lehmann and deLateur 1999).

      2. Be aware that local temperature elevation produces many responses: increase in blood flow, increased extensibility of collagen tissues, increased capillary permeability, and enzymatic activity (Lehmann and deLateur 1999).

      3. Know that short-wave diathermy is a high-frequency electro-magnetic current operating at frequencies of between 13 and 27.12 MHz that is converted into heat (Draper et al. 1999).

      4. Microwave diathermy is a device that applies to specific areas of the body, electromagnetic energy in the microwave frequency bands of 915 MHz to 2,450 MHz. Be aware that short-wave diathermy and microwave diathermy selectively heat muscle (Cameron 2003).

      5. Locally applied thermal treatments (ice and heat packs) are commonly used in painful conditions and can be easily applied by the patient at home. There is no evidence to demonstrate that treatment by a practitioner is better than treatment by patients themselves (Robinson et al. 2003).

      6. Know that superficial heat includes hot packs, heating pads, paraffin wax, fluidotherapy, hydrotherapy, and radiant heat (heat lamps). Superficial heat produces heating of only the superficial tissues up to 0.5 cm from the surface of the skin, whereas deep heating modalities heat to the depth of 3–5 cm (Linchitz and Sorrell 2003).

      7. Know that in ice massage a block of ice is rubbed over the skin surface. The initial phase of cooling is followed by analgesia (Linchitz and Sorrell 2003).

8. Know that temperature modalities should rarely be used alone, but rather in conjunction with appropriate exercises, such as stretching, for increasing range of motion and for strengthening (Watson 2000; Linchitz and Sorrell 2003).

9. Heating modalities should not be used for patients with impaired consciousness, over anesthetized areas, or where circulation is decreased (Lehmann and deLateur 1999). Deep heating modalities should not be used over active malignancies, over gonads, or over a developing fetus (Lehmann and deLateur 1999; Lerman 2001).

10. Know that thermal electrotherapy modalities are contraindicated in the presence of metal implants and cardiac pacemakers. Short-wave diathermy should not be used if either the patient or operator might be pregnant (Lerman et al. 2001).

D. Ultrasound

1. Ultrasound is produced from electromagnetic energy with a frequency of 0.5 to 3.5 MHz, which is converted by a transducer to mechanical energy with similar frequency and intensity of up to 3 W/cm^2 (Ebenbichler and Resch 1994).

2. Pulsed or continuous ultrasound increases cell permeability by setting up cavitation; stable cavitation reduces the nerve conduction velocity of C fibers, thus decreasing pain (Casimiro et al. 2002).

3. Ultrasound is most commonly used in the treatment of acute tendonitis and calcific tendonitis (Lehman and de Latour 1999; Robertson and Baker 2001).

4. Ultrasound is commonly used in the management of musculoskeletal pain. The therapeutic effects of ultrasound are presumed to come from its thermal effects. The evidence for the efficacy for ultrasound in the management of musculoskeletal pain conditions remains weak (Van der Windt et al. 1999; Robertson and Baker 2001; Wright and Sluka 2001).

5. Ultrasound is effective for the treatment of pain and improvement of range of motion in rheumatoid disease of the hands (Casimiro et al. 2003).

6. Ultrasound is contraindicated over areas containing fluid such as the eyes over amniotic fluid in pregnant women and over joints with active effusion (Lehmann and deLateur 1999).

II. Manipulation mobilization, massage, and traction

A. Manipulation mobilization

1. Be aware that massage, manipulation, and mobilization are widely used for treating pain problems, especially spinal pain (Battie et al. 1994; Haldemann and Hooper 1999; Gracey et al. 2002).

2. Know that peripheral joint mobilization and manipulation are frequently used to treat pain (Jette and Delitto 1997; Broome 2000).

3. Understand that manipulation, massage, and mobilization are rarely applied in isolation, but are often used in combination with education and exercise therapy (Grieve 1994; Gracey et al. 2002).

4. Know the difference between joint mobilization and manipulation.

    a. Spinal adjustment or manipulation involves small-amplitude and high-velocity thrusts; the exact physiological effect of this action is still unknown, but it is hypothesized that correction of dysfunctions leads to improved biomechanical function (Grieve 1994; Haldemann and Hooper 1999; Broome 2000).

    b. Mobilization includes those procedures in which a therapist uses hands and fingers to handle tissues. The mobilization is used to increase range of motion beyond the resistance that limits passive range of motion or exercise. Mobilization differs from manipulation or adjustment in that there is no forceful thrust (Grieve 1994; Haldeman and Hooper 1999).

5. Be aware that there is evidence that manipulation reduces pain in acute and chronic spinal conditions but that the long-term effectiveness and advantage over other established treatments is less clear. There is conflicting evidence on the efficacy of manipulation for the management of disability and long-term work loss (Hoving et al. 2002; Assendelft et al. 2003).

B. Massage

1. Be aware that massage is the application of touch or force to soft tissues, usually muscles, tendons, or ligaments, without causing movement or change of joint position (De Domenico and Wood 1997; Clay and Pounds 2002).
2. Know that massage includes several types and techniques, but the relative effectiveness of each of these is not established; massage focusing on specific points (acupoints) may be more effective than traditional Swedish massage techniques (De Domenico and Wood 1997; Furlan et al. 2002).
3. Be aware that there is evidence that massage is effective in the treatment of subacute and chronic spinal pain, especially if combined with exercises and education (Furlan et al. 2002).
4. Understand that deep friction massage therapy is commonly used to treat tendonitis and epicondylitis (Brosseau et al. 2002) and involves firm and sustained manipulation of the tissues over an underlying bony surface, mobilizing the soft tissue by reducing adhesions (Cyriax 1975; Brosseau et al. 2002).

C. Traction

1. Know that manual stretching techniques improve the range of joint motion and the extensibility of soft tissues. Sustained progressive stretching is included in the stretch and spray technique to inactivate trigger points. This technique often is used in conjunction with spraying with a vapocoolant (Travell and Simons 1998; Hanten et al. 2000).
2. Know that traction is a mechanical distraction of tissues, done manually or mechanically. It is an adjunct to treatment of spinal problems. There is little evidence to support the use of mechanical traction as an outpatient treatment for simple low back and neck pain (Swenson 2003).

III. Exercise: Know the purpose of using exercises in the management of pain.

A. Know that immobilization can reduce strength and function of muscles, ligaments, and tendons. Prescribed exercises that increase the forces being transmitted to muscles, ligaments, tendons, and bones will maintain and gradually increase the strength and functional capacity of these structures (Mujika and Padilla 2001a).

B. Know that reduced physical activity reduces cardiovascular fitness (Mujika and Padilla 2001a) and that graded aerobic exercises increase cardiovascular fitness (Mujika and Padilla 2001a,b).

C. Be aware that aerobic exercises to increase cardiopulmonary capacity fitness and endurance include rhythmic, repetitive, dynamic activities such as brisk walking, running, cycling, and swimming. These activities involve large muscle groups and should be performed for at least 20 minutes three times weekly (Wittink and Hoskins 2002).

D. Stretching exercises should be done slowly, steadily, and sustained at the limit of range. Ballistic stretching exercises, involving bouncing and jerking, should not be used (Watson 2000).

E. Know that exercises include passive, active assisted, resistive, progressive resistive, and stretching exercises.

1. Passive movements can reduce pain and stiffness and improve range of motion (Chiarello et al. 1997).
2. General exercise programs are effective in reducing pain and disability for both subacute and chronic pain problems (Liddle et al. 2004).
3. Specific exercises can be used to target specific tissues and joints to maintain and increase muscle strength, increase range of motion, and promote general physiological conditioning (Watson 2000).

F. Understand that physical exercise can be used with other therapies such as manipulation and TENS.

G. Understand that the goals of therapeutic exercises include increased strength, endurance, range of motion, co-ordination and balance; reduction of pain, spasm, edema, and postural deviations; and the promotion of activities of daily living (Watson 2000).

H. Understand that goals for physical exercises should be agreed, maintained, and reviewed regularly. Gains in physical exercise targets must translate into targeted increases in physical activities of daily living and return to normal activity (including work), and goals should be set accordingly (Harding and Watson 2000).

I. Understand that fear of physical activity can limit participation in physical exercise and activity (Vlaeyen and Linton 2000). Participation in physical activity, when introduced appropriately, can reduce fear of exercise and perception of pain (Vlaeyen and Linton 2000; Vlaeyen et al. 2002).

J. Know that there is evidence that patients with herniated nucleus pulposus with low back and leg pain can benefit from a physical exercise program (Saal 1990).

K. Know that general exercise regimes involving stretching exercises and aerobic conditioning exercises can help patients with chronic pain of musculoskeletal origin by reducing pain report and self-reported disability (Harding et al. 1998; Mannion et al. 2001; Liddle et al. 2004).

L. Know that there is little evidence to support the use of specific exercises over general exercise in the management of low back pain (van Tulder et al. 2003).

M. Understand that routine general physical exercise programs improve mood (Brosse et al. 2002).

N. Be aware that patient compliance with physical exercise reduces after treatment ceases. Supervised exercise is likely to result in better compliance and maintenance of effect than unsupervised exercise (American College of Sports Medicine 2000; Liddle et al. 2004). Specific strategies are required to ensure that exercise is continued to promote a healthy lifestyle (Watson 2000).

REFERENCES

American College of Sports Medicine. *ACSM's Guidelines for Exercise Testing and Prescription,* 6th ed. Philadelphia: Lippincott Williams and Wilkins, 2000.

Assendelft WJ, Morton SC, Yu EI, Suttorp MJ, Shekelle PG. Spinal manipulative therapy for low back pain. A meta-analysis of effectiveness relative to other therapies. *Ann Intern Med* 2003; 138:871–881. CD003528

Battie M, Cherkin D, Dunn R. Managing LBP: attitudes and treatment preferences of physical therapists. *Phys Ther* 1994; 74:219–226.

Broome RT. *Chiropractic Peripheral Joint Technique.* Boston: Butterworth Heinemann, 2000.

Brosse AL, Sheets ES, Lett HS, Blumenthal JA. Exercise and the treatment of clinical depression in adults: recent findings and future directions. *Sports Med* 2002; 32:741–760.

Brosseau L, Casimiro L, Milne S, et al. Deep transverse friction massage for treating tendinitis. *Cochrane Database Syst Rev* 2002; 4:CD003528.

Cameron MH. *Physical Agents in Rehabilitation.* New York: WB Saunders, 2003.

Casimiro L, Brosseau L, Robinson V, et al. Therapeutic ultrasound for the treatment of rheumatoid arthritis. *Cochrane Database Syst Rev* 2002; 3:CD003787.

Chiarello CM, Gundersen L, O'Halloran T. The effect of continuous passive motion duration and increment on range of motion in total knee arthroplasty patients. *J Orthop Sports Phys Ther* 1997; 25:119–127.

Clay JH, Pounds DM. *Basic Clinical Massage Therapy: Integrating Anatomy and Treatment.* Philadelphia: Lippincott Williams and Wilkins, 2002.

Cyriax J. *Textbook of Orthopaedic Medicine,* Vol. 2, 9th ed. Baltimore: Williams and Wilkins, 1975.

Dandy DJ, Edwards DJ. *Essential Orthopaedics,* 4th ed. Edinburgh: Churchill Livingstone 1999; 273–281.

De Domenico G, Wood EC. *Beard's Massage.* New York: WB Saunders, 1997.

Draper DO, Knight K, Fujiwara T, Castel JC. Temperature change in human muscle during and after pulsed shortwave diathermy. *J Orthop Sports Phys Ther* 1999; 24:13–22.

Ebenbichler G, Resch KL. Kritische Überprüfung des therapeutischen Ultraschalls. (In German.) *Wien Med Wochenschr* 1994; 3:51–53.

Furlan AD, Brosseau L, Imamura M, Irvin E. Massage for low back pain. *Cochrane Database Syst Rev* 2002; 2:CD001929.

Gracey JH, McDonough SM, Baxter GD. Physiotherapy management of low back pain: a survey of current practice in Northern Ireland. *Spine* 2002; 27:406–411.

Grieve GP. *Modern Manual Therapy of the Vertebral Column.* Edinburgh: Churchill Livingstone, 1994.

Haldeman S, Hooper P. Mobilisation, manipulation massage and exercise for the relief of musculoskeletal pain. In: Wall PD, Melzack R (Eds). *Textbook of Pain,* 4th ed. Edinburgh: Churchill Livingstone, 1999, pp 1399–1418.

Hanten WP, Olson SL, Butts NL, Nowicki AL. Effectiveness of a home program of ischemic pressure followed by sustained stretch for treatment of myofascial trigger points. *Phys Ther* 2000; 80:997–1003.

Harding V, Watson PJ. Increasing activity & improving function in chronic pain management. *Physiotherapy* 2000; 86:619–630.

Harding VR, Simmonds MD, Watson PJ. Physical therapy for chronic pain. *Pain Clin Updates* 1998; 6:3:1–4.

Hoving JL, Koes BW, de Vet HC, et al. Manual therapy, physical therapy, or continued care by a general practitioner for patients with neck pain. A randomized, controlled trial. *Ann Intern Med* 2002; 136:713–722.

Jette AM, Delitto A. Physical therapy treatment choices for musculoskeletal impairments. *Phys Ther* 1997; 77:145–154.

Lehmann JF, de Lateur BJ. Ultrasound, shortwave, microwave, laser and superficial eat and cold in the treatment of pain. In: Wall PD, Melzack R (Eds). *Textbook of Pain,* 4th ed. Edinburgh: Churchill Livingstone, 1999, pp 1383–1397.

Lerman Y, Jacubovich R, Green MS. Pregnancy outcome following exposure to shortwaves among female physiotherapists in Israel. *Am J Ind Med* 2001 39:499–504.

Liddle SD, Baxter DG, Gracey JH. Exercise and chronic back pain: what works? *Pain* 2004; 107:176–190.

Linchitz RM, Sorrell PJ. Physical therapy techniques. In: Raj PP (Ed). *Pain Medicine: A Comprehensive Review.* Philadelphia: Mosby, 2003, pp 327–333.

Mannion AF, Junge A, Taimela S, et al. Active therapy for chronic low back pain: Part 3. Factors influencing self-rated disability and its change following therapy. *Spine* 2001; 26:920–929.

Mujika I, Padilla S. Cardiorespiratory and metabolic characteristics of detraining in humans. *Med Sci Sport Exerc* 2001a; 33:413–421.

Mujika I, Padilla S. Muscular characteristics of detraining in humans. *Med Sci Sport Exerc* 2001b; 33:1297–1303.

Robertson VJ, Baker KG. A review of therapeutic ultrasound: effectiveness studies. *Phys Ther* 2001; 81:1339–1350.

Robinson V, Brosseau L, Casimiro L, et al. Thermotherapy for treating rheumatoid arthritis (Cochrane Review). In: *The Cochrane Library*, Issue 4. Chichester: John Wiley & Sons, Ltd., 2003.

Saal JA. Dynamic muscular stabilization in the nonoperative treatment of lumbar pain syndromes. *Orthop Rev* 1990; 19:691–700.

Swenson RS. Therapeutic modalities in the management of nonspecific neck pain. *Phys Med Rehabil Clin N Am* 2003; 14:605–627.

Travell G, Simons DG. *Myofascial Pain and Dysfunction: The Trigger Point Manual,* 2nd ed. Lippincott Williams and Wilkins, 1998.

Van der Windt DAW, Van der Heijden GJM, Van den Berg SGM, et al. Ultrasound therapy for musculoskeletal disorders: a systematic review. *Pain* 1999; 81:257–271.

van Tulder MW, Malmivaara A, Esmail R, Koes BW. Exercise therapy for low back pain. *Cochrane Database Syst Rev* 2000; 2:CD000335.

Vlaeyen JWS, Linton SJ. Fear avoidance and its consequence in chronic musculoskeletal pain: state of the art. *Pain* 2000; 85:317–332.

Vlaeyen JWS, de Jong J, Geilen M, Heuts PHTG, van Breukelen G. The treatment of fear of movement/(re)injury in chronic low back pain: further evidence on the effectiveness of exposure in vivo. *Clin J Pain* 2002; 18:251–261.

Watson PJ. The pain management programme: physical activities programme content. In: Main CJ, Spanswick CC (Eds). *Pain Management: An Interdisciplinary Approach.* Edinburgh: Churchill Livingstone, 2000, pp 285–301.

Wittink H, Hoskins MT. *Chronic Pain. Management for Physical Therapists,* 2nd ed. Boston: Butterworth Heinemann, 2002.

Wright A, Sluka KA. Nonpharmacological treatments for musculoskeletal pain. *Clin J Pain 2001;* 17:33–46.

Core Curriculum for Professional Education in Pain, edited by J. Edmond Charlton, IASP Press, Seattle, © 2005.

23

Work Rehabilitation

I.   Know that the longer workers remain absent from work the more likely they are to remain off work, and appreciate the importance of, and need for, early intervention (Waddell 1998).

II. Understand that workers presenting with painful back conditions require a clinical examination and screening for the potential presence of serious spinal diseases and for nerve root pain. Radiological imaging is not normally indicated at an initial assessment (Veterans Health Administration 1999; Waddell et al. 1999). Examination findings suggestive of poor outcome (return to work) include:

   A.   Age greater than 50

   B.   More severe symptoms

   C.   Long duration of symptoms

   D.   Symptoms that affect the ability to work

   E.   Poor response to previous treatments or rehabilitation

III. Know that appropriate early management of mechanical (nonspecific) spinal pain includes the provision of adequate analgesia and advice on remaining at or returning to work as soon as possible (Carter and Birrell 2000).

IV. Know that most workers are able to remain at work with symptoms of pain and that although work may exacerbate symptoms, in most cases it is unlikely to cause harm (Andersson 1997; Dionne 1999).

V.   Understand that the decision by a worker to be absent from work is not directly predicted by clinical features or the physical demands of work, but is a complex interaction among occupational, individual, and psychosocial factors (Dionne 1999; Burton and Main 2000; Waddell et al. 2003).

VI. Know that, in the case of low back pain, a simple stepped care approach should be applied starting with simple, low-intensity, low-cost measures and "stepping up" the intensity of intervention until the patient does manage to return to his or her normal activities (Von Korff and Moore 2001; Haldorsen et al. 2002).

VII. Understand that psychosocial factors are the main determinants of disability and are significant predictors of prolonged work absence in painful conditions (Burton and Main 2000; Main and Burton 2000; Waddell and Burton 2000).

VIII. Know that those who remain absent from work for more than 3–6 weeks require a specific assessment of psychosocial and occupational risk factors.

   A.   This assessment should include:

      1.   The workers' attributions about the cause of their pain.
      2.   Their assumption about continuing work.
      3.   Their attitude to their workplace, including safety.
      4.   Their perception of the attitudes of others, including coworkers and supervisors.

   B.   Know that in this context, equating work-related symptoms with work-related injury is counterproductive (Kendall et al. 1997; Marhold et al. 2002; Waddell et al. 2003).

IX.   Be able to identify obstacles to recovery (Kendall et al. 1997; Burton and Main 2000; Main and Burton 2000; Nachemson and Vingard 2000), including:

    A.   Fear of (re-)injury associated with physical activity and working.

    B.   Low expectations of recovery/return to work.

    C.   Low mood, anxiety, and withdrawal from normal social interaction including work.

    D.   Reliance on passive treatments.

    E.   Negative attitude to physical activity and self-management.

    F.   Poor relationships with coworkers and supervisors.

X.   Understand that a successful, comprehensive rehabilitation program includes general exercise, cognitive therapy, and vocational elements (Waddell and Burton 2000; Waddell and Watson 2004).

XI.   Understand that early intervention strategies lead to quicker return to work and reduced long-term disability. Simple low-intensity interventions (advice, information, activity management) are appropriate for with those with work loss of short duration or those who do not demonstrate factors associated with poor outcome (Wood 1987; Linton and Andersson 2000; Marhold et al. 2001; Haldorsen et al. 2002).

XII.   Know that simple low-intensity interventions are not suitable for workers with significant barriers to recovery or for those with prolonged (more than 6 months') work absence (Marhold et al. 2001; Haldorsen et al. 2002).

XIII.   Understand that clinical management is more effective if combined with a rehabilitation strategy and promotion of self-management techniques. Rehabilitation requires a combination of therapeutic, psychosocial, and work-related interventions that address both the clinical problem and issues in the individual's physical and social environment (Waddell and Watson 2004).

XIV.   Understand that those who do not return to work within a few weeks require intensive multidisciplinary approaches, which should include active exercise, addressing distorted beliefs about pain, enhancing positive coping strategies, and promoting self-management (Haldorsen et al. 2002). Such approaches should be delivered as near to the worker's place of work as possible; removing workers from their workplace for rehabilitation may, in some cases, prolong work loss (Loisel et al. 1997; Waddell and Watson 2004).

XV.   Know that managing the risk factors associated with poor outcome assists return to work (Haldorsen et al. 2002).

XVI.   Understand that even those who have been absent from work for many months can be rehabilitated successfully through a comprehensive work rehabilitation program (Jordan et al. 1998; Watson et al. 2004.

XVII.   Be aware that managing the worker's workload and physical workspace may facilitate earlier return to work, provided this is an initiative provided by the employer and that it is time-limited and regularly reviewed (Krause et al. 1998).

XVIII. Know that positive management of the workplace environment, including managing occupational risks (including stress management), monitoring sickness absence, and promoting job satisfaction and good industrial relations can reduce the incidence and duration of work absences. Joint employer and employee approaches to the management of pain in the workplace may be beneficial.

XIX.   Know that modification of the physical workplace alone is ineffective in reducing sickness absence. Modified work programs can be effective in returning workers with pain problems to work (Krause et al. 1998: Marnetoft and Selander 2000). These programs include:

    A.   Modified work programs including light duties (a temporary or permanent restriction in work activity that is less than full duties),

B. Graded work exposure, in which the hours of lighter duties or usual duties are gradually increased until the worker return to full duties.

C. Work trials, in which a worker is give the opportunity to work in a job at the discretion of an employer.

D. Supported employment, which involves paid work with the support of a vocational coach or advisor in the workplace.

XX. Understand that there is little evidence to demonstrate that evidence-based guidelines are implemented in practice (van der Weide et al. 1997, 1999; Volinn 1999).

XXI. Know that a Functional Capacity Assessment (FCA) is a "detailed examination and evaluation that objectively measures the client's current level of function in terms of the demands of competitive employment" (American Physical Therapy Association 1997).

XXII. Know that FCAs are often used to monitor the progress of the workers and to make decisions about the worker's suitability to return to work (King et al. 1998; Mooney 2002). FCAs are used to inform about a person's progress in rehabilitation and to direct treatment to improve performance (Mooney 2002).

XXIII. Understand that FCAs are measures of physical performance and not of physical capacity. Physical performance measures are assessments of both physiological states (physical capacity) and psychological (behavioral) states (Kaplan et al. 1996; Watson 1999).

XXIV. Know that although some FCAs have been found to be reliable and valid, commercially available FCAs vary widely with respect to their validity and reliability (Innes and Straker 1999a,b). FCAs are most reliable when the domains tested are limited (Innes and Straker 1999a; Renneman et al. 2002a,b).

XXV. Understand that there is little research into the ability of FCAs to predict return to and retention in work (Jones and Kumar 2003; Reneman and Dijkstra 2003). The ability of FCAs to predict return to work is less robust than other variables such as age, duration of symptoms, and gender (Matheson et al. 2002).

REFERENCES

American Physical Therapy Association. *Occupational Health Guidelines: Evaluating Functional Capacity.* Alexandria, VA: American Physical Therapy Association, 1997, p 48.

Andersson GBJ. The epidemiology of spinal disorders. In: Frymoer JW (Ed). *The Adult Spine: Principles and Practice.* Philadelphia: Lippincott-Raven, 1997, pp 93–141.

Burton AK, Main CJ. Obstacles to recovery from work-related musculoskeletal disorders. In: Karwowski W (Ed). *International Encyclopedia of Ergonomics and Human Factors.* London: Taylor & Francis, 2000, pp 1542–1544.

Carter JT, Birrell LN (Eds). *Occupational Health Guidelines for the Management of Low Back Pain at Work: Principal Recommendations.* London: Faculty of Occupational Medicine, 2000.

Dionne CE. Low back pain. In: Crombie IK, Croft PR, Linton SJ, Le Resche L, Von Korff M (Eds). *Epidemiology of Pain.* Seattle: IASP Press, 1999, pp 283–297.

Haldorsen EMH, Grasdal AL, Skouen JS, et al. Is there a right treatment for a particular patient group? Comparison of ordinary treatment, light multidisciplinary treatment, and extensive multidisciplinary treatment for long-term sick-listed employees with musculoskeletal pain. *Pain* 2002; 95:49–63.

Innes E, Straker L. Reliability of work-related assessments. *Work* 1999a; 13:107–124.

Innes E, Straker L. Validity of work-related assessments. *Work* 1999b; 13:1025–1152.

Jones T, Kumar S. Functional capacity evaluation of manual materials handlers: a review. *Disabil Rehabil* 2003; 25:179–191.

Jordan KD, Mayer TG, Gatchel RJ. Should extended disability be an exclusion criterion for tertiary rehabilitation? Socioeconomic outcomes of early versus late functional restoration in compensation spinal disorders. *Spine* 1998; 23:2110–2116.

Kaplan GM, Wurtele SK, Gillis D. Maximal effort during functional capacity evaluations: an examination of psychological factors. *Arch Phys Med Rehabil* 1996; 77:161–164.

Kendall NAS, Linton SJ, Main CJ. *Guide to Assessing Psychosocial Yellow Flags in Acute Low Back Pain: Risk Factors for Long Term Disability and Workloss.* Accident and Rehabilitation and Compensation Insurance Corporation of New Zealand and the National Health Committee. New Zealand, 1997.

King PM, Tuckwell N, Barrett TE. A critical review of functional capacity evaluations. *Phys Ther* 1998; 78:852–866.

Krause N, Dasinger LK, Neuhauser F. Modified work and return to work: a review of the literature. *J Occup Rehabil* 1998; 8:113–139.

Linton SJ, Andersson T. Can chronic disability be prevented? A randomized trial of a cognitive-behavior intervention and two forms of information for patents with spinal pain. *Spine* 2000; 25:2855–2831.

Loisel P, Abenhaim L, Durand P, et al. A population-based, randomized clinical trial on back pain management. *Spine* 1997; 22:2911–2918.

Main CJ, Burton AK. Economic and occupational influences on pain and disability. In: Main CJ, Spanswick CC (Eds). *Pain Management: An Interdisciplinary Approach.* Edinburgh: Churchill Livingstone, 2000, pp 63–87.

Marhold C, Linton SJ, Melin L. A cognitive-behavioral return-to-work program: effects on pain patients with a history of long-term versus short-term sick leave. *Pain* 2001; 91:155–163.

Marhold C, Linton SJ, Melin L. Identification of obstacles for chronic pain patients to return to work: evaluation of a questionnaire. *J Occup Rehabil* 2002; 12:65–75.

Marnetoft SU, Selander J. Multidisciplinary vocational rehabilitation focusing on work training and case management for unemployed sick-listed people. *Int J Rehabil Res* 2000; 234:271–279.

Matheson LN, Isernhagen SJ, Hart DL. Relationships among lifting ability, grip force, and return to work. *Phys Ther* 2002; 82:249–256.

Mooney V. Functional capacity evaluation. *Orthopedics* 2002; 25:1094–1099.

Nachemson AL, Vingard. Assessment of patients with neck and back pain: a best evidence synthesis. In: Nachemson AL, Jonsson E (Eds). *Neck and Back Pain: The Scientific Evidence of Cause, Diagnosis and Treatment.* Philadelphia: Lippincott Williams and Wilkins,2000, pp 189–235.

Reneman MF, Dijkstra PU. Introduction to the special issue on functional capacity evaluations: from expert based to evidence based. *J Occup Rehabil* 2003; 13:203–204.

Reneman MF, Dijkstra PU, Westmaas M, Goeken LN. Test-retest reliability of lifting and carrying in a 2-day functional capacity evaluation. *J Occup Rehabil* 2002a; 12:269–275.

Reneman MF, Jaegers SM, Westmaas M, Goeken LN. The reliability of determining effort level of lifting and carrying in a functional capacity evaluation. *Work* 2002b; 18:23–27.

Van der Weide WE, Verbeek JHAM, van Dijk FJH. An audit of occupational health care for employees with low back pain. *Scand J Work Environ Health* 1997; 23:165–178.

Van der Weide WE, Verbeek JHAM, van Dijk FJH. Relation between indicators of quality of occupational rehabilitation of employees with low back pain. *Occup Environ Med* 1999; 56:488–493.

Veterans Health Administration. *Clinical Practice Guideline for the Management of Low Back Pain or Sciatica in the Primary Care Setting.* Washington, DC: Department of Veterans Affairs, 1999.

Volinn E. Do workplace interventions prevent low-back disorders? If so why? a methodological commentary. *Ergonomics* 1999; 42:258–272.

von Korff M, Moore JC. Stepped care for back pain: activating approaches for primary care. *Ann Intern Med* 2001; 134:911–917.

Waddell G. *The Back Pain Revolution.* Edinburgh: Churchill Livingstone, 1998.

Waddell G, Burton AK. *Occupational Health Guidelines for the Management of Low Back Pain at Work—Evidence Review.* London: Faculty of Occupational Medicine, 2000.

Waddell G, Watson PJ. Rehabilitation. In: Waddell G (Ed). *The Back Pain Revolution,* 2nd ed. Edinburgh: Churchill Livingstone, 2004.

Waddell G, McIntosh A, Hutchinson A, Feder G, Lewis M. *Low Back Pain Evidence Review.* London: Royal College of General Practitioners, 1999.

Waddell G, Burton AK, Main CJ. *Screening for Risk of Long-Term Incapacity: A Conceptual and Scientific Review.* London: Royal Society of Medicine Press, 2003.

Watson PJ. Non-physiological determinant of physical performance in musculoskeletal pain. Max M (Ed). *Pain 1999—An Updated Review—Refresher Course Syllabus.* Seattle: IASP Press, 1999, pp 153–158.

Watson PJ, Booker CK, Moores L, Main CJ. Returning the chronically unemployed with low back pain to employment. *Eur J Pain* 2004: 8(4):359–369.

Wood DJ. Design and evaluation of a back injury prevention program within a geriatric hospital. *Spine* 1987; 97–82.

Core Curriculum for Professional Education in Pain, edited by J. Edmond Charlton, IASP Press, Seattle, © 2005.

24

Complementary Therapies

I. Definition

A. Understand that there is no definition for complementary and alternative therapies (CATs).

B. Complementary and alternative therapies are therapies and beliefs that currently are not accepted as part of conventional medicine. Complementary therapies may be considered as those that are used alongside conventional medicine, and alternative therapies as those used instead of conventional medicine.

II. What are complementary and alternative therapies?

A. Be aware that the distinction is unclear between therapies considered to be CATs as opposed to mainstream medicine. Behavioral and cognitive therapy, counseling, and dietary advice are considered mainstream. Transcutaneous electrical nerve stimulation (TENS) and acupuncture are both covered in the chapter on stimulation-produced analgesia and lie partly in each camp.

B. Be aware that CATs cover a wide spectrum of interventions that vary greatly in their methods, age, and philosophies. The list of therapies is constantly changing.

C. The National Center for Complementary and Alternative Medicine (NCCAM), part of the National Institutes of Health, classifies CATs into five categories:

1. Alternative medical systems are built upon complete systems of theory and practice. Some are much older than conventional medicine (e.g., traditional Chinese medicine), and others have developed within Western culture (e.g., homeopathic medicine).
2. Mind-body interventions use techniques designed to enhance the mind's capacity to affect bodily function and symptoms. Some have become mainstream (e.g., cognitive-behavioral therapy), while others are still considered CAM (e.g., mental healing).
3. Biologically based therapies use substances found in nature, such as herbs, foods, and vitamins. Some supplements are used in conventional medicine.
4. Manipulative and body-based methods are based on manipulation and/or movement of one or more parts of the body (e.g., osteopathy).
5. Energy therapies involve the use of energy fields. Biofield therapies affect energy fields that purportedly surround and penetrate the human body (e.g., Reiki and Therapeutic Touch). Bioelectromagnetics-based therapies involve the unconventional use of electromagnetic fields (e.g., magnetic fields).

III. Where to collect information

A. Know where to access information with regard to CATs and understand how to interpret it.

B. Know that there are a large number of Internet sites advertising different therapies to which patients have access.

C. Remember that Internet sites may inform about what a therapy involves and its philosophy, but few have evidence of benefit beyond that of patient reports or individual opinion. Interpretation of information from Internet sites must be approached with caution because the evidence often fails to stand up to currently accepted levels of scrutiny (Morris and Avorn 2003).

D. Use an evidence-based approach to assess CATs (Ernst 2001; Moore et al. 2003a) and natural medicines (Jellin 2003).

E. Understand that patients also have access to this information and may want to discuss it. Maintaining an open mind is important until clear evidence of benefit or otherwise is demonstrated (Ernst et al. 1995).

IV. The size of the CAT market

A. Be aware of the proportion of the population using CATs. Many patients will have tried or be trying CATs on their own or alongside conventional management (Eisenberg et al. 1998; Millar 2001; Haetzman et al. 2003; Barnes et al. 2004).

B. Understand that CATs are often used in situations in which conventional medicine fails to provide adequate relief (Weintraub 2003). Common examples include back pain, arthritis, and fibromyalgia. Estimates suggest that millions of visits are made each year for neck and back pain alone (Wolsko et al. 2003).

C. Be aware that the financial implications of CATs run into billions of dollars, with more being spent out of pocket on CATs than on hospitalizations or physician visits (Eisenberg et al. 1998; Barnes et al. 2004; NCCAM).

V. The evidence base

A. Know the evidence base for CATs is currently weak or nonexistent despite their common usage (Ernst et al. 1995; Pittler et al. 2000; Moore et al. 2003b).

B. Know there is limited beneficial evidence for using supplements and herbal remedies for some painful conditions, and that side effects are uncommon and minor (Moore et al. 2003b).

C. Be aware that despite the difficulties designing good trials, more are being performed with realistic conclusions (Licciardone et al. 2003).

D. Be aware that claims on Internet sites are often misleading or have unproven health claims (Morris and Avorn 2003). It is important to assess each site critically.

E. Appreciate the difficulties developing, funding, and performing high-quality studies into CATs. Understand that a research agenda should be developed (Berman and Swyers 1997; Ernst 2004; Smith 2004).

F. Know that the evidence for homeopathy is generally poor, with the better trials suggesting no benefit (Ernst and Pittler 1998, 2000).

G. Be aware that women of childbearing age use CATs for obstetric and gynecological reasons. The evidence is inconclusive, and further studies are required (Fugh-Berman and Kronenberg 2003; Smith et al. 2003; Huntley et al. 2004).

H. Appreciate that increasingly, children are using CATs (Spigelblatt et al. 1994; Kemper and Barnes 2003; Kemper and Gardiner 2003) and that the efficacy of complementary therapies for treating children's pain is unknown as the research base is even weaker than in adults.

I. Know that musculoskeletal pain is common in older adults and that no specific recommendations can be made about the role of CATs (Weiner and Ernst 2004).

VI. Implications, costs, and side effects

A. Be aware that the agents used in some complementary therapies are active (e.g., traditional Chinese medicine).

1. The relative doses are not regulated in the same way as pharmaceutically produced drugs.

2. There are interactions between complementary medications and pharmaceutically produced drugs (Ernst 2001; Jellin 2003; Mills et al. 2004).

B. Patients may be seeing medical practitioners concurrently with CAT therapists. They may not disclose this information.

C. Patients may stop or delay conventional treatments that are of proven benefit. Others believe that conventional treatments will not be of benefit (Malik and Gopalan 2003; Moore et al. 2003a; Barnes et al. 2004).

D. Remember that conventional medical practitioners, nursing staff, and other allied practitioners have national licensing bodies and training programs often embodied in statute, but that this is not the case for many CATs (Mills and Peacock 1997; Mills and Budd 2000).

E. The market for CATs is not regulated formally, and many claims are made in their favor. Clients anticipate successful outcomes based on these claims and are prepared to pay for them.

F. Understand that the relationship between doctor and patient may be changing in today's society with the increasing role of the Internet (Tyson 2000).

G. Understand the psychological interactions between therapist and client. The therapist-client relationship may have a powerful effect in its own right.

H. Be aware of the vulnerability of patients in pain and the approaches of therapies that have weak or no real evidence of benefit.

REFERENCES

Barnes PM, Powell-Griner E, McFann K, Nahin RL. Complementary and alternative medicine use among adults: United States, 2002. *Adv Data* 2004; 343:1–19. Berman BM, Swyers JP. Establishing a research agenda for investigating alternative medical interventions for chronic pain. *Prim Care* 1997; 24:743–758.

Eisenberg DM, Davis RB, Ettner SL, et al. Trends in alternative medicine use in the United States, 1990–1997: results of a follow-up national survey. *JAMA* 1998; 280:1569–1575.

Ernst E. *The Desktop Guide to Complementary and Alternative Medicine: An Evidence-Based Approach.* London: Mosby, 2001.

Ernst E. The need for scientific rigor in studies of complementary and alternative medicine. *Am J Public Health* 2004; 94:1074.

Ernst E, Pittler MH. Efficacy of homeopathic arnica: a systematic review of placebo-controlled clinical trials. *Arch Surg* 1998; 133:1187–1190.

Ernst E, Pittler MH. Re-analysis of previous meta-analysis of clinical trials of homeopathy. *J Clin Epidemiol* 2000; 53:1188.

Ernst E, Resch KL, White AR. Complementary medicine. What physicians think of it: a meta-analysis. *Arch Intern Med* 1995; 155:2405–2448.

Fugh-Berman A, Kronenberg F. Complementary and alternative medicine (CAM) in reproductive-age women: a review of randomized controlled trials. *Reprod Toxicol* 2003; 17:137–152.

Haetzman M, Elliott AM, Smith BH, Hannaford P, Chambers WA. Chronic pain and the use of conventional and alternative therapy. *Fam Pract* 2003; 20:147–154.

Huntley AL, Coon JT, Ernst E. Complementary and alternative medicine for labor pain: a systematic review. *Am J Obstet Gynecol* 2004; 191:36–44.

Jellin JM. *Natural Medicines Comprehensive Database.* Stockton, CA: Therapeutic Research Faculty, 2003.

Kemper KJ, Barnes L. Considering culture, complementary medicine, and spirituality in pediatrics. *Clin Pediatr (Phila)* 2003; 42:205–208.

Kemper KJ, Gardiner P. Complementary and alternative medical therapies in pediatric pain treatment. In: Schechter N, Berde C, Yaster M (Eds). *Pain in Infants, Children and Adolescents.* Philadelphia: Lippincott, Williams and Wilkins, 2003, pp 449–461.

Licciardone JC, Stoll ST, Fulda KG, et al. Osteopathic manipulative treatment for chronic low back pain: a randomized controlled trial. *Spine* 2003; 28:1355–1362.

Malik IA, Gopalan S. Use of CAM results in delay in seeking medical advice for breast cancer. *Eur J Epidemiol* 2003; 18:817–822.

Millar WJ. Patterns of use—alternative health care practitioners. *Health Rep* 2001; 13:9–21.

Mills E, Montori VM, Wu P, et al. Interaction of St John's wort with conventional drugs: systematic review of clinical trials. *BMJ* 2004; 329:27–30.

Mills S, Budd S. Professional organisation of complementary and alternative medicine in the United Kingdom 2000: a report to the Department of Health. Exeter: University of Exeter, Centre for Complementary Health Studies, 2000.

Mills S, Peacock W. Professional organisation of complementary and alternative medicine in the United Kingdom 1997: a report to the Department of Health. Exeter: University of Exeter, Centre for Complementary Health Studies, 1997.

Moore RA, Edwards J, Barden J, McQuay H. *Bandolier's Little Book of Pain.* Oxford: Oxford University Press, 2003a.

Moore RA, Edwards J, Barden J, McQuay H. Complementary and alternative therapies. In: Moore RA, Edwards J, Barden J, McQuay H (Eds). *Bandolier's Little Book of Pain.* Oxford: Oxford University Press, 2003b, pp 344–389.

Morris CA, Avorn J. Internet marketing of herbal products. *JAMA* 2003; 290:1505–1509.

National Center for Complementary and Alternative Medicine. *Get the Facts.* National Institutes of Health. Available online: nccam.nih.gov.

Pittler MH, Abbot NC, Harkness EF, Ernst E. Location bias in controlled clinical trials of complementary/alternative therapies. *J Clin Epidemiol* 2000; 53:485–489.

Smith CA, Collins CT, Cyna AM, Crowther CA. Complementary and alternative therapies for pain management in labour. *Cochrane Database Syst Rev* 2003; CD003521.

Smith WB. Research methodology: implications for CAM pain research. *Clin J Pain* 2004; 20:3–7.

Spigelblatt L, Laine-Ammara G, Pless IB, Guyver A. The use of alternative medicine by children. *Pediatrics* 1994; 94811–94814.

Tyson TR. The Internet: tomorrow's portal to non-traditional health care services. *J Ambul Care Manage* 2000; 23:1–7.

Weiner DK, Ernst E. Complementary and alternative approaches to the treatment of persistent musculoskeletal pain. *Clin J Pain* 2004; 20:244–255.

Weintraub MI. Complementary and alternative methods of treatment of neck pain. *Phys Med Rehabil Clin N Am* 2003; 14:659–674.

Wolsko PM, Eisenberg DM, Davis RB, Kessler R, Phillips RS. Patterns and perceptions of care for treatment of back and neck pain: results of a national survey. *Spine* 2003; 28:292–297; discussion 298.

Part IV
Clinical States

Core Curriculum for Professional Education in Pain, edited by J. Edmond Charlton, IASP Press, Seattle, © 2005.

25

Taxonomy of Pain Systems

I.   Be familiar with the IASP classification of chronic pain syndromes, the principles upon which it is based, and the application to cases that are most commonly seen.

   A.   Know the five axes in the IASP classification system

   B.   Demonstrate ability to utilize the classification system

II.   Be able to allocate the majority of patients to a specific diagnostic code or codes within the system.

III.   Understand the applications of the definitions of pain terms.

   A.   Know the IASP definition of pain

   B.   Know the definition of commonly utilized pain terms: allodynia, analgesia, dysesthesia, hyperalgesia, hyperesthesia, paresthesia, pain threshold, pain tolerance.

REFERENCE

Merskey H, Bogduk N (Eds.), *Classification of Chronic Pain: Descriptions of Chronic Pain Syndromes and Definitions of Pain Terms,* 2nd ed. Seattle: IASP Press, 1994.

Core Curriculum for Professional Education in Pain, edited by J. Edmond Charlton, IASP Press, Seattle, © 2005.

26

Acute and Postoperative Pain

I. Be aware of the epidemiology and magnitude of the problem of inadequate pain control after operations, medical procedures and conditions, or trauma (including burns) (Cousins and Power 1999; Svensson et al. 2000; NHMRC 2005). Know the numbers and prevalence rates of moderate to severe pain in each of these contexts: the burden upon subpopulations such as infants and children, older patients, pregnant or breast-feeding patients, ethnic minorities, and patients with psychiatric illness or those unable to communicate (NHMRC 2005).

A. Managing pain in the older patient. Know that:

1. Experimental pain thresholds to a variety of noxious stimuli are increased in older people.
2. Patient-controlled analgesia (PCA) and epidural analgesia are more effective in older people than conventional opioid regimens.
3. Reported frequency and intensity of acute pain in clinical situations may be reduced in the older person.
4. Common unidimensional self-report measures of pain can be used in the older patient in the acute pain setting; in the clinical setting, the verbal descriptor scale may be more reliable than others.
5. There is an age-related decrease in opioid requirements, but significant interpatient variability persists.
6. The use of nonsteroidal anti-inflammatory drugs (NSAIDs) and COX-2 inhibitors in older people requires extreme caution; acetaminophen (paracetamol) is the preferred non-opioid analgesic.
7. The assessment of pain and evaluation of pain relief therapies in the older patient may present problems arising from differences in reporting, cognitive impairment, and difficulties in measurement.
8. Measures of present pain may be more reliable than those of past pain, especially in patients with some cognitive impairment.
9. The physiological changes associated with aging are progressive. While the rate of change can vary markedly between individuals, these changes may decrease the dose (maintenance and/or bolus) of drug required for pain relief and may lead to increased accumulation of active metabolites.

B. Ethnic groups and non-English-speaking patients. Understand that:

1. Multilingual printed information and pain measurement scales are useful in managing patients from different cultural or ethnic backgrounds.
2. With appropriate instruction, PCA may help overcome some of the barriers to postoperative analgesia provision in a multicultural environment.
3. Ethnic and cultural background can affect significantly the ability to assess and treat acute pain.

C. Managing acute pain during pregnancy (see Chapter 36). Know that:

1. Use of NSAIDs during pregnancy does not seem to increase the risk of adverse birth outcome, but is associated with increased risk of miscarriage.
2. Use of opioids in pregnancy does not cause fetal malformations, but results in neonatal abstinence syndrome.
3. Meralgia paresthetica is a nerve entrapment syndrome with significantly increased incidence in pregnancy.

4. For pain management in pregnancy, nonpharmacological treatment options should be considered where possible before analgesic medications are used.

5. Use of medications for pain in pregnancy should be guided by published recommendations; ongoing analgesic use requires close liaison between the obstetrician and the medical practitioner managing the pain.

D. Managing pain in the puerperium. Know that:

1. Routine episiotomy does not reduce perineal pain; perineal wounds due to birth trauma should be sutured using continuous subcuticular absorbable sutures.

2. Acetaminophen and rectal NSAIDs are effective in perineal pain after childbirth.

3. The application of cooling, in particular cooling gel pads, and the use of warm baths is effective in treatment of perineal pain after childbirth.

4. Codeine should be avoided in treatment of perineal pain after childbirth.

5. Bromocriptine should be avoided for the treatment of breast pain in the puerperium because of possible serious adverse effects.

6. Acetaminophen and NSAIDs are equally, but only modestly, effective in treating uterine pain.

7. Pain after childbirth requires appropriate treatment as it coincides with new emotional, physical, and learning demands and may trigger postnatal depression.

8. Management of breast and nipple pain should target the cause.

9. Prescribing of medications during lactation requires consideration of transfer into breast milk, uptake by the baby, and potential adverse effects for the baby; available prescribing guidelines should be followed.

10. Acetaminophen and several NSAIDs, in particular ibuprofen, seem safe non-opioids in lactation.

11. Parenteral morphine, fentanyl, and other oral opioids including oxycodone are considered safe in lactation and should be preferred over meperidine (pethidine).

12. Local anesthetics appear safe in lactation.

II. Be aware of adverse physiological and psychological effects of acute pain and their modification for anesthetic (regional versus general) and analgesic techniques (Cousins and Power 1999; Kehlet 1998, 1999).

A. Metabolic: substrate mobilization, catabolism (particularly protein wasting) mediated largely by hormone secretion (from the anterior and posterior pituitary, adrenal cortex and medulla, and pancreas) (Barratt et al. 2002).

B. Cardiovascular: hypertension, tachycardia, myocardial ischemia (if coronary artery disease present), lowered fibrillation threshold (neurally and humorally mediated) (Cousins and Power 1999).

C. Hypercoagulability: risks of thrombotic or embolic disease from immobilization, tissue injury, and hormonal (e.g., epinephrine) actions.

D. Pulmonary compromise due to splinting and intrinsic diaphragmatic muscle impairment (Cousins and Power 1999; Rigg et al. 2002).

E. Gastrointestinal dysfunction due to pain and pain therapies (especially opioids) (Kehlet 1999).

F. Psychological distress and cognitive dysfunction due to pain and stress hormonal responses (e.g., hypoxia from splinting or hyponatremia due to excessive antidiuretic hormone secretion), anxiety, helplessness, insomnia, and pain therapies (Cousins and Power 1999).

G. Predisposition to chronic pain due to central neuronal sensitization.

III. Be familiar with the pharmacological properties of the major classes of drugs used for acute pain management, beginning with usual starting doses, frequencies, and comparative (equivalent) doses (Cousins and Power 1999; MacIntyre and Ready 2003; Moore et al. 2003; ANZCA 2005; NHMRC 2005).

A. For opioids, know:

    1. Major chemical types, receptor selectivity, and agonist features (see Chapter 13) of compounds used, to permit rational drug substitution in the presence of adverse reaction or side effects from an agent of one type (e.g., a full agonist versus a mixed agonist-antagonist or partial agonist, or phenylpiperidine versus alkaloid versus peptide) (Moore et al. 2003).

    2. The wide range of durations of actions available through selection of ultra-short-acting (alfentanil, remifentanil) to ultra-long-acting (methadone) compounds.

    3. Common adverse effects (respiratory depression, sedation, constipation, nausea, pruritus, and urinary retention), including predisposing patient factors (e.g., prostatism, chronic lung disease) and concurrent drug therapies (e.g., anticholinergics, benzodiazepines), and how to evaluate and treat them.

    4. The dangers of sudden reversal of perioperative opioid therapy with naloxone (Cherny 1996).

    5. Benefits and risks of spinal opioids and evidence for and against the selection of spinal versus systemic routes of opioid administration for specific operative procedures and patients (e.g., comorbidity).

    6. How to approach the opioid treatment of acute pain in the opioid-tolerant patient, whether after deliberate, therapeutic chronic opioid therapy such as for cancer pain or in the known or suspected substance abuser (Mitra and Sinatra 2004). (See Chapter 44.)

    7. For patients able to take oral medications, and requiring ongoing management of severe acute pain, know when and how to convert from immediate-release oral opioids such as morphine and oxycodone to controlled-release (or slow-release) preparations (Ginsberg et al. 2003). Be aware of the need to educate ward staff about the differences in the use of immediate-release and controlled-release oral opioids and the dangers of confusing these two different types of preparation.

    8. Be aware of the evidence of efficacy of controlled release oral opioids in management of appropriately selected patients with acute pain (Sunshine et al. 1996; Reuben et al. 1999; Kampe et al. 2004).

    9. Acknowledge the special problems associated with opioid prescribing in patients with either opioid tolerance or substance abuse.

B. With regard to the opioid-tolerant patient (see Chapter 44), understand that:

    1. Opioid-tolerant patients report higher pain scores and have a lower incidence of opioid-induced nausea and vomiting.

    2. Usual preadmission opioid regimens should be maintained, where possible, or appropriate substitutions made.

    3. Opioid-tolerant patients are at risk of opioid withdrawal if non-opioid analgesic regimens or tramadol are used.

    4. PCA settings may need to include a background infusion to replace the usual opioid dose and a higher bolus dose.

    5. Neuraxial opioids can be used effectively in opioid-tolerant patients, although higher doses may be required, and these doses may be inadequate to prevent withdrawal.

    6. Ketamine may reduce opioid requirements in opioid-tolerant patients.

    7. Liaison with all clinicians involved in the treatment of the opioid-tolerant patient is important.

C. With regard to patients with a substance abuse disorder (see Chapter 44):

    1. Naltrexone should be stopped at least 24 hours prior to elective surgery.

    2. Patients who have completed naltrexone therapy should be regarded as opioid naive; in the immediate post-treatment phase they may be opioid-sensitive.

    3. Maintenance methadone regimens should be continued where possible.

    4. Buprenorphine maintenance may be continued; if buprenorphine is ceased prior to surgery, conversion to an alternative opioid is required.

    5. There is no cross-tolerance between central nervous system stimulants and opioids.

D. For nonselective NSAIDs and acetaminophen, know:

1. Different routes and dosage forms (e.g., oral, intravenous, rectal).
2. How to modify doses or withhold NSAIDs in the presence of patient comorbidity (congestive heart failure, renal disease, ulcer disease, coagulopathy) (ANZCA 2005; NHMRC 2005).
3. How to select particular NSAIDs to lessen the risk of specific side effects (e.g., nonacetylated compounds for platelet sparing; nabumetone to lessen gastrointestinal blood loss).
4. That there is a "plateau effect" such that dosage increases beyond the recommended range increase the incidence of side effects but do not improve analgesia (Souter et al. 1994).
5. The efficacy and utility of NSAIDs when administered via intra-articular, topical, and local infiltration routes (Tramer et al. 1998).
6. Pharmacokinetic profiles of the NSAIDs.
7. Controversies concerning NSAIDs and orthopedic surgery (Dumont et al. 2000).
8. Efficacy of NSAIDs for acute pain: aspirin, ibuprofen, diclofenac, piroxicam, naproxen, and ketorolac (ANZCA 2005).

E. For local anesthetics, know:

1. The anatomy of commonly used nerve blocks.
2. The major classes of agents, to guide drug substitution in the presence of allergy to one class (i.e., amino-ester versus amide).
3. The risks and benefits of addition of epinephrine, or combination analgesia (i.e., local anesthetic plus an opioid or NSAIDs).
4. The signs, symptoms, and treatment of systemic local anesthetic toxicity; the risk of toxicity in relation to selection of agent and site of administration; and how to distinguish such toxicity from other common adverse effects of local anesthesia (e.g., hypotension).
5. The indications, risks, benefits, and efficacy of local anesthetic application at common peripheral sites (brachial plexus, intercostal nerve, interpleural space) and epidurally.
6. Chirality in local anesthetic formulations. Additives in local anesthetic preparations and their clinical significance.

F. For tramadol, know:

1. Basic pharmacology
2. Adverse effects especially risk of serotonin syndrome
3. Drug interactions of importance
4. Dosage strategies
5. Efficacy in neuropathic pain

G. For ketamine, know:

1. Basic pharmacology (Schmid et al. 1999).
2. Side-effect profile
3. Dosage strategies
4. Difference between anesthetic and analgesic doses
5. Usefulness in nociceptive pain states

H. For the spinal and epidural routes of analgesia, know:

1. The risks and benefits of these routes of analgesia (Carr and Cousins 1998), noting especially the risks associated with using drugs by these routes, which were not designed for such use.
2. In particular, know the risks, and minimization of such risks, in patients under treatment with drugs altering the coagulation system (Horlocker et al. 1995, 2003; Horlocker and Wedel 1998).
3. The rationale for combinations of drugs used by the spinal and epidural routes (Walker et al. 2002).

4. The evidence for efficacy and side effects of individual agents (Carr and Cousins 1998) and combinations of agents (Walker et al. 2002). For example, be aware that there is weak and inconsistent evidence that the addition of clonidine to an epidural or intrathecal opioid is more effective than clonidine or the opioid alone.

5. Epidural and intrathecal clonidine prolong the effects of local anesthetics.

6. Epidural epinephrine in combination with a local anesthetic improves the quality of postoperative thoracic epidural analgesia. Intrathecal midazolam prolongs the analgesic effect of intrathecal opioids.

7. Intrathecal neostigmine prolongs the analgesic effect of intrathecal morphine or bupivacaine.

8. Intrathecal neostigmine is associated with an increased incidence of nausea and vomiting except at low doses.

9. There is conflicting evidence of analgesic efficacy for the addition of clonidine to local anesthetic plexus blocks.

10. The importance of protocols and procedures for safe management, pre-, intra-, and postoperatively, including the education and training of all staff involved.

11. The key diagnostic features and appropriate management of important complications or concurrent problems that may arise in conjunction with such treatments including:

    a. Epidural hematoma
    b. Epidural abscess
    c. Spinal nerve root(s) lesion(s)
    d. Cauda equina syndrome
    e. Transient neurological symptoms
    f. Meningitis
    g. Headache associated with intracranial hypotension
    h. Limb compartment syndrome, potentially masked by excessive epidural analgesia
    i. Temporary impairment of bladder function leading to a stretched bladder (Carr and Cousins 1998)

G. For epidural analgesia, understand that:

1. For epidural analgesia, all techniques of epidural analgesia for all types of surgery provide better postoperative pain relief compared with parenteral opioid administration.

2. Epidural local anesthetics improve oxygenation and reduce pulmonary infections and other pulmonary complications compared with parenteral opioids.

3. Thoracic epidural analgesia utilizing local anesthetics improves bowel recovery after abdominal surgery.

4. Thoracic epidural analgesia extended for more than 24 hours reduces the incidence of postoperative myocardial infarction.

5. Epidural analgesia is not associated with increased risk of anastomotic leakage after bowel surgery.

6. Thoracic epidural analgesia reduces the incidence of pneumonia and the need for ventilation in patients with multiple rib fractures.

7. Lumbar epidural analgesia reduces graft occlusion rates after peripheral vascular surgery.

8. Combinations of low concentrations of local anesthetics and opioids provide better analgesia than that provided by the individual compounds.

9. The risk of permanent neurological damage in association with epidural analgesia is small; the incidence is higher where there have been diagnostic delays; and if indicated, immediate decompression (within 8 hours of the onset of neurological signs) increases the likelihood of partial or good neurological recovery.

10. The provision of epidural analgesia by continuous infusion or patient-controlled administration of local anesthetic-opioid mixtures is safe on general hospital wards, as long as it is supervised by an anesthesia-based pain service with 24-hour medical staff coverage and monitored by well-trained nursing staff.

H. For intrathecal analgesia, understand that:

    1. The combination of spinal opioids with local anesthetics reduces dose requirements when compared to either drug given alone.

    2. Intrathecal morphine at doses of 100–200 µg offers effective analgesia with a low risk of adverse effects.

    3. Clinical experience with morphine, fentanyl, and sufentanil has shown no neurotoxicity or behavioral changes at normal clinical intrathecal doses.

I. For regional analgesia and concurrent anticoagulant medications, know that:

    1. Anticoagulation is the most important risk factor for the development of epidural hematoma after neuraxial blockade.

J. For the COX-2 inhibitors (see Chapter 14), know:

    1. Structural differences between these agents and conventional NSAIDs.

    2. Selectivity for the COX-2 enzyme between different agents.

    3. Comparisons between COX-2 inhibitors and nonselective NSAIDs in terms of analgesic activity and side-effect profile.

    4. The pharmaco-economic impact of COX-2 inhibitors.

    5. Opioid-sparing effects.

    6. Controversies concerning COX-2 inhibitors (Kharasch 2004).

IV. Be able to formulate a comprehensive plan for optimal perioperative pain management based on the diagnosis of the type of pain and its cause, patient preference, physical and mental status, and available expertise and technology (ANZCA 2005; NHMRC 2005).

A. Know the indications and contraindications for use of the major drug classes available for acute pain management, and evidence for their costs and effectiveness when delivered by varied routes (e.g., systemic, spinal) and infusion patterns (e.g., bolus doses, continuous infusion, patient-controlled).

    1. Local anesthetics

    2. NSAIDs, COX-2 inhibitors, and acetaminophen

    3. Opioids

    4. Alpha-agonists

    5. Others (e.g., tramadol, ketamine, lignocaine, anticonvulsants, and antidepressants)

B. For patient-controlled analgesia:

    1. Know how to write a "PCA prescription" for opioid administration via systemic (intravenous, subcutaneous) or epidural routes

        a. Bolus dose

        b. Lockout interval

        c. Basal infusion rate

        d. Dosage limit per time interval (e.g., 4 or 8 hours)

    1. Know how to titrate a PCA prescription according to clinical need.

    2. Be familiar with the pros and cons (including expense) of different devices and drugs for systemic PCA used currently (electrical, mechanical) or by other routes of delivery (transbuccal, intranasal, transdermal iontophoretic, inhaled).

    3. Know how to manage common problems associated with PCA use, such as: patients' reluctance to use PCA, pruritus, and mechanical difficulties with button devices.

    4. Appreciate the importance of preoperative education to maximize PCA effectiveness.

    5. Appreciate problems associated with drug combinations used in PCA devices.

C. Be able to manage analgesia during the transitions from "nil by mouth" to oral intake, and from inpatient care through hospital discharge (Macintyre and Ready 2003).

D. Be able to select drugs, and to adjust doses and delivery techniques, according to the specific needs of the particular patient under treatment (e.g., considering age, physical status, and mental status) and the available resources (e.g., personnel, expertise, budget, and monitoring) of the setting in which treatment will be provided.

E. Be able to diagnose acute neuropathic pain (Cousins and Power 1999; NHMRC 2005) and select appropriate treatment options, alone or in combination, such as:
    1. Oral administration of anticonvulsant drugs such as carbamazepine, sodium valproate, and gabapentin (ANZCA 2005; NHMRC 2005)
    2. Oral tricyclic antidepressants, e.g., amitriptyline, nortriptyline (ANZCA 2005; NHMRC 2005)
    3. Oral membrane stabilizers e.g., mexiletine, flecainide
    4. Subcutaneous or intravenous lignocaine infusion (Brose and Cousins 1991)
    5. Subcutaneous or intravenous ketamine infusion
    6. Supplementary use of appropriate agents/routes from III–IV above depending upon the relative contributions of nociceptive, neuropathic, psychological, and environmental factors (Cousins and Power 1999; ANZCA 2005; NHMRC 2005).

F. Be aware that any sudden or gradual increase in analgesic requirements postoperatively could be a warning that:

    1. A complication of the surgery has occurred such as leaking bowel anastomosis, compartment syndrome, or infection.
    2. A complication of the pain relief technique has occurred, such as epidural hematoma or abscess.
    3. The nature of the pain has changed, e.g., a neuropathic component has evolved, or psychological/environmental factors have assumed greater importance.

G. Understand the need for increased opioid doses in patients with preexisting opioid treatment for cancer pain and chronic noncancer pain. There is a need for:

    1. Calculation of equivalent systemic dose for existing oral (or other route) opioids.
    2. Calculation of additional dose of opioid to cover new stimulus of postoperative pain.

H. Understand the limitations of some alternative routes of opioid administration:

    1. Transdermal "skin patch." There are long lag times to attain and recover from effective blood concentrations (note: standard opioid patches are not currently approved for acute pain).
    2. Sublingual, e.g., buprenorphine tablets: effective but with long duration effects. However, a partial agonist drug with a ceiling to side effects (e.g., oral transmucosal fentanyl citrate) is effective but has the potential for high peak concentrations and thus is not currently recommended for acute pain in opioid-naive patients.
    3. Transpulmonary: an experimental method, with the potential of virtually 100% bioavailability for drugs such as morphine and fentanyl delivered by a computer-controlled system (Ward et al. 1997; Mather et al. 1998).
    4. Intranasal: an experimental method that has been reported for fentanyl, butorphanol, and meperidine (ANZCA 2005). Insufficient data are available for routine clinical use in acute pain.

I. Nitrous oxide:

    1. Understand that nitrous oxide (N_2O) is an effective analgesic during labor and is an effective analgesic agent in a variety of other acute pain situations.
    2. Neuropathy and bone marrow suppression are rare but potentially serious complications of nitrous oxide use, particularly in at-risk patients.
    3. The information about the complications of nitrous oxide comes from case reports only. There are no controlled studies that evaluate the safety of repeated intermittent exposure to nitrous oxide in humans and no data to guide the appropriate maximum duration or number of times a patient can safely be exposed to nitrous oxide.

4. The suggestions for the use of nitrous oxide are extrapolations only from the information above. Consideration should be given to duration of exposure and supplementation with vitamin B_{12}, methionine, and folic or folinic acid.

5. If nitrous oxide is used with other sedative or analgesic agents, appropriate clinical monitoring should be used.

J. Progression from acute to chronic pain:

1. Chronic postsurgical pain is common, may be severe, and may lead to significant disability (Macrae 2001).
2. Risk factors that predispose patients to the development of chronic postsurgical pain include the severity of pre and postoperative pain, intra-operative nerve injury, and psychological vulnerability.
3. Specific early analgesic interventions may reduce the incidence of chronic pain after surgery.
4. Many patients suffering chronic pain relate the onset to an acute incident.

K. Preemptive and preventive analgesia:

1. Understand that the timing of a single analgesic intervention (pre- versus postincisional), defined as preemptive analgesia, does not have a clinically significant effect on postoperative pain relief. Evidence for and against preemptive analgesia to avert central sensitization (Kissen 2000; Perkins and Kehlet 2000; Ballantyne 2001; Katz and McCartney 2002; Moiniche et al. 2002; Siddall and Cousins 2004).
2. There is evidence that some analgesic interventions have an effect on postoperative pain or on analgesic consumption that exceeds the expected duration of action of the drug, defined as preventive analgesia.
3. NMDA (*N*-methyl-D-aspartate) receptor antagonist drugs in particular may show preventive analgesic effects.

V. Be familiar with nonpharmacological methods of acute pain control.

A. Know that:

1. Combined sensory-procedural information is effective in reducing pain and distress.
2. Training in coping methods or behavioral instruction prior to surgery reduces pain, negative affect and analgesic use.
3. Hypnosis and attentional techniques reduce procedure-related pain.

B. Transcutaneous electrical nerve stimulation (TENS):

1. Be aware of evidence for and against its efficacy (compared to sham TENS or no TENS).
2. Know techniques of its use (electrode placement and stimulation parameters).
3. Know that certain stimulation patterns of TENS may be effective in some acute pain settings.

C. Acupuncture:

1. Know that acupuncture may be effective in some acute pain settings.

D. Cognitive-behavioral treatment:

1. For cognitive-behavioral methods (including patient education, relaxation, distraction), know the major approaches, techniques, limitations (e.g., severe pain intensity, or cognitive impairment) and clinical research that favors or opposes their use for acute pain (Carr and Goudas 1999).

VI. Know the clinical outcomes (e.g., length and cost of hospitalization, complications due to untreated pain or pain treatments, readmission due to inadequate pain control, patient satisfaction, and staff satisfaction) to be evaluated in an organized approach to acute pain management (Miaskowski 1994).

A. Know the types of monitoring (e.g., sedation level, respiratory rate, and vital signs), including the frequency of assessment and institutional assignment of responsibility for performance that have been recommended by major professional organizations concerned with control of acute pain (ANZCA 2005).

B. Know how to organize an acute pain service that supervises the quality of pain management within an institution, documents institutional performance, ensures the quality of this function, and (if shortfalls arise) recognizes them and prevents their recurrence (Werner et al. 2002).

VII. Assessment and measurement of acute pain and its treatment

A. Understand that there is good correlation between the categorical and numerical rating scales, including the visual analogue scale.

B. Understand that pain intensity should be recorded as "the fifth vital sign" in all patients because regular assessment of pain leads to improved acute pain management. Self-reporting of pain should be used whenever appropriate because pain is by definition a subjective experience.

C. Understand that the pain measurement tool chosen should be appropriate to the individual patient. Developmental, cognitive, emotional, and cultural factors should be considered.

D. Scoring should incorporate different components of pain. In the postoperative patient this should include static pain (pain at rest) and dynamic pain (e.g., pain on sitting or coughing).

E. Uncontrolled or unexpected pain requires a reassessment of the diagnosis and consideration of alternative causes for the pain (e.g., a new surgical/ medical diagnosis, neuropathic pain).

VIII. Educational objectives

A. Appreciate the importance of preoperative education to reduce patient anxiety and improve the efficacy of postoperative analgesic strategies.

B. Understand that patients, unless told otherwise, generally have an expectation that they will have to endure postoperative pain and that it will be severe (Warfield and Kahn 1995).

C. Understand that preoperative education improves patient or parent knowledge of pain and enhances positive attitudes toward pain relief.

D. Staff education and the use of guidelines improve pain assessment, pain relief, and prescribing practices.

E. Appreciate that even "simple" techniques of pain relief can be more effective if attention is given to education documentation, patient assessment, and provision of appropriate guidelines and policies.

F. Understand that successful management of acute pain requires close liaison with all personnel involved in the care of the patient and that the major impediment to effective acute pain management is the lack of organization and delivery of pain relief rather than the analgesic techniques themselves.

IX. Nonsurgical (medical) pain. Understand that acute pain management is not restricted to the treatment of postsurgical pain. There are several nonsurgical and medical conditions that require specialized acute pain management (NHMRC 2005):

A. Pain associated with acute spinal cord injury (Attal et al. 2000; Cardenas et al. 2002; Sindrup and Jensen 1999; Siddall et al. 2002).

1. Understand that intravenous opioids, ketamine, and lignocaine decrease acute spinal cord injury pain.
2. Know gabapentin can be effective in the treatment of acute spinal cord injury pain. Treatment of acute spinal cord pain is largely based on evidence from studies of other neuropathic and nociceptive pain syndromes.

B. Pain associated with acute burns and burns dressings (Jonsson et al. 1991; Choiniere et al. 1992; Long et al. 2001).

   1. Understand that opioids, particularly via PCA, are effective in burn pain, including procedural pain.
   2. Acute pain following burn injury can be nociceptive and/or neuropathic in nature and may be constant (background pain), intermittent, or procedure-related.
   3. Acute pain following burn injury requires aggressive multimodal and multidisciplinary treatment.
   4. Despite adequate treatment, pain after burns may become chronic.

C. Acute lower back pain (Kendall et al. 1997; NHMRC 2005).

   1. It is important to rule out serious causes ("red flags").
   2. Acute low back pain is nonspecific in about 95% of cases, and serious causes are rare; common findings also occur in asymptomatic controls and may not be the cause of pain.
   3. Advice to stay active, heat wrap therapy, "activity-focused" printed and verbal information, and behavioral therapy interventions are beneficial in acute low back pain.
   4. Advice to stay active, exercises, multimodal therapy, and pulsed electromagnetic therapy are effective in acute neck pain.
   5. Soft collars are not effective for acute neck pain.

D. Acute herpes zoster infection (Wood et al. 1996; Jackson et al. 1997; Hwang et al. 1999).

   1. Understand that antiviral agents started within 72 hours of onset of rash accelerate acute pain resolution and may reduce the severity and duration of postherpetic neuralgia.
   2. Amitriptyline given in low doses from the onset of rash for 90 days reduces the incidence of postherpetic neuralgia.
   3. Topical aspirin is an effective analgesic in acute zoster.
   4. Sympathetic blocks are effective in acute zoster pain in provision of early and appropriate analgesia as an important component of the management of acute zoster and may have benefits in reducing postherpetic neuralgia.

E. Pain associated with acute myocardial ischaemia and infarction (O'Leary et al. 1987; Baumann et al 2000; Schifferdecker and Spodick 2003).

   1. Morphine, beta blockers, and nitroglycerin are effective and appropriate agents in the treatment of acute ischemic chest pain.
   2. The mainstay of analgesia in acute coronary syndrome is the restoration of adequate myocardial oxygenation, including the use of supplemental oxygen, nitroglycerin, beta blockers, and strategies to improve coronary vascular perfusion.

F. Acute cancer pain (McQuay and Jadad 1994; Soares et al. 2003).

   1. Understand that oral transmucosal fentanyl is effective in treating acute breakthrough pain in cancer patients.
   2. Analgesic medications prescribed for cancer pain should be adjusted to alterations of pain intensity.
   3. Opioid doses for individual patients with cancer pain should be titrated to achieve maximum analgesic benefit with minimal adverse effects Acute pain in patients with cancer often signals disease progression; sudden severe pain in patients with cancer should be recognized as a medical emergency and assessed and treated immediately.
   4. Cancer patients on opioid analgesia need access to immediate-release opioids for breakthrough analgesia; if the response is insufficient after 30 minutes, administration should be repeated.
   5. Breakthrough analgesia should be one-sixth of the total regular opioid dose in patients with cancer pain. If nausea and vomiting accompany acute pain, parenteral opioids are needed to treat acute cancer pain.

G. Pain syndromes in patients with HIV/AIDS (Kaplan et al. 1996; Shlay et al. 1998). Know that:

1. Neuropathic pain is common in patients with HIV/AIDS.
2. In the absence of specific evidence, the treatment of pain in patients with HIV/AIDS should be based on similar principles to those for the management of cancer pain.
3. Interaction between antiretroviral and antibiotic medications and opioids should be considered in this population.

H. Pain associated with hematological disorders such as sickle cell disease and hemophilia (Ballas and Delengowski 1993; Yaster et al. 1994; Weiner et al. 2003). Know that:

1. Hydroxyurea is effective in decreasing the frequency of acute crises and life-threatening complications.
2. Know transfusion requirements in sickle cell disease.
3. Intravenous opioid loading optimizes analgesia in the early stages of an acute sickle cell crisis. Effective analgesia may be continued with intravenous (including PCA) opioids such as morphine; however, meperidine should be avoided.
4. Intravenous ketorolac or methylprednisolone may decrease acute pain in sickle cell crises.
5. Oxygen supplementation during a sickle cell crisis does not decrease pain.

I. Abdominal pain of nonsurgical origin such as dysmenorrhoea, renal and biliary colic, and irritable bowel syndrome (Larkin and Prescott 1992; Labrecque et al. 1994; Poynard et al. 2001; Kim et al. 2002; Marjoribanks et al. 2003). Know that:

1. Analgesics do not interfere with the diagnostic process in acute abdominal pain.
2. NSAIDs are superior to opioids in the treatment of renal colic.
3. The onset of analgesia is fastest with intravenous NSAIDs in renal colic.
4. Antispasmodics and peppermint oil are effective in the treatment of acute pain in irritable bowel syndrome.
5. NSAIDS and vitamin B_1 are effective in the treatment of primary dysmenorrhoea.
6. There is no difference between meperidine and morphine in the treatment of renal colic.
7. Ketorolac is as effective as meperidine in the treatment of biliary colic.

J. Pain associated with acute orofacial conditions such as sinusitis and oral ulceration.

1. NSAIDs, COX-2 selective inhibitors, acetaminophen, opioids, and tramadol provide effective analgesia after dental extraction.
2. NSAIDS and COX-2-selective inhibitors provide better analgesia with fewer adverse effects than acetaminophen, acetaminophen/opioid combinations, acetaminophen/tramadol combinations, tramadol, or weaker opioids after dental extraction.
3. Rofecoxib has an extended duration of analgesia following dental extraction.
4. Perioperative local anesthetic infiltration does not improve analgesia after tonsillectomy.
5. Aspirin and NSAIDs increase the likelihood of reoperation for post-tonsillectomy bleeding.
6. PCA opioids may treat pain effectively in acute mucositis.
7. Perioperative dexamethasone administration reduces acute pain, nausea, and swelling after third-molar extraction.
8. Topical treatments may provide analgesia in acute oral ulceration.
9. Recurrent or persistent orofacial pain requires biopsychosocial assessment and appropriate multidisciplinary approaches.
10. Neuropathic orofacial pain (atypical odontalgia, phantom pain) may be exacerbated by repeated dental procedures, incorrect drug therapy, or psychological factors.

K. Pain management of acute headache including the management of migraine, cluster headache and post-dural puncture headache (PDPH) (see Chapter 37). Know that:

1. Triptans are effective in the treatment of severe migraine.

2. Aspirin-metoclopramide is effective in the treatment of migraine with mild symptoms.
3. The addition of caffeine to aspirin or acetaminophen improves analgesia in acute tension-type headache.
4. The incidence of PDPH may be reduced by using small-gauge needles with a non-cutting edge.
5. There is no evidence that bed rest is beneficial in the treatment and prevention of PDPH.
6. Further high-quality trials are required to determine the efficacy of epidural blood patch administration in the treatment of PDPH.
7. Ibuprofen and acetaminophen are effective in the treatment of migraine with mild symptoms.
8. A "stratified care strategy" is effective in treating migraine.
9. Simple analgesics such as aspirin, acetaminophen, and NSAIDs, either alone or in combination, are effective in the treatment of episodic tension-type headache.
10. Sumatriptan is effective in the treatment of cluster headache.
11. Oxygen is effective in the treatment of cluster headache.
12. Opioids should be used with extreme caution in the treatment of headache, and meperidine should be avoided.

L. Acute musculoskeletal pain:

1. Understand that topical and oral NSAIDs improve acute shoulder pain.
2. Subacromial corticosteroid injection relieves acute shoulder pain in the early stages.
3. Exercises improve acute shoulder pain in patients with rotator cuff disease. Therapeutic ultrasound may improve acute shoulder pain in calcific tendonitis.
4. Advice to stay active, exercises, injection therapy, and foot orthoses are effective in acute patellofemoral pain.
5. Low-level laser therapy is ineffective in the management of patellofemoral pain.
6. A management plan for acute musculoskeletal pain should comprise the elements of assessment (history and physical examination, but ancillary investigations are not generally indicated), management (information, assurance, advice to resume normal activity, and pain management), and review to reassess pain and revise the management plan.
7. Information should be provided to patients in correct but neutral terms, avoiding alarming diagnostic labels to overcome inappropriate expectations, fears, or mistaken beliefs.
8. Treat pain with acetaminophen; if it is ineffective, NSAIDs may be used.
9. Oral opioids, preferably short-acting agents at regular intervals, may be necessary to relieve severe acute musculoskeletal pain; any ongoing need for such treatment requires reassessment.
10. Adjuvant agents such as anticonvulsants, antidepressants, and muscle relaxants are not recommended for the routine treatment of acute musculoskeletal pain.

M. Acute pain management in intensive care. Know that:

1. Pain relief needs should be considered and assessed in all patients throughout their stay in intensive care.
2. Daily interruptions of sedative infusions reduce the duration of ventilation and length of stay in the intensive care unit without causing adverse psychological outcomes.
3. Gabapentin and carbamazepine are effective in reducing the pain associated with Guillain-Barré syndrome.
4. Patients should be provided with appropriate sedation and analgesia during potentially painful procedures.
5. Observation of behavioral and physiological responses permits assessment of pain in unconscious patients.
6. When painful procedures are performed on sedated patients in intensive care, appropriate efforts should be made to deepen sedation or provide analgesia or local anesthesia.

REFERENCES

ANZCA (Australian and New Zealand College of Anaesthetists). *Acute Pain Management: Scientific Evidence,* 2005. Available at: www.anzca.edu.au/publications/acutepain.htm. Accessed 24 July, 2005.

Attal N, Gaude V, Brasseur L, et al. Intravenous lignocaine in central pain; a double blind, placebo controlled, psychophysical study. *Neurology* 2000; 54:564–574.

Ballantyne J. Pre-emptive analgesia: an unsolved problem. *Curr Opin Anesthesiol* 2001; 14:499–504.

Ballas SK, Delengowski A. Pain measurement in hospitalised adults with sickle cell painful episodes. *Ann Clin Lab Sci* 1993; 23:358–361.

Barratt SM, Smith RC, Kee AJ, et al. Multimodal analgesia and intravenous nutrition preserves total body protein following major upper gastrointestinal surgery. *Reg Anesth Pain Med* 2002; 27:15–22.

Baumann BM, Perrone J, Hornig SE, et al. Randomized, double blind, placebo controlled trial of diazepam, nitroglycerin or both for the treatment of patients with potential cocaine-associated acute coronary syndromes. *Acad Emerg Med* 2000; 7:878–885.

Brose WG, Cousins MJ. Subcutaneous lidocaine for treatment of neuropathic cancer pain. *Pain* 1991; 45:145–148.

Cardenas DD, Warms CA, Turner JA, et al. Efficacy of amitriptyline for relief of pain in spinal cord injury: results of a randomised controlled trial. *Pain* 2002; 95:365–373.

Carr DB, Cousins MJ. Spinal route of analgesia: opioids and future options. In: Cousins MJ, Bridenbaugh PO (Eds). *Neural Blockade in Clinical Anesthesia and Management of Pain,* 3rd ed. Philadelphia: Lippincott-Raven, 1998, pp 915–984.

Carr DB, Goudas LC. Acute pain. *Lancet* 1999; 353:2051–2058.

Cherny NI. Opioid analgesics: comparative features and prescribing guidelines. *Drugs* 1996; 51:713–737.

Choiniere M, Grenier R, Paquette C. Patient-controlled analgesia: a double-blind study in burn patients. *Anaesthesia* 1992; 47:467–472.

Cousins MJ, Power I. Acute and postoperative pain. In: Wall PD, Melzack R (Eds). *Textbook of Pain,* 4th ed. Edinburgh: Churchill Livingstone, 1999, pp 447–491.

Dumont AS, Verma S, Dumont RJ, Hurlbert RJ. Nonsteroidal anti-inflammatory drugs and bone metabolism in spinal fusion surgery: a pharmacological quandary. *J Pharmacol Toxicol Methods* 2000; 43:31–39.

Ginsberg B, Sinatra RS, Adler LJ, et al. Conversion to oral controlled-release oxycodone from intravenous opioid analgesic in the postoperative setting. *Pain Med* 2003; 4:31–38.

Horlocker TT, Wedel DJ. Spinal and epidural blockade and perioperative low molecular weight heparin: smooth sailing on the Titanic. *Anesth Analg* 1998; 86:115–136.

Horlocker TT, Wedel DJ, Schroeder DR, et al. Pre-operative antiplatelet therapy does not increase the risk of spinal haematoma associated with regional anaesthesia. *Anesth Analg* 1995; 80:303–309.

Horlocker TT, Wedel DJ, Benzon H, et al. Regional anesthesia in the anticoagulated patient—defining the risks. The second ASRA consensus conference on neuraxial anesthesia and anticoagulation. *Reg Anesth Pain Med* 2003; 28:172–197.

Hwang SM, Kang YC, Lee YB, et al. The effects of epidural blockade on the acute pain in herpes zoster. *Arch Dermatol* 1999; 135:1359–1364.

Jackson JL, Gibbons R, Meyer G, et al. The effect of treating herpes zoster with oral acyclovir in preventing postherpetic neuralgia. A meta-analysis. *Arch Intern Med* 1997; 157:909–912.

Jonsson A, Cassuto J, Hanson B. Inhibition of burn pain by intravenous lignocaine infusion. *Lancet* 1991; 338:151–152.

Kampe S, Warm M, Kaufmann J, et al. Clinical efficacy of controlled-release oxycodone 20 mg administered in a 12-hour dosing schedule on the management of postoperative pain after breast surgery for cancer. *Curr Med Res Opin* 2004; 20:199–202.

Kaplan R, Conant M, Cundiff D, et al. Sustained-release morphine sulfate in the management of pain associated with acquired immunodeficiency syndrome. *J Pain Symptom Manage* 1996; 12:150–160.

Katz J, McCartney CJL. Current status of pre-emptive analgesia. *Curr Opin Anaesthesiol* 2002; 15:435–441.

Kehlet H. Modification of responses to surgery by neural blockade. In: Cousins MJ, Bridenbaugh PO (Eds). *Neural Blockade in Clinical Anesthesia and Management of Pain,* 3rd ed. Philadelphia: Lippincott-Raven, 1998, pp 129–175.

Kehlet H. Acute pain control and accelerated postoperative surgical recovery. *Surg Clin North Am* 1999; 79:431–443.

Kendall NAS, Linton SJ, Main CJ. *Guide to Assessing Psychosocial Yellow Flags in Acute Low Back Pain: Risk Factors for Long Term Disability and Workloss.* Accident and Rehabilitation and Compensation Insurance Corporation of New Zealand and the National Health Committee, 1997.

Kharasch ED. Peri-operative COX-2 inhibitors: knowledge and challenges. *Anesth Analg* 2004; 98:1–3.

Kim MK, Strait RT, Sato TT, et al. A randomised clinical trial of analgesia in children with acute abdominal pain. *Acad Emerg Med* 2002; 9:281–287.

Kissen I. Preemptive analgesia. *Anesthesiology* 2000; 93(4): 1138–1143.

Labrecque M, Dostaler LP, Roussell R et al. Efficacy of non steroidal anti-inflammatory drugs in the treatment of acute renal colic. A meta-analysis. *Arch Intern Med* 1994;154:1381–1387.

Larkin GL, Prescott JE. A randomized, double-blind, comparative study of the efficacy of ketorolac tromethamine versus meperidine in the treatment of severe migraine. *Ann Emerg Med* 1992; 21:919–924.

Long TD, Cathers TA, Twillman R, et al. Morphine-infused silver sulfadiazine (MISS) cream for burn analgesia: a pilot study. *J Burn Care Rehabil* 2001; 22:118–123.

Macintyre PE, Ready LB. *Acute Pain Management: A Practical Guide,* 2nd ed. London: Saunders, 2003.

Macrae WA. Chronic pain after surgery. *Br J Anaesth* 2001; 87:88–98.

Marjoribanks J, Proctor ML, Farquhar C. Nonsteroidal anti-inflammatory drugs for primary dysmenorrhoea. *Cochrane Database Syst Rev* 2003; 4: CD001751.

Mather LE, Woodhouse A, Ward ME. Pulmonary administration of aerosolised fentanyl: pharmacokinetic analysis of systemic delivery. *Br J Clin Pharmacol* 1998; 46:37–43.

McQuay HJ, Jadad AR. Incident pain. *Cancer Surv* 1994; 21:17–24.

Miaskowski C. Pain management: quality assurance and changing practice. In: Gebhart GF, Hammond DL, Jensen TS (Eds). *Proceedings of the 7th World Congress on Pain,* Progress in Pain Research and Management, Vol. 2. Seattle: IASP Press, 1994, pp 75–96.

Mitra S, Sinatra RS. Perioperative management of acute pain in the opioid-dependent patient. *Anesthesiology* 2004; 101:212–227.

Moinche S, Kehlet H, Dahl JB. A qualitative and quantitative systematic review of preemptive analgesia for postoperative pain relief: the role of timing of analgesia. *Anesthesiology* 2002; 96:725–741.

Moore A, Edwards J. Barden J, McQuay H. *Bandolier's Little Book of Pain.* New York: Oxford University Press, 2003.

NHMRC (National Health and Medical Research Council of Australia). Acute pain management: scientific evidence. Available at: www.nhmrc.gov.au/publications/synopses/cp57syn.htm. Accessed 26 July, 2005.

O'Leary U, Puglia C. Friehling TD, et al. Nitrous oxide anaesthesia in patients with ischaemic chest discomfort: effect on beta endorphin levels. *J Clin Pharmacol* 1987; 27:957–961.

Perkins FM, Kehlet H. Chronic pain as an outcome of surgery: a review of predictive factors. *Anesthesiology* 2000; 93:1123–1133.

Poynard T, Regimbeau C, Benhamou Y. Meta-analysis of smooth muscle relaxants in the treatment of irritable bowel syndrome. *Aliment Pharmacol Ther* 2001; 15:355–361.

Reuben SS, Connelly HR, Maciolek H. Postoperative analgesia with controlled-release oxycodone for outpatient anterior cruciate ligament surgery. *Anesth Analg* 1999; 88:1286–1291.

Rigg JR, Jamrozik K, Myles PS, et al. Epidural anaesthesia and analgesia and outcome of major surgery: a randomised trial. *Lancet* 2002; 359:1276–1282.

Schifferdecker B, Spodick DH. Nonsteroidal anti-inflammatory drugs in the treatment of pericarditis. *Cardiol Rev* 2003; 11:211–217.

Schmid RL, Sandler AN, Katz J. Use and efficacy of low-dose ketamine in the management of acute postoperative pain: a review of current techniques and outcomes. *Pain* 1999; 82:111–125.

Shlay JC, Chaloner K, Max MB, et al. Acupuncture and amitriptyline for pain due to HIV-related peripheral neuropathy: a randomized controlled trial. Terry Beirn Community Programs for Clinical Research on AIDS. *JAMA* 1998; 280:1590–1595.

Siddall PJ, Cousins MJ. Persistent pain as a disease entity: implications for clinical management. *Anesth Analg* 2004; 99:510–520.

Siddall PJ, Yezierski RP, Loeser JD. Taxonomy and epidemiology of spinal cord injury pain. In: Burchiel KJ, Yezierski RP (Eds). *Spinal Cord Injury Pain: Assessment, Mechanisms, Management,* Progress in Pain Research and Management, Vol. 23. Seattle: IASP Press, 2002.

Sindrup SH, Jensen TS. Efficacy of pharmacological treatment of neuropathic pain: an update and effect related mechanism of drug action. *Pain* 1999; 83:389–400.

Soares LG, Martins M, Uchoa R. Intravenous fentanyl for cancer pain: a fast titration protocol for the emergency room. *J Pain Symptom Manage* 2003; 26:876–881.

Souter AJ, Fredman B, White PF. Controversies in the perioperative use of anti inflammatory drugs. *Anesth Analg* 1994; 79:1178–1190.

Sunshine AS, Olson NZ, Colon A, et al. Analgesic efficacy of controlled-release oxycodone in postoperative pain. *J Clin Pharmacol* 1996; 36:595–603.

Svensson I, Sjostrom B, Haljamae H. Assessment of pain experiences after elective surgery. *J Pain Symptom Manage* 2000; 20:193–201.

Tramer M, Williams JE, Carroll D, et al. Comparing analgesic efficacy of nonsteroidal anti-inflammatory drugs given by different routes for acute and chronic pain: a qualitative systematic review. *Acta Anaesthesiol Scand* 1998; 42:71–79.

Walker SM, Goudas LC, Cousins MJ, Carr DB. Combination spinal analgesic chemotherapy: a systematic review. *Anesth Analg* 2002; 95:674–715.

Ward ME, Woodhouse A, Mather LE, et al. Morphine pharmacokinetics after pulmonary administration from a novel aerosol delivery system. *Clin Pharmacol Ther* 1997; 6:596–609.

Warfield CA, Kahn CH. Acute pain management: programs in US hospitals and experiences and attitudes among US adults. *Anesthesiology* 1995; 83:1090–1094.

Weiner DL, Hibberd PL, Betit P, et al. Preliminary assessment of inhaled nitric oxide for acute vaso-occlusive crisis in pediatric patients with sickle cell disease. *JAMA* 2003; 289:1136–1142.

Werner MU, Soholm L, Rotball-Nielsen P, Kehlet H. Does an acute pain service improve postoperative outcome? *Anesth Analg* 2002; 95:1361–1321.

Wood MJ, Kay R, Dworkin RH, et al. Oral acyclovir therapy accelerates pain resolution in patients with herpes zoster: a meta-analysis of placebo-controlled trials. *Clin Infect Dis* 1996; 22:341–347.

Yaster M, Tobin JR, Billett C, et al. Epidural analgesia in the management of severe vaso-occlusive sickle cell crisis. *Pediatrics* 1994; 93:310–315.

Core Curriculum for Professional Education in Pain, edited by J. Edmond Charlton, IASP Press, Seattle, © 2005.

27

Cancer Pain

I. General principles (Twycross 1994, 1997; Hanks et al. 1998; Regnard and Tempest 1998; Cherny and Portenoy 1999a,b; Hillier et al. 2000, 2002)

  A. Recognize that pain management is part of a broader therapeutic endeavor known as palliative care. Know that palliative care is defined as the active, total care of the patient with active, progressive, life threatening disease. Recognize that palliative care involves a variety of health care professionals. Know that palliative care provides a model for continuing management including control of pain and symptoms, maintenance of function, psychosocial and spiritual support for the patient and family, and comprehensive care at the end of life.

  B. Know that pain is common in cancer and that many patients have more than one site of pain. Know that the prevalence of pain in cancer varies with the nature of the cancer, the stage of the disease, and the methods used for assessment. Know that more than 50% of patients in hospitals and hospices have pain. Know that advanced cancer is more likely to be painful. Know that breakthrough and incident pain are common in cancer pain (McQuay and Jadad 1994; Addington-Hall and McCarthy 1995; Vainio and Auvinen 1996; Portenoy et al. 1999).

  C. Understand that adequate pain relief can be achieved by at least 75% of cancer patients who receive optimal analgesic management using simple techniques such as those suggested by the World Health Organization analgesic ladder. Know the difficulties in interpreting validation studies (Jadad and Browman 1995; Zech et al. 1995; World Health Organization 1998a).

  D. Know about the barriers to cancer pain treatment, including patient related barriers, health care provider barriers, and health policy and reimbursement barriers. Recognize the importance of health care provider education in removing these barriers.

  E. Recognize the need to assess the quality of analgesia in terms of effectiveness, efficacy, efficiency, humanity, and equity.

  F. Know the importance of developing evidence-based practice in the management of cancer pain. Realize that much of the evidence about cancer pain management is incomplete. Know that clinicians often need to make analgesic treatment decisions based on less robust evidence. Know the importance of balancing benefits and burdens of treatment in this situation (McQuay and Moore 1998).

II. Evaluation of patients with cancer pain (McGuire 1995; Higginson 1997)

  A. Recognize the importance of assessing the need for primary anticancer therapies. Recognize the need to assess for other medical problems (e.g., anemia, infection, and hypercalcemia).

  B. Recognize the importance of comprehensive pain assessment. Know that optimal pain management within the broader context of palliative care depends on detailed information about the pain, comorbid and premorbid medical problems, and physical function. Recognize the importance of psychosocial and spiritual factors. Be aware of the role of the family and significant others (Steifel 1993; Derrickson 1996; Grond et al. 1996; Gatchel and Turk 1999; Twycross 1999).

  C. Know that cancer pain is associated with structural pathology. Realize that definition of the extent of the disease and the nature of the underlying etiology of the pain is essential to pain assessment. Know the roles of radiological investigations into the etiology of pain. Know the importance of assessment of the contribution of skeletal, neural and soft-tissue pathology to pain (Gonzales et al. 1991).

D. Know that the comprehensive evaluation of cancer pain requires an accurate history, a full physical examination, a review of laboratory and radiographic tests and appropriate further investigations. Know specific methods of investigating cancer pain, e.g., ultrasound, radioisotope, single photon emission computed tomography, computed tomography, positron emission tomography, and magnetic resonance imaging scanning, with biopsy if necessary. Know about the need for surgical staging in some cases (Irvine 2000).

E. Know that syndrome recognition is an essential part of pain assessment. Recognize that this may provide information relevant to treatment and prognosis. Know the characteristics of common pain syndromes. Know that these can be direct effects of tumor (e.g., bone metastases) or may result from anticancer therapies (e.g., surgery, drugs), from general debility (e.g., pressure sores), or from factors unrelated to the disease or its treatment (e.g. osteoarthritis) (Cherny and Portenoy 1999a).

F. Know the importance of an accurate characterization of the pain or pains including location, severity, quality, temporal factors, and aggravating/relieving factors.

G. Recognize the significance of different temporal patterns of pain (e.g., continuous, intermittent, acute pain superimposed on continuous pain). Know how to assess these different clinical presentations when making treatment decisions (e.g., use of supplemental doses of an opioid to treat "breakthrough pain"). Know that rapidly escalating pain is an emergency that requires prompt assessment and intervention (Portenoy 1997).

H. Know that the consistent use of a valid pain measurement scale (e.g., verbal categorical, numerical, or visual analogue) can help inform clinical practice. Be aware of the need to use appropriate pain measurement approaches for children, elderly patients and those with learning disabilities or cognitive impairment. Know the inherent problems with the use of these tools in different circumstances, e.g., the frail or confused patient (De Conno et al. 1994; Smith et al. 1998; De Wit 1999).

I. Understand the importance of inferring a pathophysiological mechanism for each pain and recognize the implications that this has for therapy. Know that "nociceptive pains" are sustained by continuing injury to somatic structures ("somatic pain") or visceral structures ("visceral pain"). Know that abnormal processes in the peripheral or central nervous system sustain "neuropathic pains." Neuropathic pains may include painful peripheral mononeuropathy and polyneuropathy, plexopathies, pain from spinal cord compression, complex regional pain syndrome, and deafferentation pain.

J. Recognize that an increase in pain intensity following a stable period necessitates new evaluation of the underlying etiology and pain syndrome.

K. Know the common emergencies in cancer patients that present with pain (e.g., back pain due to spinal cord compression, pathological fracture). Be aware of the need for prompt evaluation and treatment of these conditions.

L. Know the issues involved in the assessment and treatment of pain at the end of life (Saunders and Platt 1999).

M. Know the importance of assessment of factors other than pain. These include physical symptoms (e.g., fatigue, nausea, anorexia and constipation), coexisting psychological symptoms and psychiatric disorders (e.g., anxiety and depression), functional status, family dynamics, spirituality, social support systems, medical support systems, and financial resources (Breitbart et al. 1999).

N. Know that cancer pain and distress affects activities of daily living, family life, and social functioning. Realize that it is important to assess and address these issues during pain management (Lancee et al. 1994; Strang 1998).

O. Recognize that the patient's and family's health beliefs and previous experiences affect the presentation of pain and its management (Ward et al. 1993; Glajchen et al. 1995).

P. Recognize that pain predominantly sustained by psychological factors appears to be rare in the cancer population. Know that psychological factors are important in determining the impact of the pain on the patient's life and response to pain. Appreciate the difficulties that can be faced if a patient with long-standing chronic pain from a benign condition develops pain from cancer. Know about the differences in behavioral response that may be seen. Know that psychological and psychiatric problems may accompany pain. Realize that it is important to treat distress as well as pain (Massie and Holland 1992; Glover et al. 1995; Holland 1997; Passik et al. 1998; Strang 1998).

Q. Know about the need for psychoeducational care that involves a program of educational, psychological and social strategies aimed at treatment and support (Ferrell et al. 1993; Devine and Westlake 1995).

III. Principles of cancer pain treatment (Patt 1993; Cleeland et al. 1994; Jacox et al. 1994; Cherny and Portenoy 1999b; Hillier et al. 2000; Simpson and Budd 2000)

A. Recognize that therapies for pain must be integrated into the oncological management of the patient. Know that management may include both primary anticancer therapy—intended to prolong life—and palliative care.

B. Recognize that treatments aimed at the underlying pathology may also be useful in the management of cancer pain. Know that these treatments may include radiotherapy, pharmacotherapy (including chemotherapy and hormonal, biological and antibiotic therapy), and surgery. Know that the use of any of these strategies for analgesic purposes requires careful evaluation. Realize that the appropriateness, feasibility, benefits, burdens, and risks of such treatment must be carefully considered (Ashby and Stoffell 1991).

C. Know that analgesic pharmacotherapy is the mainstay of cancer pain management. Know that most patients with cancer pain can be managed effectively with an optimal oral opioid regimen. Know the principles of opioid switching. Recognize the importance of expertise in opioid therapeutics for all practitioners who treat patients with cancer (Hanks et al. 2001).

D. Know that the use of other drugs e.g., nonsteroidal anti inflammatory drugs (NSAIDs), cyclooxygenase-2 inhibitors (coxibs), antidepressants, and anticonvulsants may be useful in the management of cancer pain.

E. Recognize the importance of other modalities for the treatment of cancer pain. Know that many patients achieve better pain control if opioid therapy is integrated with other analgesic modalities (multimodal therapy). Know that some patients who are unable to achieve a favorable balance between opioid analgesia and side effects require an alternative approach.

F. Know that alternatives may include invasive techniques such as nerve blocks, spinal drug delivery and neurostimulation, and surgery, as well as physical treatments and psychological approaches.

G. Know that patients must receive a full explanation of the procedure and risks of any invasive procedure before giving consent. Where there is no evidence base to indicate likely benefit, the patient should be made aware of this.

IV. Pharmacological approaches to cancer pain (Jacox et al. 1994; World Health Organization 1998a; Cherny and Portenoy 1999b; Hillier et al. 2000; Hanks et al. 2001)

A. Understand the "analgesic ladder" approach to drug selection. Know the indications and dosing guidelines for non-opioid analgesics, including acetaminophen (paracetamol), NSAIDs, and coxibs (step one). Know the therapeutics of opioids that are used orally for moderate pain, including codeine, oxycodone (combined with a non-opioid analgesic in a single preparation), propoxyphene, hydrocodone, and dihydrocodeine (step two). Know the therapeutics of opioids that are used for severe cancer pain, including morphine, hydromorphone, oxycodone (used alone), levorphanol, methadone, fentanyl, buprenorphine, and diamorphine (step three). Know the rationale for sometimes omitting step 2 analgesics from the ladder.

B. Understand the pharmacokinetics of opioid analgesics given by different routes including the relationships between kinetics and efficacy. Know the importance of active metabolites for some opioids (specifically morphine and meperidine [pethidine]) and that this factor may be important in those with renal impairment.

C. Know the reasons why meperidine (pethidine) should not be used for cancer pain management.

D. Know the rationale for oral administration of drugs whenever feasible.

E. Know the availability other routes of opioid administration. Know the indications for sublingual, oral transmucosal, rectal, transdermal, subcutaneous, intramuscular, and intravenous use. Know that intravenous drugs may be given by repeated injection, continuous infusion, and patient-controlled delivery. Know the pharmacology and availability of drugs given directly into the central nervous system, e.g., by epidural, intrathecal, or intraventricular routes. Know that drugs can be given by repeated administration, continuous infusion, and patient-controlled analgesia. Know that drugs may be delivered via a percutaneous catheter, an implanted subcutaneous port, or a fully implanted pump.

F. Know the appropriate dosing intervals for different drugs by different routes. Know that some routes may not be appropriate in certain situations e.g., transdermal drug delivery for rapidly changing pain.

G. Know about the value of "around the clock" dosing, but be aware of the importance of supplemental "rescue" doses offered on an as needed basis for pain exacerbations (Coluzzi 1998).

H. Know the critical importance of dose titration to individualize opioid therapy. Know that dose titration is based on the principle that the dose should be increased until adequate analgesia occurs or intolerable and unmanageable side effects supervene. Recognize that the absolute dose is not important as long as a favorable balance between analgesia and side effects is maintained.

I. Know the concept of opioid switching in some patients who develop tolerance to, or side effects from, the first-line opioid, when it may be beneficial to try an alternative opioid (de Stoutz et al. 1995; Hawley et al. 1998).

J. Know that patients may become tolerant to some opioid side effects, e.g., nausea, but not usually to others, e.g., constipation. Know the importance of prompt management of common opioid side effects in optimizing therapy. Know the pharmacology, therapeutics, and side effects of drugs used for the treatment of opioid induced emesis. Know about different types of aperients (bulking, stool-softening, and stimulant agents). Know the potential adverse effects of aperients. Know treatments that are used for refractory constipation, e.g., regular aperients that are titrated to effect bowel lavage. Be aware of the use of psychostimulants for opioid induced sedation and how to prescribe them (Dalal and Melzack 1998).

K. Know that the risk of ventilatory depression is extremely low when opioid doses are gradually titrated. Know that a new cardiopulmonary insult in a patient who is receiving opioids may produce ventilatory depression that is, in part, naloxone reversible. As a consequence, know that a response to naloxone is not evidence for a primary opioid effect.

L. Know about the concept of equianalgesic doses and the many factors affecting this. Know that the use of equianalgesic dose tables, when switching opioids or changing from one route of administration to another, is a guide to therapy rather than definitive. Realize that opioid switching and changes of route of administration, e.g., oral to spinal, must be individualized (Ripamonti et al. 1998).

M. Know the concept of tolerance and its importance in cancer pain management. Be aware that cancer patients with stable disease seldom escalate opioid dose. Know that patients who do escalate the opioid dose probably do so because of recurrent or progressive disease.

N. Know about physical dependence on opioids and its implications for cancer pain management. Know that all patients on opioids will develop withdrawal symptoms if the drugs are stopped abruptly. Be aware of the need to prevent this problem by tapering opioids prior to discontinuation of therapy and avoiding antagonist drugs.

O. Know the definitions of problem drug use, tolerance and dependence. Know that problem drug use is fundamentally a psychological and behavioral disorder characterized by loss of control over drug use, compulsive drug use, and continued drug use despite harm. Know that iatrogenic addiction during opioid treatment for cancer pain is very rare.

P. Know the indications, pharmacological properties, therapeutic guidelines and side effects of other analgesics used to treat cancer pain, including drugs used for neuropathic pain such as antidepressants, anticonvulsants, local anesthetics, corticosteroids, and miscellaneous drugs such as ketamine, baclofen, and clonidine (McQuay et al. 1995, 1996; Mercadante et al. 1995).

Q. Know the indications, pharmacological properties, therapeutic guidelines and side effects of other analgesics used to treat cancer pain, including NSAIDs, coxibs, calcitonin, bisphosphonates, and radiopharmaceuticals (e.g., strontium 89).

R. Know about the use of drugs for malignant bowel obstruction, e.g., corticosteroids, anticholinergic drugs (e.g., scopolamine), and octreotide (Doyle et al. 1998).

V. Anesthesiologic approaches to cancer pain (Wall and Melzack 1999; Simpson and Budd 2000)

A. Know about the important aspects of explanation and consent when considering anesthesiologic techniques for pain management. Know how to explain the benefits and burdens of such interventions to patients, caregivers, medical staff and other health care professionals.

B. Understand the common nerve blocks used to manage cancer pain. Know about their indications and risks.

C. Recognize that sympathetic nerve blocks with local anesthetic may be valuable in some types of cancer pains. Know about other procedures that may be useful in selected patients with cancer pain, e.g., myofascial trigger point injection or injection of a neuroma or metastasis.

D. Know about the use of prolonged temporary blocks using local anesthetic infusions.

E. Know the role of neurolytic blocks in some cases, e.g., celiac plexus block in the management of abdominal pain due to cancer of the upper gastrointestinal tract.

F. Understand the indications, risks and practical implications of intraspinal therapies for cancer pain. These may include epidural or intrathecal drugs delivered by percutaneous or implanted systems. Be aware of the organizational structures required for the ongoing care of patients receiving spinal drug delivery.

G. Know about the use of nitrous oxide for transitory analgesia.

H. Know the strengths and weaknesses of using modern technology in palliating cancer pain (Seely and Mount 1999).

VI. Surgical and interventional radiological approaches to cancer pain (Simpson and Budd 2000)

A. Recognize that some types of surgery can provide analgesia for those with cancer, e.g., repair of bowel obstruction, stabilization of pathological fracture, and vertebrectomy for metastatic disease.

B. Know about patient preparation. Realize the importance of adequate explanation and consent when considering surgery in this situation.

C. Be aware of the common neurosurgical procedures that may be useful for cancer pain, e.g., rhizotomy and cordotomy. Know about ventricular drug delivery. Know the indications and risks for these procedures.

VII. Neurostimulatory approaches to cancer pain (Hansson and Lundberg 1999; Simpson 1999)

    A. Know that some noninvasive or minimally invasive stimulatory approaches, including counterirritation, transcutaneous electrical nerve stimulation, and acupuncture, are used empirically for some patients with cancer pain. Know that a strong evidence base does not support these interventions at present.

    B. Recognize that invasive neurostimulatory approaches, including spinal cord stimulation and deep brain stimulation, are rarely used for cancer pain.

VIII. Physical therapy for cancer pain (Doyle et al. 1998; Wall and Melzack 1999; O'Gorman and Elfred 2000)

    A. Know that physical therapy can be useful in cancer pain management, e.g., prevention of secondary painful myofascial or joint complications in patients with weakened limbs.

    B. Recognize that physical modalities, such as the use of heat or cold, can be used to treat some patients with cancer pain.

IX. Psychological approaches to cancer pain (Doyle et al. 1998; Breitbart et al. 1999; Skevington 2000)

    A. Recognize the range of psychological and psychosocial concerns that may be identified through a comprehensive assessment. Know about the need to select therapy appropriately.

    B. Know that psychiatric disorders, most often depression and anxiety, are common in those with cancer pain.

    C. Recognize that caregivers also suffer distress.

    D. Recognize the importance of spiritual problems in some patients and families (Stoter 2000).

    E. Be aware of the types of problems that should be referred to mental health care providers.

    F. Be aware of the cognitive interventions, such as relaxation training, that may be used to improve pain control or coping with pain. Recognize that some patients with cancer pain can benefit from these techniques (Carroll and Seers 1998).

X. Special populations with cancer pain

    A. Be aware of the needs of children with cancer pain. These include age appropriate assessment techniques, appropriate staff training and availability of interventions for procedure related pain. Be aware that there is a lack of specific research into cancer pain in children. Know about appropriate drugs and adjustment of doses for age and weight. Know the use of drugs not licensed for use in children. Know the use of nondrug pain management therapies. Know the psychological adaptation of the dying child and his or her family (Doyle et al. 1998; World Health Organization 1998b; Berde and Collins 1999).

    B. Be aware of the needs of those with learning difficulties with cancer pain. Know about the difficulties in assessment and communication.

    C. Be aware of the needs of the elderly with cancer pain. These include psychosocial concerns and changes in drug selection and dosing associated with age related variation in pharmacokinetics and pharmacodynamics. Know the importance of cognitive impairment in the elderly. Know the effects of comorbidity on drug handling and the problems of polypharmacy.

    D. Be aware of the needs of problem drug users. These may include the requirement for closer monitoring of drug use and the increased likelihood of undertreatment. Know how to manage drug withdrawal. Know when to refer to appropriate specialists in addiction medicine.

    E. Be aware of possible cultural differences in the presentation of painful disease, reaction to life - threatening illness, and response to therapies.

F.   Be aware of the issues of adequate explanation and consent in these groups.

XI.   Ethical issues (Ashby and Stoffell 1998; Randall and Downie 1999)

A.   Understand that the acceptable ratio of benefit to burden in the therapeutics of cancer pain may vary according to the stage of illness.

B.   Critically appraise the ethical issues regarding physician-assisted suicide and euthanasia.

C.   Know about the doctrine of double effect, including the fundamental importance of intent, when prescribing in end-of-life care.

REFERENCES

Addington-Hall J, McCarthy M. Dying from cancer: results of a national population-based survey. *Palliat Med* 1995; 9:295–303.

Ashby M. Stoffell B. Therapeutic ratio and defined phases: proposal of ethical framework for palliative care. *BMJ* 1991; 302:1322–1324.

Berde CB, Collins JJ. Cancer pain and palliative care in children. In: Wall PD, Melzack R (Eds). *Textbook of Pain,* 4th ed. Edinburgh: Churchill Livingstone, 1999, pp 967–999.

Breitbart W, Passik SD, Rosenfield BT. Cancer, mind and spirit. In: Wall PD, Melzack R (Eds). *Textbook of Pain,* 4th ed. Edinburgh: Churchill Livingstone, 1999, pp 1065–1113.

Carroll D, Seers K. Relaxation for the relief of chronic pain: a systematic review. *J Adv Nurs* 1998; 27:476–487.

Cherny NI, Portenoy RK. Cancer pain: principles of assessment and pain syndromes. In: Wall PD, Melzack R (Eds). *Textbook of Pain,* 4th ed. Edinburgh: Churchill Livingstone, 1999a, pp 1017–1065.

Cherny NI, Portenoy RK. Practical issues in the management of cancer pain. In: Wall PD, Melzack R (Eds). *Textbook of Pain,* 4th ed. Edinburgh: Churchill Livingstone, 1999b, pp 1479–1523.

Cleeland CS, Gonin R, Hatfield AK, et al. Pain and its treatment in outpatients with metastatic cancer. *N Engl J Med* 1994; 330:592–596.

Coluzzi PH. Cancer pain management: new perspectives on opioids and episodic pain. *Am J Hospice Palliat Care* 1998; 15:13–22.

Dalal S, Melzack R. Potentiation of opioid analgesia by psychostimulant drugs: a review. *J Pain Symptom Manage* 1998; 164:245–253.

De Conno F, Caracenim A, Gamba A, et al. Pain measurement in cancer patients: a comparison of six methods. *Pain* 1994; 57:161–166.

Derrickson NA. The spiritual work of the dying: a framework and case studies. *Hosp J* 1996; 11:11–30.

De Stoutz ND, Bruera E, Suarez-Almazor M. Opioid rotation for toxicity reduction in terminal cancer patients. *J Pain Symptom Manage* 1995; 10:378–384.

Devine EC, Westlake SK. The effects of psychoeducational care provided to adults with cancer; meta-analysis of 116 studies. *Oncol Nurs Forum* 1995; 22:1369–1381.

De Wit R, Van Dan F, Hanneman M, et al. Evaluation of the use of a pain diary in chronic cancer pain patients at home. *Pain* 1999; 79:89–99.

Doyle D, Hanks GWC, MacDonald N (Eds). *Oxford Textbook of Palliative Medicine.* Oxford: Oxford University Press, 1998.

Ferrell BR, Rhiner M, Ferrell BA. Development and implementation of a pain education program. *Cancer* 1993; 72:3426–3432.

Gatchel RJ, Turk DC. Psychosocial factors in pain: critical perspectives. London: Guilford Press, 1999.

Glajchen M, Fitzmartin RD, Blom D, Swanton R. Psychosocial barriers to cancer pain relief. *Cancer Pract* 1995; 3:76–82.

Glover J, Dibble SL, Dodd MJ, Miaskowski C. Mood states in oncology outpatients: does pain make a difference? *J Pain Symptom Manage* 1995; 10:120–128.

Gonzales GR, Elliott KJ, Portenoy RK, Foley KM. The impact of a comprehensive evaluation in the management of cancer pain. *Pain* 1991; 47:141–144.

Grond S, Zech D, Diefenbach C, Radbruch L, Lehmann KA. Assessment of cancer pain: a prospective evaluation in 2266 cancer patients referred to a pain service. *Pain* 1996; 64:107–114.

Hanks G, Portenoy RK, MacDonald N, Forbes K. Difficult pain problems. In: Doyle D, Hanks GWC, MacDonald N (Eds). *Oxford Textbook of Palliative Medicine.* New York: Oxford University Press, 1998.

Hanks GW, de Conno F, Cherny N, et al. Morphine and alternative opioids in cancer pain: the EAPC recommendations. *Br J Cancer* 2001; 84:587–593.

Hansson P, Lundeberg T. TCNS, vibration and acupuncture as pain-relieving measures. In: Wall PD, Melzack R (Eds). *Textbook of Pain,* 4th ed. Edinburgh: Churchill Livingstone, 1999, pp 1341–1353.

Hawley P, Forbes K, Hanks GW. Opioids, confusion and opioid rotation. *Palliat Med* 1998; 12:63–64.

Higginson IJ. Innovations in assessment: epidemiology and assessment of pain in advanced cancer. In: Jensen TS, Turner JA, Wiesenfeld-Hallin Z (Eds). *Proceedings of the 8th World Congress on Pain,* Progress in Pain Research and Management, Vol. 8. Seattle: IASP Press, 1997, pp 707–716.

Hillier R, Finlay I, Welsh J, Miles A (Eds). *The Effective Management of Cancer Pain.* London: Aesculapius Medical Press, 2000.

Hillier R, Finlay I, Miles A (Eds). *Effective Management of Cancer Pain,* 2nd ed. London: Aesculapius Medical Press, 2002.

Holland JC. Preliminary guidelines for the treatment of distress. *Oncology* 1997; 11:109–117.

Irvine A. Establishing the aetiology of pain: the role of radiological investigations and diagnosis. In: Hillier R, Finlay I, Welsh J, Miles A (Eds). *The Effective Management of Cancer Pain.* London: Aesculapius Medical Press, 2000.

Jacox A, Carr DB, Payne R. *Management of Cancer Pain,* Clinical Practice Guideline No. 9, AHCPR Publication No. 940592. Rockville, MD: U.S. Department of Health and Human Services, Agency for Health Care Policy and Research, 1994.

Jadad AR, Browman GP. The WHO analgesic ladder for cancer pain management: stepping up the quality of its evaluation. *JAMA* 1995; 274:1870–1873.

Lancee WJ, Vachon ML, Ghadirian P, et al. The impact of pain and impaired role performance on distress in patients with cancer. *Can J Psychiatry* 1994; 39:617–622.

Massie MJ, Holland JC. The cancer patient with pain: psychiatric complications and their management. *J Pain Symptom Manage* 1992; 7:99–109.

McGuire D. The multiple dimensions of cancer pain: a framework for assessment and management. In: McGuire DB, Yarbro CH, Ferrell BR (Eds). *Cancer Pain Management.* Boston: Jones and Bartlett, 1995, pp 1–17.

McQuay HJ, Jadad AR. Incident pain. *Cancer Surveys* 1994; 21:17–24.

McQuay H, Moore A. *An Evidence-based Resource for Pain Relief.* Oxford: Oxford University Press, 1998.

McQuay HJ, Carroll D, Jadad AR, Wiffen PJ, Moore A. Anticonvulsant drugs for management of pain: a systematic review. *BMJ* 1995; 311:1047–1052.

McQuay HJ, Tramer M, Nye BA, et al. A systematic review of antidepressants in neuropathic pain. *Pain* 1996; 68:217–227.

Mercadante S, Lodi F, Sapio M, Calligara M, Serretta R. Long-term ketamine subcutaneous continuous infusion in neuropathic cancer pain. *J Pain Symptom Manage* 1995; 10:564–568

O'Gorman B, Elfred A. Physiotherapy. In: Simpson KH, Budd K (Eds). *Cancer Pain Management: A Comprehensive Approach.* Oxford: Oxford University Press, 2000, pp 63–74.

Passik SD, Dugan W, McDonald MV, et al. Oncologists' recognition of depression in their patients with cancer. *J Clin Oncol* 1998; 16:1594–1600.

Patt RB. *Cancer Pain.* Philadelphia: J.B. Lippincott, 1993.

Portenoy RK. Treatment of temporal variations in chronic cancer pain. *Semin Oncol* 1997; 24:S16-7–12.

Portenoy RK, Payne RD, Jacobsen P. Breakthrough pain: characteristics and impact in patients with cancer pain. *Pain* 1999; 81:129–134.

Randall F, Downie RS. *Palliative Care Ethics. A Companion for All Specialties.* Oxford: Oxford University Press, 1999.

Regnard C, Tempest S. *A Guide to Symptom Relief in Advanced Disease.* Hockland and Hochland, 1998.

Ripamonti C, Groff L, Brunelli C, et al. Switching from morphine to oral methadone in treating cancer pain: what is the equianalgesic dose ratio? *J Clin Oncol* 1998; 16:3216–3221

Saunders CM, Platt M. Pain and impending death. In: Wall PD, Melzack R (Eds). *Textbook of Pain,* 4th ed. Edinburgh: Churchill Livingstone, 1999, pp 1113–1125.

Seely JF, Mount BM. Palliative medicine and modern technology. *CMAJ* 1999; 161:1120–1125.

Skevington SM. Psychological support. In: Simpson KH, Budd K (Eds). *Cancer Pain Management: A Comprehensive Approach.* Oxford: Oxford University Press, 2000, pp 15–36.

Simpson B. Spinal cord and deep brain stimulation. In: Wall PD, Melzack R (Eds). *Textbook of Pain,* 4th ed. Edinburgh: Churchill Livingstone, 1999, pp 1353–1383.

Simpson KH, Budd K. *Cancer Pain Management. A Comprehensive Approach.* Oxford: Oxford University Press, 2000.

Smith WB, Gracely RH, Safer MA. The meaning of pain: cancer patient's ratings and recall of pain intensity and affect. *Pain* 1998; 78:123–129.

Stiefel F. Psychosocial aspects of cancer pain. *Support Care Cancer* 1993; 1:130–134.

Stoter D. Spiritual help. In: Simpson KH, Budd K (Eds). *Cancer Pain Management: A Comprehensive Approach.* Oxford: Oxford University Press, 2000, pp 36–48.

Strang P. Cancer pain: a provoker of emotional, social and existential distress. *Acta Oncol* 1998; 37:641–644.

Twycross RG. *Pain Relief in Advanced Cancer.* Edinburgh: Churchill Livingstone, 1994.

Twycross RG. *Symptom Management in Advanced Cancer.* Oxford: Radcliffe Medical Press, 1997.

Twycross RG. *Pain and Suffering: Introducing Palliative Care.* Oxford: Radcliffe Medical Press, 1999.

Vainio A, Auvinen A. Prevalence of symptoms among patients with advanced cancer: an international collaborative study. Symptom Prevalence Group. *J Pain Symptom Manage* 1996; 12:3–10.

Wall PD, Melzack R (Eds). *Textbook of Pain,* 4th ed. Edinburgh: Churchill Livingstone, 1999.

Ward SE, Goldberg N, Miller-McCauley V, et al. Patient-related barriers to management of cancer pain. *Pain* 1993; 52:319–324.

World Health Organization. *Cancer Pain Relief: with a Guide to Opioid Availability,* 2nd ed. Geneva: World Health Organization, 1998a.

World Health Organization. *Cancer Pain and Palliative Care in Children.* Geneva: World Health Organization/IASP, 1998b.

Zech DFJ, Grond S, Lynch J, Hertel D, Lehmann KA. Validation of the WHO guidelines for cancer pain relief: a 10-year prospective study. *Pain* 1995; 63:65–76.

Core Curriculum for Professional Education in Pain, edited by J. Edmond Charlton, IASP Press, Seattle, © 2005.

28

Cervical Radicular Pain

I.   Know the structure of the cervical intervertebral foramina (Bogduk 2003a).

II.   Know the disposition of the cervical spinal nerves and their roots in the intervertebral foramina, and understand their dural, skeletal, and articular relations (An 1996).

III.   Understand, and be able to explain, how radicular pain and radiculopathy differ from neck pain and somatic referred pain (Merskey and Bogduk 1994; Bogduk 1999, 2002, 2003b).

IV.   Understand the difference between radicular pain and radiculopathy, and understand their respective, different mechanisms (Merskey and Bogduk 1994; Bogduk 1999).

V.   Be able to list systematically the possible causes of cervical radicular pain and of radiculopathy, and be aware of their relative prevalences (Bogduk 1999).

VI.   Appreciate the reliability and validity of history and neurological examination for diagnosis of radiculopathy, but understand their limitations in the diagnosis of cervical radicular pain (Viikara-Juntura 1989; Bogduk 1999, 2002, 2003b).

VII.   Know the indications and validity of medical imaging in the assessment of cervical radicular pain (Bogduk 1999).

VIII. Understand the lack of validity of electrodiagnostic tests for the investigation of cervical radicular pain (Dvorak 1998; Bogduk 1999).

IX.   Understand the natural history of acute cervical radicular pain and its relevance to management (Bogduk 1999).

X.   Appreciate the lack of any proven or demonstrated physiological basis for commonly used interventions for cervical radicular pain (Bogduk and Mercer 1995).

XI.   Be aware of the cardinal evidence for the efficacy, or lack thereof, of interventions commonly used for acute or chronic cervical radicular pain, such as:

A. Drugs

B. Exercises

C. Manual therapy

D. Traction

E. Epidural steroid injections

F. Transforaminal injections of steroids

(British Association of Physical Medicine 1966; Goldie and Landquist 1970; Purkis 1986; Rowlingson et al. 1986; Shulman 1986; Cicala et al. 1989; Klaber Moffett et al. 1990; Mangar and Thomas 1991; Ferrante et al. 1993; Castagnera et al. 1994; Bush and Hillier 1996; Persson et al. 1997; Bogduk 1999; Slipman et al. 2000; Vallee et al. 2001).

XII.   Be aware of the potential complications of injection therapies for cervical radicular pain (Bogduk 1999; Brouwers et al. 2001; Baker et al. 2002; Rathmell et al. 2004).

XIII. Understand the indications and efficacy of surgical treatment for cervical radicular pain (Chestnut et al. 1992; Brigham and Tsahakis 1995; Ahlgren and Garfin 1996; Persson et al. 1997; Gore and Sepic 1998; Bogduk 1999).

    A. Ensure the patient has a clear understanding of the reason(s) for any diagnostic test or procedure and the likely benefit to be derived. Where there is no evidence base to indicate likely benefit, the patient should be made aware of this.

    B. Be aware that outcome of any treatment should be assessed by more than one method if appropriate.

REFERENCES

Ahlgren BR, Garfin SR. Cervical radiculopathy. *Orthop Clin North Am* 1996; 27:253–263.

An HS. Cervical root entrapment. *Hand Clinics* 1996; 12:719–730.

Baker R, Dreyfuss P, Mercer S, Bogduk N. Cervical transforaminal injection of corticosteroids into a radicular artery: a possible mechanism for spinal cord injury. *Pain* 2002; 103:211–215.

Bogduk N. *Medical Management of Acute Cervical Radicular Pain: An Evidence-Based Approach.* Newcastle: Newcastle Bone and Joint Institute, 1999.

Bogduk N. Cervical pain. In: Ashbury AK, McKhann GM, McDonald WI, Goadsby PJ, MacArthur JC (Eds). *Disease of the Nervous System: Clinical Neuroscience and Therapeutic Principles.* Cambridge: Cambridge University Press, 2002, pp 742–759.

Bogduk N. Anatomy and biomechanics of the spine. In: Hochberg MC, Silman AJ, Smolen JS, Weinblatt ME, Weisman MH (Eds). *Rheumatology,* 3rd ed, Vol. 1. Philadelphia: Mosby, 2003a, pp 545–566.

Bogduk N. Neck and arm pain. In: Aminoff MJ, Daroff RB (Eds). *Encyclopedia of the Neurological Sciences,* Vol. 3. Amsterdam: Academic Press, 2003b, pp 390–398.

Brigham CD, Tsahakis PJ. Anterior cervical foraminotomy and fusion: surgical technique and results. *Spine* 1995; 20:766–770.

British Association of Physical Medicine. Pain in the neck and arm: a multicentre trial of the effects of physiotherapy. *BMJ* 1966; 1:253–258.

Brouwers PJAM, Kottnik EJBL, Simon MAM, Prevo RL. A cervical anterior spinal artery syndrome after diagnostic blockade of the right C6 nerve root. *Pain* 2001; 91:397–399.

Bush K, Hillier S. Outcome of cervical radiculopathy treated with periradicular/epidural corticosteroid injections: a prospective study with independent clinical review. *Eur Spine J* 1996; 5:319–325.

Castagnera L, Maurette P, Paintillart V, et al. Long-term results of cervical epidural steroid injection with and without morphine in chronic cervical radicular pain. *Pain* 1994; 58:239–243.

Chestnut RM, Abitbol JJ, Garfin SR. Surgical management of cervical radiculopathy. *Orthop Clin North Am* 1992; 23:461–474.

Cicala RS, Thoni K, Angel JJ. Long-term results of cervical epidural steroid injections. *Clin J Pain* 1989; 5:143–145.

Dvorak J. Epidemiology, physical examination and neurodiagnostics. *Spine* 1998; 23:2663–2673.

Ferrante FM, Wilson SP, Iacabo C, et al. Clinical classification as a predictor of therapeutic outcome after cervical epidural steroid injection. *Spine* 1993; 18:730–736.

Goldie I, Landquist A. Evaluation of the effects of different forms of physiotherapy in cervical pain. *Scand J Rehab Med* 1970; 2–3:117–121.

Gore DR, Sepic SB. Anterior discectomy and fusion for painful cervical disc disease: a report of 50 patients with an average follow-up of 21 years. *Spine* 1998; 23:2047–2051.

Klaber Moffett JA, Hughes GI, Griffiths P. An investigation of the effects of cervical traction. Part 1: Clinical effectiveness. *Clin Rehab* 1990; 4:205–211.

Mangar D, Thomas PB. Epidural steroid injections in the treatment of cervical and lumbar pain syndromes. *Regional Anesth* 1991; 16:246.

Merskey H, Bogduk N (Eds). *Classification of Chronic Pain. Descriptions of Chronic Pain Syndromes and Definitions of Pain Terms,* 2nd ed. Seattle: IASP Press, 1994.

Persson LCG, Carlsson CA, Carlsson JY. Long-lasting cervical radicular pain managed with surgery, physiotherapy or a cervical collar: a prospective, randomized study. *Spine* 1997; 22:751–758.

Purkis IE. Cervical epidural steroids. *Pain Clinic* 1986; 1:3–7.

Rathmell JR, Aprill C, Bogduk N. Cervical transforaminal injection of steroids. *Anesthesiology* 2004; 100:1595–1600.

Rowlingson JC, Kirschenbaum LP. Epidural analgesic techniques in the management of cervical pain. *Anesth Analg* 1986; 65:938–942.

Shulman M. Treatment of neck pain with cervical epidural steroid injection. *Regional Anesth* 1986; 11:92–94.

Slipman CW, Lipetz JS, Jackson HB, Rogers DP, Vresilovic EJ. Therapeutic selective nerve root block in the nonsurgical treatment of atraumatic cervical spondylotic radicular pain: a retrospective analysis with independent clinical review. *Arch Phys Med Rehabil* 2000; 81:741–746.

Vallee JN, Feydy A, Carlier RY, et al. Chronic cervical radiculopathy: lateral-approach periradicular corticosteroid injection. *Radiology* 2001; 218:886–892.

Viikari-Juntura E, Porras M, Laasonen EM. Validity of clinical tests in the diagnosis of root compression in cervical disc disease. *Spine* 1989; 14:253–257.

Core Curriculum for Professional Education in Pain, edited by J. Edmond Charlton, IASP Press, Seattle, © 2005.

29

Neck Pain

I.   Know the structure of the cervical spine, and understand how it normally operates.

    A.   Know the component parts of the cervical vertebrae and the structure of the intervertebral disks and zygapophysial joints (Bogduk 2003a).

    B.   Appreciate the disposition, actions, and functions of the paravertebral muscles of the cervical spine (Bogduk 2003a).

    C.   Know the innervation of the bones, disks, joints, ligaments, muscles, and dura mater of the cervical spine (Bogduk 2002a).

    D.   Understand how the cervical spine moves (Bogduk and Mercer 2000).

II.   Appreciate the limitations of evidence concerning the possible causes of acute neck pain, and the controversial status of causes of chronic neck pain. Be able to explain the reason for this controversy (Bogduk 2003b,c; Bogduk and Yoganandan 2001).

III. Understand, and be able to explain, how neck pain and somatic referred pain differ from radicular pain and radiculopathy (Merskey and Bogduk 1994). Understand how the investigation and treatment of these conditions differ, and how they are subject to different bases of evidence (Bogduk 2002b,c).

IV.   Appreciate how disorders of the cervical spine may cause referred pain that is perceived as headache (Bogduk 2004).

V.   Understand the lack of validity of diagnostic labels commonly applied to acute and chronic neck pain (Bogduk 2003b,d). Be aware of the evidence that refutes diagnoses such as spondylosis, osteoarthrosis, and congenital anomalies as causes of neck pain (Bogduk 1999, 2003b,d). Be able to apply diagnostic labels according to recommended criteria (Merskey and Bogduk 1994).

VI.   Appreciate the significance and utility of history in the assessment of patients with neck pain (Nachemson and Jonsson 2000; Australian Acute Musculoskeletal Pain Guidelines Group 2003; Bogduk 2003d). Be able to obtain a comprehensive history of neck pain.

VII. Appreciate the lack of reliability and validity of physical examination in the assessment of patients with neck pain (Bogduk 1999, 2003d; Nachemson and Jonsson 2000).

VIII. Appreciate the lack of validity of conventional medical imaging in the assessment of neck pain (Bogduk 1999, 2003d; Nachemson and Jonsson 2000).

IX.   Be aware of the etiological and prognostic risk factors for neck pain (Bogduk 1999, 2003d; Australian Acute Musculoskeletal Pain Guidelines Group 2003). Understand that the evidence indicates that psychological factors are of far less significance for neck pain than they are for back pain, but that psychosocial factors in the work environment are often associated with complaints of neck pain (Bogduk 1999, 2003d).

X.   Be aware of the favorable natural history of neck pain after whiplash, but understand how some patients may be injured and develop symptoms (Bogduk 1999, 2003d; Barnsley et al. 2002).

XI.   Understand the rationale for invasive tests such as diagnostic joint blocks and diskography for the investigation of neck pain, and be aware of both the evidence for these procedures and the basis for controversies concerning them (Bogduk and Lord 1998; Bogduk 1999, 2002c, 2003d,e; Nachemson and Jonsson 2000).

XII. Appreciate the lack of any proven or demonstrated physiological basis for commonly used interventions for neck pain (Bogduk and Mercer 1995).

XIII. Be aware of the cardinal evidence for the efficacy of reassurance, maintaining activity, and exercise for the treatment of acute neck pain (Nachemson and Jonsson 2000; Australian Acute Musculoskeletal Pain Guidelines Group 2003; Bogduk 2003d).

XIV. Be aware of the lack of evidence of efficacy of commonly used treatments for either acute or chronic neck pain. (Bogduk 1999, 2003d; Nachemson and Johnson 2000; Australian Acute Musculoskeletal Pain Guidelines Group 2003). This applies to:

A. Drugs

B. Manual therapy

C. Acupuncture

D. Traction

E. TENS

F. Massage

G. Biofeedback

H. Neck school

I. Patient education

J. Behavioral therapy

K. Multidisciplinary therapy

L. Injections, including:

  1. Epidural steroids
  2. Prolotherapy
  3. Trigger point injections
  4. Botulinum toxin

M. Intra-articular steroids

XV. Understand the reasons for the limited efficacy of surgical treatment of neck pain (Nachemson and Jonsson 2000; Bogduk 2003d):

A. Valid and non-valid indications

B. Appropriate and inappropriate procedures

C. Complications and side effects

D. Ensure that the patient has a clear understanding of the reason(s) for any diagnostic test or procedure and the likely benefit to be derived. Where there is no evidence base to indicate likely benefit, the patient should be made aware of this.

E. Be aware that outcome of any treatment should be assessed by more than one method if appropriate.

XVI. Be aware of the evidence concerning the rationale and efficacy of medial branch neurotomy for neck pain (Lord et al. 1996, 1998; Centre for Health Services and Policy Branch 2001; Lord and Bogduk 2002; Bogduk 2003d).

REFERENCES

Australian Acute Musculoskeletal Pain Guidelines Group. *Evidence-Based Management of Acute Musculoskeletal Pain.* Brisbane: Australian Academic Press, 2003. Available at: www.nhmrc.gov.au.

Barnsley L, Lord SM, Bogduk N. The pathophysiology of whiplash. In: Malanga GA, Nadler SF (Eds). *Whiplash.* Philadelphia: Hanley & Belfus, 2002, pp 41–77.

Bogduk N. The neck. *Bailliere's Clin Rheumatol* 1999; 13:261–285.

Bogduk N. Innervation and pain patterns of the cervical spine. In: Grant R (Ed). *Physical Therapy of the Cervical and Thoracic Spine,* 3rd ed. New York: Churchill Livingstone, 2002a, pp 61–72.

Bogduk N. Cervical pain. In: Ashbury AK, McKhann GM, McDonald WI, Goadsby PJ, MacArthur JC (Eds). *Disease of the Nervous System: Clinical Neuroscience and Therapeutic Principles.* Cambridge: Cambridge University Press, 2002b, pp 742–759.

Bogduk N. Diagnostic nerve blocks in chronic pain. *Best Practice Res Clin Anaesth* 2002c: 16:565–578.

Bogduk N. Anatomy and biomechanics of the spine. In: Hochberg MC, Silman AJ, Smolen JS, Weinblatt ME, Weisman MH (Eds). *Rheumatology,* 3rd ed, Vol. 1. Philadelphia: Mosby, 2003a, pp 545–466.

Bogduk N. The anatomy and pathophysiology of neck pain. *Phys Med Rehabil Clin N Am* 2003b; 14:455–472.

Bogduk N. Neck and arm pain. In: Aminoff MJ, Daroff RB (Eds). *Encyclopedia of the Neurological Sciences,* Vol. 3. Amsterdam: Academic Press, 2003c, pp 390–398.

Bogduk N. Neck pain and whiplash. In: Jensen TS, Wilson PR, Rice ASC. *Clinical Pain Management: Chronic Pain.* London: Arnold, 2003d, pp 504–519.

Bogduk N. Diagnostic procedures in chronic pain. In: Jensen TS, Wilson PR, Rice ASC (Eds). *Clinical Pain Management: Chronic Pain.* London: Arnold, 2003e, pp 125–144.

Bogduk N. The neck and headaches. *Neurol Clin N Am* 2004; 22:151–171.

Bogduk N, Lord SM. Cervical zygapophysial joint pain. *Neurosurg Q* 1998; 8:107–117.

Bogduk N, Mercer S. Selection and application of treatment. In: Refshauge KM, Gass EM (Eds). *Musculoskeletal Physiotherapy: Clinical Science and Practice.* Oxford: Butterworth Heinemann, 1995, pp 169–181.

Bogduk N, Mercer SR. Biomechanics of the cervical spine. 1: Normal kinematics. *Clin Biomech* 2000; 15:633–648.

Bogduk N, Yoganandan N. Biomechanics of the cervical spine. 3: Minor injuries. *Clin Biomech* 2001; 16:267–275.

Centre for Health Services and Policy Branch. Percutaneous radiofrequency neurotomy treatment of chronic cervical pain following whiplash injury. Vancouver: University of British Columbia, British Columbia Office of Health Technology Assessment, 2001.

Lord SM, Bogduk N. Radiofrequency procedures in chronic pain. *Best Pract Res Clin Anaesth* 2002; 16:597–617.

Lord SM, Barnsley L, Wallis BJ, McDonald GJ, Bogduk N. Percutaneous radio-frequency neurotomy for chronic cervical zygapophysial-joint pain. *N Engl J Med* 1996; 335:1721–1726.

Lord SM, McDonald GJ, Bogduk N. Percutaneous radiofrequency neurotomy of the cervical medial branches: a validated treatment for cervical zygapophysial joint pain. *Neurosurg Q* 1998; 8:288–308.

Merskey H, Bogduk N (Eds). *Classification of Chronic Pain: Descriptions of Chronic Pain Syndromes and Definitions of Pain Terms,* 2nd ed. Seattle: IASP Press, 1994.

Nachemson A, Jonsson E (Eds). *Neck and Back Pain: The Scientific Evidence of Causes, Diagnosis, and Treatment.* Philadelphia: Lippincott, Williams & Wilkins, 2000.

Core Curriculum for Professional Education in Pain, edited by J. Edmond Charlton, IASP Press, Seattle, © 2005.

30

Lumbar Radicular Pain

I.   Know the structure of the lumbar vertebral canal and intervertebral foramina (Bogduk 1997, Chapter 5).

II.   Know the disposition of the lumbar and sacral nerve roots in the cauda equina and their dural, skeletal, and articular relations (Bogduk 1997, Chapter 10).

III. Know the disposition of the lumbar and sacral nerve roots in the intervertebral foramina and their dural, skeletal, and articular relations (Bogduk 1997, Chapter 10).

IV.   Understand, and be able to explain, how radicular pain and radiculopathy differ from low back pain and somatic referred pain (Merskey and Bogduk 1994).

V.   Understand the difference between radicular pain and radiculopathy and understand their respective, different mechanisms (Smyth and Wright 1959; Howe et al. 1977; Howe 1979; Devor 1996; Kawakami et al. 1996a,b; Olmarker 1996; Bogduk 1997).

VI.   Be able to list systematically the possible causes of radicular pain and of radiculopathy, and be aware of their relative prevalences (Bogduk and Govind 1999, Chapter 3).

VII. Appreciate the reliability and validity of history and neurological examination for diagnosis of radiculopathy, but understand their limitations in the diagnosis of radicular pain (Norlen 1944; Knutsson 1961; Spangfort 1972; Nelson et al. 1979; Kosteljanetz et al. 1984, 1988; Morris et al. 1986; Deyo et al. 1987; Haldeman et al. 1988; McCombe et al. 1989; Thelander et al. 1992).

VIII. Know the indications and validity of medical imaging in the assessment of lumbar radicular pain (Weisel 1986; Boden et al. 1990; Jensen et al. 1994; Albeck et al. 1995; Brant-Zawadzki et al. 1995; Andersson et al. 1996; Herzog 1996).

IX.   Understand the lack of validity of electrodiagnostic tests for the investigation of lumbar radicular pain (Knutsson 1961; Haldeman et al. 1988; Andersson et al. 1996; Dvorak 1996).

X.   Understand the natural history of acute lumbar radicular pain and its relevance to management (Saal et al. 1990; Bozzao et al 1992; Bush et al. 1992; Delauche-Cavalier et al. 1992; Maigne et al. 1992; Weber et al. 1993; Dullerud and Nakstad 1994; Matsubara et al. 1995).

XI.   Appreciate the lack of any proven or demonstrated physiological basis for commonly used interventions for lumbar radicular pain (Bogduk and Mercer 1995).

XII. Be aware of the cardinal evidence for the efficacy, or lack thereof, of interventions commonly used for acute low back pain and for chronic low back pain (Matthews and Hickling 1975; Larsson et al. 1980; Coxhead et al. 1981; Fraser 1984; Kepes and Duncalf 1985; Bogduk and Govind 1999, Chapters 9, 11, 12; Pal et al. 1986; Haimovic and Beresford 1986; Gogan and Fraser 1992; Bogduk 1995; Bogduk et al. 1995; Koes et al. 1995; Watts and Silagy 1995; McQuay and Moore 1996; Saal 1996; Carette et al. 1997; Vroomen et al. 1999; Riew et al. 2000; Karppinen et al. 2001a,b; Vad et al. 2002), such as:

   A. Bed rest

   B. Staying active

   C. Drugs

    D.   Exercises

    E.   Manual therapy

    F.   Traction

    G.   Epidural steroid injections

    H.   Transforaminal injections of steroids

    I.   Chemonucleolysis

XIII.   Understand the indications and efficacy of surgical treatment for lumbar radicular pain (Gibson et al. 1999; Waddell et al. 2000).

REFERENCES

Albeck MJ, Hilden J, Kjaer L, et al. A controlled comparison of myelography, computed tomography, and magnetic resonance imaging in clinically suspected lumbar disc herniation. *Spine* 1995; 20:443–448.

Andersson GBJ, Brown MD, Dvorak J, et al. Consensus summary on the diagnosis and treatment of lumbar disc herniation. *Spine* 1996; 21(Suppl 24S):75S–78S.

Boden SD, Davis DO, Dina TS, Patronas NJ, Wiesel SW. Abnormal magnetic-resonance scans of the lumbar spine in asymptomatic subjects. *J Bone Joint Surg* 1990; 72A:403–408.

Bogduk N. Spine update: epidural steroids. *Spine* 1995; 20:845–848.

Bogduk N. *Clinical Anatomy of the Lumbar Spine and Sacrum,* 3rd ed. Edinburgh: Churchill Livingstone, 1997.

Bogduk N, Govind J. *Medical Management of Acute Lumbar Radicular Pain: An Evidence-Based Approach.* Newcastle: Newcastle Bone and Joint Institute, 1999.

Bogduk N, Aprill C, Derby R. Epidural steroid injections. In: White AH (Ed). *Diagnosis and Conservative Treatment,* Spine Care, Vol. 1. St. Louis: Mosby, 1995, pp 322–343.

Bozzao A, Galluci M, Masciocchi C, et al. Lumbar disc herniation: MR imaging assessment of natural history in patients treated without surgery. *Radiology* 1992; 185:135–141.

Brant-Zawadzki M, Jensen MC, Obuchowski N, Ross JS, Modic MT. Interobserver and intraobserver variability in interpretation of lumbar disc abnormalities. *Spine* 1995; 20:1257–1264.

Bush K, Cowan N, Katz DE, Gishen P. The natural history of sciatica associated with disc pathology: a prospective study with clinical and independent radiologic follow-up. *Spine* 1992; 17:1205–1210.

Carette S, LeClaire R, Marcoux S, et al. Epidural corticosteroids injections for sciatica due to herniated nucleus pulposus. *N Engl J Med* 1997; 336:1634–1640.

Coxhead CE, Inskip H, Meade TW, North WRS, Troup JDG. Multicentre trial of physiotherapy in the management of sciatic symptoms. *Lancet* 1981; 1:1065–1068.

Delauche-Cavallier M-C, Budet C, Laredo J-D, et al. Lumbar disc herniation: computed tomography scan changes after conservative treatment of nerve root compression. *Spine* 1992; 17:927–933.

Devor M. Pain arising from the nerve root and the dorsal root ganglion. In: Weinstein JN, Gordon SL (Eds). *Low Back Pain: A Scientific and Clinical Overview.* Rosemont, IL: American Academy of Orthopaedic Surgeons, 1996, pp 187–208.

Deyo RA, Tsui-Wu YJ. Descriptive epidemiology of low-back pain and its related medical care in the United States. *Spine* 1987; 12:264–268.

Dullerud R, Nakstad PH. CT changes after conservative treatment for lumbar disc herniation. *Acta Radiol* 1994; 35:415–419.

Dvorak J. Neurophysiologic tests in diagnosis of nerve root compression caused by disc herniation. *Spine* 1996; 21(Suppl 24S):39S–44S.

Fraser RD. Chymopapain for the treatment of intervertebral disc herniation; the final report of a double blind study. *Spine* 1984; 9:815–818.

Gibson JNA, Grant IC, Waddell G. The Cochrane review of surgery for lumbar disc prolapse and degenerative lumbar spondylosis. *Spine* 1999; 24:1820–1832.

Gogan WJ, Fraser RD. Chymopapain: a 10-year, double-blind study. *Spine* 1992; 17:388–394.

Haimovic IC, Beresford HR. Dexamethasone is not superior to placebo for treating lumbosacral radicular pain. *Neurology* 1986; 36:1593–1594.

Haldeman S, Shouka M, Robboy S. Computed tomography, electrodiagnostic and clinical findings in chronic workers' compensation patients with back and leg pain. *Spine* 1988; 13:345–350.

Herzog RJ. The radiologic assessment for a lumbar disc herniation. *Spine* 1996; 21(Suppl 24S):19S–38S.

Howe JF. A neurophysiological basis for the radicular pain of nerve root compression. In: Bonica JJ. Liebeskind JC, Albe-Fessard DG (Eds). *Proceedings of the Second World Congress on Pain,* Advances in Pain Research and Therapy, Vol. 3. New York: Raven Press, 1979, pp 647–657.

Howe JF, Loeser JD, Calvin WH. Mechanosensitivity of dorsal root ganglia and chronically injured axons: a physiological basis for the radicular pain of nerve root compression. *Pain* 1977; 3:25–41.

Jensen MC, Bran-Zawadzki MN, Obucjowski N, et al. Magnetic resonance imaging of the lumbar spine in people without back pain. *N Engl J Med* 1994; 331:69–73.

Karppinen J, Malmivaara A, Kurunlahti M, et al. Periradicular infiltration for sciatica: a randomized controlled trial. *Spine* 2001a; 26:1059–1067.

Karppinen J, Ohinmaa A, Malmivaara A, et al. Cost-effectiveness of periradicular infiltration for sciatica: subgroup analysis of a randomized controlled trial. *Spine* 2001b; 26:2587–2595.

Kawakami M, Weinstein JN, Tamaki T, Hashizue H. The difference in nociceptive potential of the nucleus pulposus and the anulus fibrosus. In: Weinstein JN, Gordon SL (Eds). *Low Back Pain: A Scientific and Clinical Overview.* Rosemont, IL: American Academy of Orthopaedic Surgeons, 1996a, pp 209–213.

Kawakami M, Tamaki T, Weinstein JN, et al. Pathomechanism of pain-related behavior produced by allografts of intervertebral disc in the rat. *Spine* 1996b; 21:2101–2107.

Kepes ER, Duncalf D. Treatment of backache with spinal injections of local anesthetics, spinal and systemic steroids: a review. *Pain* 1985; 22:33–47.

Knutsson B. Comparative value of electromyographic, myelographic and clinical-neurological examination in diagnosis of lumbar root compression syndrome. *Acta Orthop Scand* 1961; Suppl 49.

Koes BW, Scholten RJPM, Bouter LM. Efficacy of epidural steroid injections for low back pain and sciatica: a systematic review of randomized clinical trials. *Pain* 1995; 63:279–288.

Kosteljanetz M, Espersen JO, Halaburt H, Miletic T. Predictive value of clinical and surgical findings in patients with lumbago-sciatica: a prospective study (Part I). *Acta Neurochir* 1984; 73:67–76.

Kosteljanetz M, Bang F, Schmidt-Olsen S. The clinical significance of straight-leg raising (Lasegue's sign) in the diagnosis of prolapsed lumbar disc: interobserver variation and correlation with surgical finding. *Spine* 1988; 13:393–395.

Larsson U, Choler U, Lidstrom A, et al. Auto-traction for treatment of lumbago-sciatica. *Acta Orthop Scand* 1980; 51:791–798.

Maigne JY, Rime B, Delinge B. Computed tomographic follow-up study of forty-eight cases of nonoperatively treated lumbar intervertebral disc herniation. *Spine* 1992; 17:1071–1074.

Matsubara Y, Kato F, Mimatsu K, Kajino G, Nakamura S, Nitta H. Serial changes on MRI in lumbar disc herniations treated conservatively. *Neuroradiology* 1995; 37:378–383.

Matthews JA, Hickling J. Lumbar traction: a double-blind controlled study for sciatica. *Rheumatol Rehab* 1975; 14:222–225.

McCombe PF, Fairbank JCT, Cockersole BC, Punsent PB. Reproducibility of physical signs in low-back pain. *Spine* 1989;14:908–918.

McQuay HJ, Moore A. Epidural steroids for sciatica. *Anaesth Intensive Care* 1996; 24:284–286.

Merskey H, Bogduk N (Eds). *Classification of Chronic Pain: Descriptions of Chronic Pain Syndromes and Definitions of Pain Terms,* 2nd ed. Seattle: IASP Press, 1994.

Morris EW, Di Paola M, Vallance R, Waddell G. Diagnosis and decision making in lumbar disc prolapse and nerve entrapment. *Spine* 1986; 11:436–439.

Nelson MA, Allen P, Clamp SE, de Dombal FT. Reliability and reproducibility of clinical findings in low-back pain. *Spine* 1979; 4:97–101.

Norlen G. On the value of the neurological symptoms in sciatica for the localization of a lumbar disc herniation. *Acta Chir Scand* 1944; 95(Suppl):1–96.

Olmarker K. Mechanical and biochemical injury of spinal nerve roots: an experimental perspective. In: Weinstein JN, Gordon SL (Eds). *Low Back Pain: A Scientific and Clinical Overview.* Rosemont, IL: American Academy of Orthopaedic Surgeons, 1996, pp 215–233.

Pal B, Mangion P, Hossain MA, Diffey BL. A controlled trial of continuous lumbar traction in the treatment of back pain and sciatica. *Br J Rheumatol* 1986; 25:181–183.

Riew KD, Yin Y, Gilula L, et al. The effect of nerve-root injections on the need for operative treatment of lumbar radicular pain: a prospective, randomized, controlled, double-blind study. *J Bone Joint Surg* 2000; 82A:1589–1593.

Saal JA. Natural history and nonoperative treatment of lumbar disc herniation. *Spine* 1996; 21(Suppl 24S):2S–9S.

Saal JA, Saal JS, Herzog RJ. The natural history of lumbar intervertebral disc extrusions treated nonoperatively. *Spine* 1990; 15:683–686.

Smyth MJ, Wright V. Sciatica and the intervertebral disc: an experimental study. *J Bone Joint Surg* 1959; 40A:1401–1418.

Spangfort EV. The lumbar disc herniation: a computer-aided analysis of 2,504 operations. *Acta Orthop Scand* 1972; (Suppl 142).

Thelander U, Fagerlund M, Friberg S, Larsson S. Straight leg raising test versus radiological size, shape, and position of lumbar disc hernias. *Spine* 1992; 17:395–399.

Vad VB, Bhat AL, Lutz GE, Cammisa F. Transforaminal epidural steroid injections in lumbosacral radiculopathy. *Spine* 2002; 27:11–16.

Vroomen PCAJ, de Krom CTFM, Wilmink JT, Kester ADM, Andre KJ. Lack of effectiveness of bed rest for sciatica. *N Engl J Med* 1999; 340:418–423.

Waddell G, Gibson JNA, Grant I. Surgical treatment of lumbar disc prolapse and degenerative lumbar disc disease. In: Nachemson A, Jonsson E (Eds). *Neck and Back Pain: The Scientific Evidence of Causes, Diagnosis, and Treatment.* Philadelphia: Lippincott, Williams & Wilkins, 2000, pp 305–325.

Watts RW, Silagy CA. A meta-analysis on the efficacy of epidural steroids in the treatment of sciatica. *Anaesth Intensive Care* 1995; 23:564–569.

Weber H, Holme I, Amlie E. The natural course of acute sciatica with nerve root symptoms in a double-blind placebo-controlled trial evaluating the effect of piroxicam. *Spine* 1993; 18:1433–1438.

Wiesel SW. A study of computer- assisted tomography. 1. The incidence of positive CAT scans in an asymptomatic group of patients. *Spine* 1986; 9:549–551.

Core Curriculum for Professional Education in Pain, edited by J. Edmond Charlton, IASP Press, Seattle, © 2005.

31

Low Back Pain

I. Know the structure of the lumbar spine and sacrum, and understand how they normally operate.

   A. Know the component parts of the lumbar vertebrae and the structure of the intervertebral disks and zygapophysial joints (Bogduk 1997, Chapters 1–4).

   B. Appreciate the disposition, actions and functions of the paravertebral muscles of the lumbar spine (Bogduk 1997, Chapter 9).

   C. Know the innervation of the bones, disks, joints, ligaments, muscles, and dura mater of the lumbar spine (Bogduk 1997, Chapter 10).

   D. Understand how the lumbar spine moves (Bogduk 1997, Chapter 8).

   E. Understand the function of the sacroiliac joint (Bogduk 1997, Chapter 14).

II. Appreciate the limitations of evidence concerning the possible causes of acute low back pain, and the controversial status of causes of chronic low back pain. Be able to explain the reason for this (Bogduk 1997, Chapter 15; Nachemson and Jonsson 2000, Chapter 7; Bogduk and McGuirk 2002, Chapters 3, 14).

III. Understand, and be able to explain, how back pain and somatic referred pain differ from radicular pain, radiculopathy, and sciatica (Merskey and Bogduk 1994). Understand how the investigation and treatment of these conditions differ, and how they are subject to totally different bases of evidence.

IV. Understand the lack of validity of diagnostic labels commonly applied to acute and chronic low back pain. Be aware of the evidence that refutes instability and radiographic diagnoses such as spondylosis, spondylolisthesis, and congenital anomalies as causes of back pain. Be able to apply diagnostic labels according to recommended criteria (Merskey and Bogduk 1994; Bogduk 2000; Nachemson and Jonsson 2000, Chapter 7; Bogduk and McGuirk 2002, Chapters 3, 14).

V. Be able to obtain a comprehensive history of low back pain. Appreciate the significance and utility of history in the assessment of patients with low back pain (Nachemson and Jonsson 2000, Chapter 9; Bogduk and McGuirk 2002, Chapters 6 and 15).

VI. Appreciate the lack of reliability and validity of physical examination in the assessment of patients with low back pain (Nachemson and Jonsson 2000, Chapter 9; Bogduk and McGuirk 2002, Chapter 7).

VII. Be able to perform a valid assessment of psychosocial factors pertinent to the management of low back pain (Waddell et al. 1980, 1993; Main et al. 1992, 1998; Fishbain et al. 1995, 1999; Keefe et al. 1999).

VIII. Appreciate the lack of validity of conventional medical imaging in the assessment of low back pain (Bogduk and McGuirk 2002, Chapter 8).

IX. Understand the rationale for invasive tests such as diagnostic joint blocks and diskography for the investigation of low back pain, and be aware of both the evidence for these procedures and the basis for controversies concerning them (Nachemson and Jonsson 2000, Chapter 9; Bogduk and McGuirk 2002, Chapters 19, 20).

X. Understand the natural history of acute low back pain back pain (Nachemson and Jonsson 2000, Chapter 8; Bogduk and McGuirk 2002, Chapter 4).

XI.   Appreciate the differences between, and the clinical significance and utility of etiological risk factors and prognostic risk factors for low back pain (Nachemson and Jonsson 2000, Chapters 2, 4; Bogduk and McGuirk 2002, Chapter 5).

XII. Understand the significance of psychosocial and occupational factors associated with complaints of low back pain and its chronicity (Nachemson and Jonsson 2000, Chapters 3, 5).

XIII. Appreciate the lack of any proven or demonstrated physiological basis for commonly used interventions for low back pain (Bogduk and Mercer 1995).

XIV. Be aware of the cardinal evidence for the efficacy, or lack thereof, of interventions commonly used for acute low back pain and for chronic low back pain (Indahl et al. 1995, 1998; Turner et al. 1995; Loisel et al. 1997; Waddell et al. 1997; Cherkin et al. 1998; van Tulder et al. 1997, 1999, 2000a, 2000b; Morley et al. 1999; Nachemson and Johnson 2000, Chapters 11, 12; Bogduk and McGuirk 2002, Chapters 11, 12, 17, 18, 21, 22; Guzman et al. 2001; Nelemans et al, 2001; McGuirk et al. 2001), such as:

A. Bed rest

B. Staying active

C. Drugs

D. Exercises

E. Manual therapy

F. Acupuncture

G. Belts and corsets

H. Traction

I. TENS

J. Massage

K. Biofeedback

L. Hydrotherapy

M. Back school

N. Patient education

O. Behavioral therapy

P. Multidisciplinary therapy

Q. Functional restoration

R. Workplace intervention

S. Injections, including:

   1. Epidural steroids
   2. Prolotherapy
   3. Trigger point injections
   4. Botulinum toxin

T. Intra-articular steroids

U. Spinal cord stimulation

V. Intraspinal opioids

XV. Understand the reasons for the limited efficacy of surgical treatment of low back pain (Turner et al. 1992; Gibson et al. 1999; Nachemson and Jonsson 2000, Chapter 13; Bogduk and McGuirk 2002, Chapters 17, 21), in terms of:

A. Valid and non-valid indications

B. Appropriate and inappropriate procedures

C. Complications and side effects

XVI. Be aware of the evidence concerning the rationale and efficacy of medial branch neurotomy and intradiskal therapies for low back pain (Bogduk and McGuirk 2002, Chapter 21).XVII. Understand the utility and limitations of multidisciplinary therapy for chronic low back pain (Morley et al. 1999; Guzman et al. 2001; Bogduk and McGuirk 2002, Chapter 18).

A. Ensure the patient has a clear understanding of the reason(s) for any diagnostic test or procedure and the likely benefit to be derived. Where there is no evidence base to indicate likely benefit, the patient should be made aware of this.

B. Be aware that the outcome of any treatment should be assessed by more than one method if appropriate.

REFERENCES

Bogduk N. *Clinical Anatomy of the Lumbar Spine and Sacrum,* 3rd ed. Edinburgh: Churchill Livingstone, 1997.

Bogduk N. What's in a name? The labelling of back pain. *Med J Aust* 2000; 173:400–401.

Bogduk N, McGuirk B. *Medical Management of Acute and Chronic Low Back Pain: An Evidence-Based Approach.* Amsterdam: Elsevier, 2002.

Bogduk N, Mercer S. Selection and application of treatment. In: Refshauge KM, Gass EM (Eds). *Musculoskeletal Physiotherapy: Clinical Science and Practice.* Oxford: Butterworth Heinemann, 1995, pp 169–181.

Cherkin DC, Deyo RA, Battie M, Street J, Barlow W. A comparison of physical therapy, chiropractic manipulation, and provision of an educational booklet for the treatment of patients with low back pain. *N Engl J Med* 1998; 339:1021–1029.

Fishbain DA, Rosomoff HL, Cutler RB, Rosomoff RS. Secondary gain concept: a review of the scientific evidence. *Clin J Pain* 1995; 11:6–21.

Fishbain DA, Cutler R, Rosomoff HL, Rosomoff RS. Chronic pain disability: exaggeration/malingering and submaximal effort research. *Clin J Pain* 1999; 15:244–274.

Gibson JNA, Grant IC, Waddell G. The Cochrane review of surgery for lumbar disc prolapse and degenerative lumbar spondylosis. *Spine* 1999; 24:1820–1832.

Guzman J, Esmail R, Karjalainen K, et al. Multidisciplinary rehabilitation for chronic back pain: systematic review. *BMJ* 2001; 322:1511–1516.

Indahl A, Velund L, Reikeraas O. Good prognosis for low back pain when left untampered: a randomized clinical trial. *Spine* 1995; 20:473–477.

Indahl A, Haldorsen EH, Holm S, Reikeras O, Ursin H. Five-year follow-up study of a controlled clinical trial using light mobilization and an informative approach to low back pain. *Spine* 1998; 23:2625–2630.

Keefe, FJ, Bradley LA, Main CJ. Psychological assessment of the pain patient for the general clinician. In: Max M (Ed). *Pain 1999—An Updated Review: Refresher Course Syllabus.* Seattle: IASP Press, 1999, pp 219–230.

Loisel P, Abenhaim L, Durand P, et al. A population-based, randomized clinical trial on back pain management. *Spine* 1997; 22:2911–2918.

Main CJ, Wood PLR, Hollis S, Spanswick CC, Waddell G. The distress and risk assessment method: a simple patient classification to identify distress and evaluate the risk of poor outcome. *Spine* 1992; 17:42–52.

Main CJ, Waddell G. Spine Update. Behavioral responses to examination: a reappraisal of the interpretation of "nonorganic signs." *Spine* 1998; 23:2367–2371.

McGuirk B, King W, Govind J, Lowry J, Bogduk N. The safety, efficacy, and cost-effectiveness of evidence-based guidelines for the management of acute low back pain in primary care. *Spine* 2001; 26:2615–2622.

Merskey H, Bogduk N (Eds). *Classification of Chronic Pain. Descriptions of Chronic Pain Syndromes and Definitions of Pain Terms,* 2nd ed. Seattle: IASP Press, 1994.

Morley S, Eccleston C, Williams A. Systematic review and meta-analysis of randomized controlled trials of cognitive behaviour therapy and behaviour therapy for chronic pain in adults, excluding headache. *Pain* 1999; 80:1013.

Nachemson A, Jonsson E (Eds). *Neck and Back Pain: The Scientific Evidence of Causes, Diagnosis, and Treatment.* Philadelphia: Lippincott, Williams and Wilkins, 2000.

Nelemans PJ, de Bie RA, deVet HCW, Sturmans F. Injection therapy for subacute and chronic benign low back pain. *Spine* 2001; 26:501–515.

Turner JA, Ersek M, Herron L, et al. Patient outcomes after lumbar spinal fusions. *JAMA* 1992; 268:907–911.

Turner JA, Loeser JD, Bell KG. Spinal cord stimulation for chronic low back pain: a systematic literature synthesis. *Neurosurgery* 1995; 37:1088–1096.

van Tulder MW, Koes BW, Bouter LM. Conservative treatment of acute and chronic nonspecific low back pain: a systematic review of randomized controlled trials of the most common interventions. *Spine* 1997; 22:2128–2156.

van Tulder MW, Cherkin DC, Berman B, Lao L, Koes BW. The effectiveness of acupuncture in the management of acute and chronic low back pain: a systematic review within the framework of the Cochrane Collaboration Back Review Group. *Spine* 1999; 24:1113–1123.

van Tulder MW, Ostelo R, Vlaeyen JWS, et al. Behavioral treatment for chronic back pain: a systematic review within the framework of the Cochrane Collaboration Back Review Group. *Spine* 2000a; 25:2688–2699.

van Tulder M, Malmivaara A, Esmail R, Koes B. Exercise therapy for low back pain: a systematic review within the framework of the Cochrane Collaboration Back Review Group. *Spine* 2000b; 21:2784–2796.

Waddell G, McCulloch JA, Kummel E, Venner RM. Nonorganic physical signs in low-back pain. *Spine* 1980; 5:117–125.

Waddell G, Newton M, Henderson I, Somerville D, Main CJ. A fear-avoidance beliefs questionnaire (FABQ) and the role of fear-avoidance beliefs in chronic low back pain and disability. *Pain* 1993;52:157–168.

Waddell G, Feder G, Lewis M. Systematic reviews of bed rest and advice to stay active for acute low back pain. *Br J Gen Pract* 1997; 47:647–652.

Core Curriculum for Professional Education in Pain, edited by J. Edmond Charlton, IASP Press, Seattle, © 2005.

32

Musculoskeletal Pain

I.   Epidemiology

   A.   Know that musculoskeletal pain is common, affects all age groups, and frequency increases with age (Kvien et al. 2003).

   B.   Know that musculoskeletal pain is a major cause of morbidity and health care costs. In particular, chronic musculoskeletal pain, often in association with rheumatic disease, is a major cause of disability (Reginster and Khaltaev 2002).

   C.   Know that there are gender differences among types and frequencies of musculoskeletal pain (Badley 2001).

   D.   Know that there are ethnic and gender disparities in health care access and treatment given (Edwards et al. 2001; Epstein and Ayanian 2001).

   E.   Know that musculoskeletal pain may be assessed and managed by multiple biomedical specialties including anesthesiology, occupational medicine, orthopedics, pain medicine, rehabilitation medicine, rheumatology, and sports medicine, with important implications for patient diagnosis and management.

   F.   Be aware that musculoskeletal pain also may be assessed and managed by a variety of nonmedical disciplines without reference to medically trained specialists, with important implications for patient diagnosis and management.

II.   Anatomy and physiology of the musculoskeletal system (Bendele 2002)

   A.   Know basic facts about collagen, elastin and adhesins, proteoglycans, and cartilage matrix turnover, degradation, and repair.

   B.   Know types and composition of bone.

   C.   Know classification of joints, and characteristics of major tissues comprising a diarthrodial (synovial) joint (hyaline cartilage, capsule, synovium/synovial fluid, and menisci).

   D.   Know the anatomy and function of ligaments and tendons, and the nature of the enthesis.

   E.   Know the anatomy and physiology of muscle(s).

III.   Mediators of inflammation, tissue destruction and repair (Calixto et al. 2000; Sutherland et al. 2000; De Leo and Yezierski 2001; Kidd and Urban 2001; Woolley 2003)

   A.   Know basic facts about cellular constituents: neutrophils, macrophages, mast cells, and platelets.

   B.   Know basic facts about growth factors and cytokines: colony-stimulating factors, growth and differentiation factors, immunoregulatory cytokines, proinflammatory cytokines, and regulation of cytokine effects.

   C.   Know basic facts about the complement system: classical and alternative pathways, complement receptors, and the nature of immune complexes.

   D.   Know basic facts about proteinases and their inhibitors, in particular metalloproteinases.

E. Know the essential nature and function of arachidonic acid derivatives, kinins, clotting factors, amines, nitric oxide, and reactive oxygen species.

IV. Molecular and cellular basis of immunity (Levite 2001; Parkin and Cohen 2001)

A. Know basic facts on antigens, antigen-presenting cells, and major histocompatibility complex (MHC) molecules, recognition of antigen by T cells, immunoglobulins and B cells, and immunoregulation in cytokines.

B. Know basic facts on immunogenetics, in particular human leukocyte antigen (HLA) association with rheumatic diseases.

C. Know basic facts on neuroendocrine influences, especially the hypothalamus-pituitary-adrenal (HPA)-gonadal axis and sex steroid influences on the immune response (Lariviere and Melzack 2000; Davidson and Diamond 2001; Straub and Cutulo 2001).

D. Know basic mechanisms of autoimmunity: self versus non-self.

E. Know that there is an emerging broad based discipline of psychoneuroimmunology (Haigh et al. 2003).

V. Anatomy and biomechanics of joints and muscles (Riley 2004)

A. Upper limbs: shoulder and arm, elbow and forearm, hand and wrist.

B. Lower limbs: hip and thigh, knee and leg, foot and ankle.

C. Spine: bones and joints, ligaments and soft tissues including intervertebral disks, muscles, nerves, and blood vessels, and sacroiliac joints.

VI. Neurophysiology of musculoskeletal pain

A. Know basic facts about peripheral receptors in relation to nociception, touch, pressure, cold, and warmth. (Costigan and Woolf 2000; Julius and Basbaum 2001; Felson et al. 2003; Jordt et al. 2003; Niv et al. 2003).

B. Be familiar with the afferent and spinal mechanisms of joint and muscle pain, including the role of descending inhibitory/facilitatory pathways from brain to spinal cord (Porreca et al. 2002; Ren and Dubner 2002; Price et al. 2003; Ru-Rong et al. 2003; Fields et al. 2005).

C. Know principles of the interactions of pain and the neuroimmune system, and understand that efferent neuronal mechanisms may contribute to joint inflammation (Schaible et al. 2002).

D. Know about the concept of neuroplasticity and the range of evidence underpinning it, in particular the nature and mechanisms of central neural sensitization (Honore et al. 2000; Watkins et al. 2001).

E. Know basic facts regarding the interaction of the sympathetic and parasympathetic nervous systems with nociception (Hogg and McLachlan 2002).

F. Know that inflammatory mediators, including neuropeptides and cytokines, are involved in the generation and persistence of inflammatory causes of musculoskeletal pain (Calixto et al. 2000; Kidd and Urban 2001; Schaible et al. 2002).

G. Be aware that pain from muscle and/or joint pathology may be referred to other structures, and know about the possible neurophysiological mechanisms of referral of pain (Arendt-Nielsen et al. 2000).

VII. Psychosocial aspects of musculoskeletal pain/disability

A. Know that personal, social and cultural influences, past and/or present, may play a significant role in the initiation, persistence, and treatment responsiveness or nonresponsiveness of musculoskeletal pain and disability.

B. Be aware of the profound effects of chronic pain on the patient (Vlaeyen and Linton 2000; Craig 2003; Greenwood et al. 2003; McCracken et al. 2004).

C. Know the role of psychiatric disorders associated with musculoskeletal pain, in relation to diatheses/stress (Woolfe 2002).

D. Know what illness behaviors are, their potential involvement in musculoskeletal pain and disability, and the implications for management.

VIII. Classification and clinical characteristics of musculoskeletal diseases

A. Recognize that there are three major groupings of musculoskeletal disease with specific clinical features and pain manifestations:

1. Inflammatory joint/muscle diseases
2. Noninflammatory joint/muscle disorders
3. Soft tissue, in particular muscle, ligament, tendon, and bursal disorders

B. Know, in the context of musculoskeletal pain, about fractures (know basic classification including stress fracture, also slipped epiphysis disorders), intra-articular mechanical derangements (such as meniscal tear, ligament rupture, loose body/bodies), infection (such as osteomyelitis and joint infection), and malignancy (know the basic classification of bone tumors with age incidence and likely bone sites) (Lew and Waldvogel 2004).

C. Be familiar with the common joint diseases (arthropathies) with or without spinal involvement: infectious arthritis, crystal arthritis (gout, pseudogout), rheumatic fever, osteoarthritis, rheumatoid arthritis, seronegative spondyloarthropathy (such as ankylosing spondylitis, reactive arthritis, inflammatory arthritis associated with ulcerative colitis and Crohn's disease), and polymyalgia rheumatica/temporal arteritis (giant cell arteritis). Know the different patterns of joint involvement in these common arthropathies, characteristic associated soft tissue abnormalities, common types of involvement of other organ systems (in particular the skin, nails, mucosa, eyes, and gastrointestinal and genitourinary systems) (Lee and Weinblatt 2001; Salvarani et al. 2002; Stafford and Youssef 2002; Underwood 2004).

D. Know that arthropathies manifest differently in children from adults, such that pediatric rheumatology is a speciality in its own right. Be aware of joint hypermobility syndrome in children and adults, and its complex interrelationship with joint pain and disability (Grahame 2001; Fitzcharles 2002).

E. Know the major research in relation to pathogenesis, diagnosis, and management of CRPS (complex regional pain syndrome) type I (reflex sympathetic dystrophy in the old nomenclature), and in particular the distinction between sympathetically maintained pain (SMP) and non-SMP along with the implications for management (Birklein and Handwerker 2001; Jänig and Baron 2002, 2003, 2004; Wasner et al. 2003; Stanton-Hicks 2003).

F. Know the nature and the principles of how to diagnose and manage the bone disorders of osteoporosis, osteomalacia, and Paget's disease (Wong et al. 2003).

G. Know the main rheumatic manifestations of malignant diseases, endocrine disorders such as hypothyroidism, HIV, and the principles of how to diagnose and manage these.

H. Know the nature and the principles of how to diagnose and manage acute compartment syndromes, fasciitis (especially necrotizing fasciitis), panniculitis, osteochondritis dissecans, osteonecrosis, and myositis ossificans progressiva (Buchbinder 2004).

I. Be familiar with the concepts and controversies generated by basic and clinical research relating to the pathogenesis, diagnosis and management of regional nonspecific pain syndromes (in which no specific pathology is identifiable), in particular myofascial pain syndromes, and widespread nonspecific musculoskeletal pain. Know that widespread nonspecific musculoskeletal pain may be associated with other pain disorders such as migraine and/or other headaches, irritable bowel or bladder syndrome, and dysmenorrhea, and be aware of the increasing evidence to suggest that the pathophysiology in relation to these disorders may be based fundamentally on a central neural sensitization disorder, i.e., an abnormality of central pain modulation (Arendt-Nielsen and Graven-Nielsen 2003; Flor 2003; Graven-Nielsen and Arendt-Nielsen 2003; Henriksson 2003; Staud et al. 2003a,b; Banic et al. 2004; Smythe 2004).

IX.   Assessment of rheumatic disease activity and severity

A. Know the GALS (gait, arms, legs, spine) locomotor screening questions and physical examination (Doherty et al. 1992; Coady et al. 2004).

B. Be able to recognize on observation joint swelling/deformity, muscle wasting, certain soft tissue pathologies. Be able to assess on examination joint tenderness, range of motion, swelling related to joints, muscle strength, muscle tenderness, muscle tone, ligament/tendon/bursal inflammation and/or structural changes, and skin color, temperature, and texture changes, and be able to recognize specific rashes such as psoriasis (Treede et al. 2002; Sarlani and Greenspan 2003).

C. Know how joint fluid aspiration and laboratory analysis may help distinguish between various causes of inflammation.

D. Know how to use laboratory analysis of blood (in particular hematology, biochemistry, microbiology, and immunology), urine, microbiological investigations of skin and body orifices, targeted tissue biopsies (such as urgent temporal artery biopsy for the diagnosis of temporal arteritis/giant cell arteritis, or muscle biopsy for the diagnosis of polymyositis/dermatomyositis), to identify specific rheumatic and/or systemic diseases, and know the possible role of arthroscopy. Be aware of the indications for referral for neurophysiological studies such as nerve conduction studies and electromyography. Know how to use acute-phase reactants (e.g. erythrocyte sedimentation rate, C-reactive protein) to monitor inflammatory disease activity (Paulus and Brahn 2004).

E. Be aware of the principles of the radiographic recognition of abnormal bones and joints, and be familiar with the range of organ-imaging techniques such as plain radiography, ultrasound, scintigraphy, CT, MRI, along with their relevance to musculoskeletal disease diagnosis and monitoring, and the use of bone densitometry to assess osteopenia (osteoporosis).

F. Understand that multiple instruments are available to evaluate and quantify different aspects of musculoskeletal disease (Scott et al. 2003), in particular:

1. Joint counts
2. Measures of function and activities of daily living (ADL)
3. Multidimensional health status instruments: arthritis impact measurement scales (AIMS) and the health assessment questionnaire (HAQ)

G. Know that pain is one of the main concerns of patients with arthritis: self-reported pain has been recommended as a core end-point measure in rheumatoid arthritis, and it is sensitive to change in arthritis activity (Minnock et al. 2003).

H. Know the types of clinical research designs (evidence-based medicine) and controversies related to these (Kvien et al. 2003; Pillemer and Tilley 2004).

X.   Treatment and rehabilitation of musculoskeletal pain/disability

A. Know the situations in which orthopedic surgical referral (such as urgent surgery for cauda equina syndrome or osteomyelitis/septic arthritis) may be required (Felson and Buckwalter 2002).

B. Know the role of local pain control measures, i.e. heat, cold, anti-inflammatory/analgesic ointments/cream application, intra-articular steroid injections with indications and contraindications, splints, passive and active movements, and massage techniques.

C. Know that there are spinal treatment techniques that may influence referred pain, such as mobilization/manipulation techniques (Fitzcharles 2002).

D. Be aware of the risks and benefits of rest and exercise (Jones and Killian 2000; Penninx et al. 2001; Pool and Axford 2001; Cotman and Berchtold 2002; Stenstrom and Minor 2003).

E. Understand the possible role of medications in musculoskeletal pain relief. Be aware that in addition to systemic pharmacology there is the possibility of local application of medication (Sawynok 2003). Know the indications, routes of administration, dose and time scheduling, and adverse effects of:

1. Simple analgesics (Altman 2004)
2. Anti-inflammatory agents: NSAIDs (including COX-2-selective inhibitors) and colchicine (Fitzgerald and Patrono 2001)
3. Corticosteroids
4. Sulfasalazine, methotrexate, leflunomide, antimalarials, and gold (O'Dell 2004)
5. Azathioprine, cyclophosphamide, and cyclosporin
6. TNF-alpha-blocking agents (Pincus et al. 2002; Olsen and Stein 2004)
7. Intra-articular hyaluronan (in joint osteoarthritis), intra-articular osmic acid and radioactive yttrium (in selected persistent noninfective synovitis) (Simkin 2000)
8. Psychotropic agents as potential pain-modulating medications
9. Membrane-stabilizing agents as potential pain-modulating medications (Vanegas and Schaible 2000)
10. Be aware of the probable importance of NMDA receptor blockade as a potential advance in analgesia (Neugebauer 2002; Mayo 2002; Scholz and Woolf 2002)
11. Opioids, noting the ongoing controversy in relation to their role in the management of chronic non malignant pain (Peloso 2001; Ballantyne and Mao 2003; von Korff and Deyo 2004)
12. Complementary and alternative medicine (Ernst 2004; Long 2001; White 2003)

F. Know the principles of management of significant osteopenia (Strewler 2004).

G. Recognize that a specific rheumatic disease, such as osteoarthritis or rheumatoid arthritis, may be associated with regional or widespread musculoskeletal pain of greater severity or extent than expected, identifiable by marked and/or extensive clinical tenderness within or outside the area of pain, indicating the presence of hyperalgesia/allodynia, which may complicate diagnosis and management. Know the clinical literature suggesting that a central neural sensitization disorder may be an important aspect of the pathophysiology in this situation (Sarkar et al. 2000; Mailis et al. 2001; Mailis-Gagnon et al. 2003).

H. Know the situations in which referral to an anesthesiologist may be required to consider spinal or other injection techniques (e.g., stellate ganglion block), diagnostic or therapeutic (Cousins and Bridenbaugh 1999; Schwartzmann 2000).

I. Know the range of nerve stimulation techniques, in particular acupuncture (dry needling), transcutaneous nerve stimulation (TNS), and spinal cord stimulation (SCS), with indications and likely mode(s) of action in pain relief (Ernst 2004).

J. Understand that musculoskeletal pain/disability management usually requires multidisciplinary team management, with an emphasis on patient education and self-management, and the circumstances in which input from a physiotherapist, occupational therapist, nurse, and psychologist may be required. Be aware that community support services are often important, with particular emphasis on the coordinating role of the family practitioner (Hadler 2001; Villemure and Bushnell 2002; Sharpe et al. 2003).

K. Be aware of recent research that raises the possibility of preventing the development of chronic musculoskeletal pain and disability.

REFERENCES

Arendt-Nielsen L, Laursen RJ, Drewes AM. Referred pain as an indicator for neural plasticity. In: Sandkuhler J, Bromm B, Gebhart GF (Eds). *Nervous System Plasticity and Chronic Pain*, Progress in Brain Research, Vol. 129. Amsterdam: Elsevier, 2000, pp 343–356.

Arendt-Nielsen L, Graven-Nielsen T. Central sensitisation in fibromyalgia and other musculoskeletal disorders. *Curr Pain Headache Rep* 2003; 7:355–361.

Altman RD. Pain relief in osteoarthritis: the rationale for combination therapy. *J Rheumatol* 2004; 31:5–7.

Badley ME. Gender differences in access and use of healthcare services. *J Rheumatol* 2001; 28:2145–2146.

Ballantyne JC, Mao J. Opioid therapy for chronic pain. *N Engl J Med* 2003; 349:1943–1953.

Banic B, Petersen-Felix S, Anderson OK, et al. Evidence for spinal cord hypersensitivity in chronic pain after whiplash injury and in fibromyalgia. *Pain* 2004; 107:7–15.

Bendele AM. Animal models of osteoarthritis in an era of molecular biology. *J Musculoskelet Neuronal Interact* 2002; 2:501–503.

Birklein F, Handwerker HO. Complex regional pain syndrome (CRPS): how to resolve the complexity? *Pain* 2001; 94:1–6.

Buchbinder R. Plantar fasciitis. *N Engl J Med* 2004; 350:2159–2166.

Calixto JB, Cabrini DA, Ferreira J, Campos MM. Kinins in pain and inflammation. *Pain* 2000; 87:1–5.

Coady D, Walker D, Kay L. Regional examination of the musculoskeletal system (REMS): a core set of clinical skills for medical students. *Rheumatology* 2004; 43:633–639.

Costigan M, Woolf CJ. Pain: molecular mechanisms. *J Pain* 2000; 1:35–44.

Cotman CW, Berchtold NC. Exercise: a behavioural intervention to enhance brain health and plasticity. *Trends Neurosci* 2002; 25:295–301.

Cousins MJ, Bridenbaugh PO (Eds). *Neural Blockade in Clinical Anesthesia and Management of Pain*, 3rd ed. Philadelphia: Lippincott-Raven.

Craig AD. A new view of pain as a homeostatic emotion. *Trends Neurosci* 2003; 26:303–307.

Davidson A, Diamond B. Autoimmune diseases. *N Engl J Med* 2001; 345:340–350.

De Leo JA, Yerzierski RP. The role of neuroinflammation and neuroimmune activation in persistent pain. *Pain* 2001; 90:1–6.

Doherty M, Dacre J, Dieppe P, Snaith M. The GALS (gait, arms, legs, spine) locomotor screen. *Ann Rheum Dis* 1992; 51:1165–1169.

Edwards CL, Fillingim RB, Keefe E. Race, ethnicity in pain. *Pain* 2001; 94:133–137.

Epstein AM, Ayanian JZ. Racial disparities in medical care. *N Engl J Med* 2001; 344:1471–1473.

Ernst E. Acupuncture: who is missing the point? *Pain* 2004; 109:203–204.

Felson DT, Buckwalter J. Debridement and lavage for osteoarthritis of the knee. *N Engl J Med* 2002; 347:132–133.

Felson DT, McLaughlin S, Goggins J, et al. Bone marrow edema and its relation to progression of knee osteoarthritis. *Ann Intern Med* 2003; 139:330–336.

Fields HL, Basbaum AI, Heinricher M. Central nervous system mechanisms of pain modulation. In: McMahon S, Koltzenburg M (Eds). *Wall and Melzack's Textbook of Pain*, 5th ed. Churchill Livingstone, 2005.

Fitzcharles MA. Is it time for rheumatologists to rethink the use of manual therapies? *J Rheumatol* 2002; 29:1117–1120.

Fitzgerald GA, Patrono C. The coxibs, selective inhibitors of cyclooxygenase-2. *N Engl J Med* 2001; 345:433–442.

Flor HJ. Cortical reorganisation and chronic pain: implications for rehabilitation. *J Rehabil Med* 2003; (41 Suppl):S66–S72.

Grahame R. Time to take hypermobility seriously (in adults and children). *Rheumatology* 2001; 40:485–487.

Graven-Nielsen T, Arendt-Nielsen L. Induction and assessment of muscle pain, referred pain, and muscular hyperalgesia. *Curr Pain Headache Rep* 2003; 7:443–451.

Greenwood KA, Thurston R, Rumble M, Walters SJ, Keefe FJ. Anger and persistent pain: current status and future direction. *Pain* 2003; 103:1–5.

Hadler NM. Rheumatology and the health of the workforce. *Arthitis Rheum* 2001; 44:1971–1974.

Haigh RC, McCabe CS, Halligan PW, Blake DR. Joint stiffness in a phantom limb: evidence of central nervous system involvement in rheumatoid arthritis. *Rheumatology (Oxford)* 2003; 42:888–892.

Henriksson KG. Hypersensitivity in muscle pain syndromes. *Curr Pain Headache Rep* 2003; 7:426–432.

Hogg PJ, McLachlan EM. Blood vessels and nerves: together or not? *Lancet* 2002; 360:1714.

Honore P, Menning PN, Rogers SD, et al. Neurochemical plasticity in persistent inflammatory pain. *Prog Brain Res* 2000; 129:357–363.

Jänig W, Baron R. Complex regional pain syndrome is a disease of the central nervous system. *Clin Auton Res* 2002; 12:150–164.

Jänig W, Baron R. Complex regional pain syndrome: mystery explained? *Lancet Neurol* 2003; 2:987–697.

Jänig W, Baron R. Experimental approach to complex regional pain syndrome (CRPS). *Pain* 2004; 108:3–7.

Jones NL, Killian KJ. Exercise limitation in health and disease. *N Engl J Med* 2000; 343:632–641.

Jordt SE, McKemy DD, Julius D. Lessons from peppers and peppermint: the molecular logic of thermosensation. *Curr Opin Neurobiol* 2003; 13:487–492.

Julius D, Basbaum AI. Molecular mechanisms of nociception. *Nature* 2001; 413:203–210.

Kidd BL, Urban LA. Mechanisms of inflammatory pain. *Br J Anaesth* 2001; 87:3–11.

Kvien TK, Mikkelsen K, Nordvag B-Y. Results from controlled clinical trials: how relevant for clinical practice? *J Rheumatol* 2003; 30:1135–1137.

Lariviere WR, Melzack R. The role of corticotropin releasing factor in pain and analgesia. *Pain* 2000; 84:1–12.

Lee DM, Weinblatt ME. Rheumatoid arthritis. *Lancet* 2001; 358:903–911.

Levite M. Nervous immunity: neurotransmitters, extracellular potassium and T-cell function. *Trends Immunol* 2001; 22:2–5.

Lew DP, Waldvogel FA. Osteomyelitis. *Lancet* 2004; 364:369–379.

Long L. Complementary therapies for osteoarthritis. *Focus Altern Comp Ther (FACT)* 2001; 6:103–107.

Mailis A, Papagapiou M, Umana M, et al. Unexplainable nondermatomal somatosensory deficits in patients with chronic non-malignant pain in the context of litigation/compensation: a role for involvement of central factors? *J Rheumatol* 2001; 28:1385–1393.

Mailis-Gagnon A, Giannoylis I, Downar J, et al. Altered central somatosensory processing in chronic pain patients with "hysterical" anaesthesia. *Neurology* 2003; 60:1501–1507.

Mayo J. Translational pain research: bridging the gap between basic and clinical research (example of NMDA receptor research). *Pain* 2002; 97:183–187.

McCracken LM, Carson JW, Eccleston C, Keefe FJ. Acceptance and change in the context of chronic pain. *Pain* 2004; 109:4–7.

Minnock P, Fitzgerald O, Bresnihan B. Women with established rheumatoid arthritis perceive pain as the predominant impairment of health status. *Rheumatology* 2003; 42:995–1000.

Neugebauer V. Metabotropic glutamate receptors—important modulators of nociception and pain behaviour. *Pain* 2002; 98:1–8.

Niv D, Gofeld M, Devor M. Causes of pain in degenerative bone and joint disease: a lesson from vertebroplasty. *Pain* 2003; 105:387–392.

O'Dell JR. Therapeutic strategies for rheumatoid arthritis. *N Engl J Med* 2004; 350:2591–2602.

Olsen NJ, Stein CM. New drugs for rheumatoid arthritis. *N Engl J Med* 2004; 350:2167–2179.

Parkin J, Cohen B. An overview of the immune system. *Lancet* 2001; 357:1777–1789.

Paulus HE, Brahn E. Is erythrocyte sedimentation rate the preferable measure of the acute phase response in rheumatoid arthritis? *J Rheumatol* 2004; 31:838–840.

Peloso PM. Opioid therapy for osteoarthritis of the hip and knee: use it or lose it? *J Rheumatol* 2001; 28:6–11.

Penninx BW, Messier SP, Rejeski WJ. Physical exercise and the prevention of disability in activities of daily living on older persons with osteoarthritis. *Arch Intern Med* 2001; 161:2309–2316.

Pillemer SR, Tilley B. Clinical trials, outcome measures, and response criteria. *J Rheumatol* 2004; 31:407–410.

Pincus T, Ferraccioli G, Sokka T, et al. Evidence from clinical trials and long-term observational studies that disease-modifying anti-rheumatic drugs slow radiographic progression in rheumatoid arthritis: updating a 1983 review. *Rheumatology* 2002; 41:1346–1356.

Pool AJ, Axford JS. The effects of exercise on the hormonal and immune systems in rheumatoid arthritis. *Rheumatology* 2001; 40:610–614.

Porreca F, Ossipov MH, Gebhart GH. Chronic pain and medullary descending facilitation. *Trends Neurosci* 2002; 25:319–325.

Price DD, Greenspan JD, Dubner R. Neurons involved in the exteroceptive function of pain. *Pain* 2003; 106:215–219.

Reginster J-Y, Khaltaev NG. Introduction and WHO perspective on the global burden of musculoskeletal conditions. *Rheumatology* 2002; 41(Suppl 1):1–2.

Ren K, Dubner R. Descending modulation in persistent pain: an update. *Pain* 2002; 100:1–6.

Riley G. Review article. The pathogenesis of tendinopathy. A molecular perspective. *Rheumatology* 2004; 43:131–142.

Ru-Rong J, Kohno T, Moore KA, Woolf CJ. Central sensitisation and long term potentiation (LTP): do pain and memory share similar mechanisms? *Trends Neurosci* 2003; 26:696–705.

Salvarani C, Cantini F, Boiardi L, Hunder GG. Polymyalgia rheumatica and giant cell arteritis. *N Engl J Med* 2002; 347:261–271.

Sarkar S, Aziz Q, Woolfe CJ, et al. Contribution of central sensitisation to the development of non-cardiac chest pain. *Lancet* 2000; 356:1154–1159.

Sarlani E, Greenspan JD. Evidence for generalised hyperalgesia in temporomandibular disorder patients. *Pain* 2003; 102:221–226.

Sawynok J. Topical and peripherally acting analgesics. *Pharmacol Rev* 2003; 55:1–20.

Schaible H-G, Ebersberger A, von Banchet GS. Mechanisms of pain in arthritis. *Ann NY Acad Sci* 2002; 66:343–354.

Scholz J, Woolf CJ. Can we conquer pain? *Nat Neurosci* 2002; 5(Suppl):1062–1067.

Schwartzman RJ. New treatments for reflex sympathetic dystrophy. *N Engl J Med* 2000; 343:654–656.

Scott DL, Antoni C, Choy HE, van Riel PCLM. Joint counts in routine practice. *Rheumatology* 2003; 42:919–923.

Sharpe L, Sensky T, Timberlake N, et al. Long-term efficacy of a cognitive behavioural treatment from a randomised controlled trial for patients recently diagnosed with rheumatoid arthritis. *Rheumatology* 2003; 42:435–441.

Simkin PA. Friction and lubrication in synovial joints. *J Rheumatol* 2000; 27:567–568.

Smythe HA. Fibromyalgia among friends. *J Rheumatol* 2004; 31:627–630.

Stafford L, Youssef PP. Spondyloarthropathies: an overview. *Intern Med J* 2002; 32:40–46.

Stanton-Hicks M. Complex regional pain syndrome. *Anaesthesiol Clin North Am* 2003; 4:733–744.

Staud R, Robinson ME, Vierck CJ Jr, Price DD. Diffuse noxious inhibitory controls (DNIC) attenuate temporal summation of second pain in normal males but not in normal females or fibromyalgia patients. *Pain* 2003a; 101:167–174.

Staud R, Cannon RC, Mauderli AP, et al. Temporal summation of pain from mechanical stimulation of muscle tissue in normal controls and subjects with fibromyalgia syndrome. *Pain* 2003b; 102:87–95.

Stenstrom CH, Minor MA. Evidence for the benefit of aerobic and strengthening exercise in rheumatoid arthritis. *Arthritis Rheum* 2003; 49:428–434.

Straub RH, Cutulo M. Involvement of the hypothalamic-pituitary–adrenal/gonadal axis and the peripheral nervous system in rheumatoid arthritis. *Arthritis Rheum* 2001; 44:493–507.

Strewler GJ. Decimal point—osteoporosis therapy at the 10-year mark. *N Engl J Med* 2004; 350:1172–1174.

Sutherland SP, Cook SP, McCleskey EW. Chemical mediators of pain due to tissue damage and ischaemia. *Prog Brain Res* 2000; 129:21–38.

Treede R-D, Rolke R, Andrews K, Magerl W. Pain elicited by blunt pressure: neurobiological basis and clinical relevance. *Pain* 2002; 98:235–240.

Underwood MR. Community management of knee pain in older people: is knee pain the new back pain? *Rheumatology* 2004; 43:2–3.

Vanegas H, Schaible H-G. Effects of antagonists to high threshold calcium channels upon spinal mechanisms of pain, hyperalgesia and allodynia. *Pain* 2000; 85:9–18.

Villemure C, Bushnell MC. Cognitive modulation of pain: how do attention and emotion influence pain processing? *Pain* 2002; 95:195–199.

Vlaeyen JWS, Linton SJ. Fear avoidance and its consequences in chronic musculoskeletal pain: a state of the art. *Pain* 2000; 85:317–332.

von Korff M, Deyo RA. Potent opioids for chronic musculoskeletal pain: flying blind? *Pain* 2004; 109:207–209.

Wasner G, Schattschneider J, Binder A, Baron R. Complex regional pain syndrome-diagnostic, mechanisms, CNS involvement and therapy. *Spinal Cord* 2003; 41:61–75.

Watkins LR, Milligan ED, Maier SF. Spinal cord glia: new players in pain. *Pain* 2001; 93:201–205.

White A. Complementary therapies for fibromyalgia. *Focus Altern Comp Ther (FACT)* 2003; 8:9–13.

Wong PKK, Spencer DG, McElduff P, et al. Secondary screening for osteoporosis in patients admitted with minimal-trauma fracture to a major teaching hospital. *Intern Med J* 2003; 33:505–510.

Woolfe F. The psychometrics of functional status questionnaires: room for improvement. *J Rheumatol* 2002; 29:865–868.

Woolley DE. The mast cell in inflammatory arthritis. *N Engl J Med* 2003; 348:1709–1711.

Core Curriculum for Professional Education in Pain, edited by J. Edmond Charlton, IASP Press, Seattle, © 2005.

33

Muscle and Myofascial Pain

I.   Know and understand the diagnostic labels appended to muscle pain, such as myalgia, nonskeletal musculoskeletal pain, chronic regional pain, regional soft tissue pain, and myofascial pain.

    A.   Understand that the term "myofascial pain" includes a general definition that refers to all muscle pain and a specific definition that refers to pain caused by myofascial trigger points (Simons et al. 1999; Tunks and Crook 1999; Mense et al. 2001).

    B.   Realize that the prevalence of muscle pain is unclear due to lack of consensus on terminology. Chronic regional pain in the general population is reported to range from 23.9% in the general adult population (Bergman et al. 2001) to 36% in internal medicine wards (Buskila et al. 2001). Muscle pain ranges from 15.2% in female sewing operators (Kaergaard and Andersen 2000) to 70% in female supermarket cashiers (Lundberg et al. 1999). Estimates of the prevalence of myofascial trigger points range from 30% in the general medical clinic (Fricton et al. 1985; Skootsky et al. 1989) to 93% (Fishbain et al. 1989; Bowsher et al. 1991; Simons 1996; Thomae et al. 1998).

II. Anatomy

    A.   Know the function and location of the muscle nociceptors (Marchettini 1993; Mense 1993, 1996; Graven-Nielsen and Mense 2001; Graven-Nielsen 2002).

    B.   Know the function of the ergoreceptors (Kniffki et al. 1981; Kaufman et al. 1983; Mense and Stahnke 1983).

    C.   Understand the function of the alpha and gamma motor neurons and how these can be affected by muscle nociception (Graven-Nielsen et al. 1997; Matre et al. 1998; Sorensen et al. 1998; Graven-Nielsen et al. 2000b; Wang et al. 2000; Svensson and Graven-Nielsen 2001).

III. Pathomechanics

    A.   Know that the underlying etiology of muscle pain is multifactorial; however, postural stresses secondary to poor ergonomic design, improper body mechanics, overload from sustained contraction, trauma, and repetitive overuse of the (upper) limbs are the most frequently described reasons for its occurrence (Lundberg et al. 1999; Madeleine et al. 1999; Westgaard 1999a,b, 2000; Kaergaard and Andersen 2000; Mense et al. 2001; Putz-Anderson et al. 2001).

    B.   Know that psychosocial factors, such as high job demands, psychological distress, poor support from colleagues, and work dissatisfaction can contribute to muscle pain (Nelson and Novy 1996; Vasseljen and Westgaard 1996; Carlson et al. 1998; McCracken et al. 1998; Lundberg 1999; Westgaard 1999a, 2000; Brulin et al. 2000; Vasseljen et al. 2001; Andersen et al. 2002; Nahit et al. 2003; Wahlstrom et al. 2003; Blangsted et al. 2004).

    C.   Know that negative thought patterns, specifically catastrophizing thoughts (Sullivan et al. 1998; Severeijns et al. 2001) and prolonged fear of movement (Vlaeyen and Linton 2000; Asmundsen et al. 2004) can contribute to the development of chronic disuse and disability with muscle pain and that measurement tools are available for assessment of these factors (Rosenstiel and Keefe 1983; McCracken et al. 1992; Waddell et al. 1993; Sullivan et al. 1995; Geisser et al. 2000; Vowles and Gross 2003; Goubert et al. 2004).

D. Know that gender differences in pain modulation may exist in muscle pain (Chesterton et al. 2003; Ge et al. 2004; 2005).

E. Understand the peripheral contributors to, and mediators of, muscle pain (e.g., sensitization through trauma or overuse by chemical, mechanical, or ischemic mechanisms) (Babenko et al. 2000; Graven-Nielsen and Mense 2001; Mense et al. 2001; Ashina et al. 2002; Rosendal et al. 2004).

F. Understand the central contributors to muscle pain (central sensitization, referred pain, and temporal summation) (Kellgren 1938; Ruch 1949; Sessle et al. 1986; Hoheisel et al. 1993; Madeleine and Lundager 1998; Sorensen et al. 1998; Koelbaek et al. 1999; Vecchiet and Vecchiet 1999; Graven-Nielsen et al. 2000a; Svensson and Graven-Nielsen 2001; Mense et al. 2001; Henriksson 2003; Kupers et al. 2004; Slater et al. 2005).

G. Understand the effects of modified muscle use (i.e. deconditioning) (Frenette 2000; Frenette et al. 2000; 2002).

H. Be aware of the hypotheses that most effectively explain trigger points (e.g., energy crisis, dysfunctional extrafusal neuromuscular junctions, and the integrated hypothesis) (Gerwin 1994; Hong and Simons 1998; Simons 2002, 2004).

IV. Clinical characteristics

A. Know the common symptoms associated with muscular pain (e.g., cramplike, diffuse, poorly localized, dull aching pain either at rest or in motion) (Kellgren 1938; Travell and Simons 1992; Arendt-Nielsen et al. 1996; Graven-Nielsen and Mense 2001).

B. Know the common signs associated with muscular pain (e.g., pain referred to distant somatic structures and modifications of superficial and deep sensitivity in the painful areas, painful loss of range of motion, and altered EMG activity in the agonist and antagonist) (Travell and Simons 1992; Arendt-Nielsen and Svensson 2001; Svensson and Graven-Nielsen 2001).

C. Know that the minimum acceptable diagnostic examination for trigger points includes "spot tenderness in a palpable band" and recognition of the pain. Additional supportive findings include eliciting the established pain pattern for that muscle, observing a twitch response, and finding painfully reduced stretch range of motion (Mense et al. 2001).

D. Be aware that trigger points are thought to be involved in pain in tension headaches (Travell and Simons 1992; Davidoff 1998; Simons and Mense 1998); low back syndromes (Simons and Travell 1983a,b; Rosomoff et al. 1989; Travell and Simons 1992; Njoo and Van der Does 1994); pelvic pain (Simons and Travell 1983b; Slocumb 1984; Schroeder 2000; Weiss 2001); intermittent claudication (Bartoli et al. 1980); and musculoskeletal diagnoses throughout the body, including bursitis, arthritis, tendinitis, and muscle tears (Travell and Simons 1992; Simons et al. 1999).

V. Assessment

Know that the lack of a formal, widely accepted, criterion-based diagnostic scheme has proved to be a serious impediment to proper diagnosis, clinical communication, and research (Simons et al. 1999; Harden et al. 2000).

A. Be able to assess abnormal posture and abnormal movement patterns from limitation of muscle strength and muscle length (Kendall et al. 1993; Sahrmann 2002). Be able to assess limitation of activities and restriction in participation due to pain.

B. Be able to identify a trigger point and know the common trigger points thought to be responsible for pain (Travell and Simons 1992). Know that the inter-rater reliability for detecting trigger points is poor in untrained and inexperienced examiners (Nice et al. 1992; Njoo and Van der Does 1994; Gerwin et al. 1997; Hsieh et al. 2000). Know that the reliability, sensitivity, and specificity of trigger points are unknown.

C. Know quantitative techniques available for assessment of local and referred pain, including pressure algometry, standardized induction and assessment of referred pain, etc. (Arendt-Nielsen 1997; Graven-Nielsen et al. 2001).

D. Know the criteria of fibromyalgia that differentiate it from myofascial pain (Wolfe et al. 1992; De Stefano et al. 2000; Harden et al. 2000).

E. Understand central pathology (such as spasticity) contributing to muscle pain (Francis et al. 1999; Elovic 2001; Hinderer and Dixon 2001; Schapiro 2001).

F. Be aware of painful muscle pathologies such as mitochondriopathies (Chelimsky et al. 1997; Andreu et al. 1999; Griggs and Karpati 1999) and other myopathies (Moxley 1996; Amato 2000; Preedy et al. 2001).

VI. Treatment

Know that the best evidence for the treatment of myofascial pain is extremely limited. Trials that are listed in the Cochrane Controlled Trials Registry show no superior effect for a particular therapy. Only a few Cochrane systematic reviews have been performed that address myofascial pain:

A. There is limited evidence that superficial needling (4 mm) inserted at trigger points is better than placebo TENS. There is limited evidence that a few sessions of dry needling, added to a regimen of physiotherapy, occupational therapy, and industrial assessments, are better than the regimen alone, immediately after treatment and at the short-term and intermediate follow-ups. There is moderate evidence that there is no difference in short-term global improvement between one session of dry needling and one session of trigger point injection with lidocaine and steroid, one session of trigger point injection with lidocaine only, or one session of cooling spray over the trigger point area followed by acupressure (Furlan et al. 2005).

B. There is no evidence of a statistically significant difference in the effectiveness of stabilization splint therapy in reducing symptoms in patients with myofascial pain syndrome compared with other active treatments. There is weak evidence to suggest that the use of stabilization splint therapy for the treatment of temporomandibular pain dysfunction syndrome may be beneficial for reducing pain severity, at rest and on palpation, when compared to no treatment (Al Ani et al. 2004; Koh and Robinson 2004).

C. Know the value of eliciting the local twitch response when injecting trigger points (Hong and Simons 1998; Chen et al. 2001; Audette et al. 2004).

D. Appreciate the importance of measuring changes in range of motion, repeated pain ratings, and functional ability to diagnose and record the progress of patients with chronic muscle and myofascial pain (Travell and Simons 1992; Simons et al. 1999).

E. Be able to educate patients about muscle pain and about the importance of self-management techniques, including a home exercise program, stretching (Travell and Simons 1992; Simons et al. 1999; Borg-Stein and Simons 2002), and ischemic pressure techniques (Hanten et al. 2000).

F. Be able to make recommendations for the workplace (Li and Buckle 1999; Muggleton et al. 1999; Stubbs 2000; Szabo and King 2000; Kumar 2001; Linton and van Tulder 2001).

G. Be able to assess whether the patient has a clear understanding of the reason(s) for the procedure and the likely benefit to be derived. Where there is no evidence base to indicate likely benefit, the patient should be made aware of this.

REFERENCES

Al Ani MZ, Davies SJ, Gray RJ, Sloan P, Glenny AM. Stabilisation splint therapy for temporomandibular pain dysfunction syndrome. *Cochrane Database Syst Rev* 2004; 1:CD002778.

Amato AA. Acid maltase deficiency and related myopathies. *Neurol Clin* 2000; 18(1):151–165.

Andersen JH, Kaergaard A, Frost P, et al. Physical, psychosocial, and individual risk factors for neck/shoulder pain with pressure tenderness in the muscles among workers performing monotonous, repetitive work. *Spine* 2002; 27(6):660–667.

Andreu AL, Hanna MG, Reichmann H, et al. Exercise intolerance due to mutations in the cytochrome b gene of mitochondrial DNA. *N Engl J Med* 1999; 341(14):1037–1044.

Arendt-Nielsen L. Induction and assessment of experimental pain from human skin, muscle and viscera. In: Jensen TS, Turner JA, Wiesenfeld-Hallin Z (Eds). *Proceedings of the 8th World Congress on Pain,* Progress in Pain Research and Management, Vol. 8. Seattle: IASP Press, 1997, pp 393–425.

Arendt-Nielsen L, Svensson P. Referred muscle pain: basic and clinical findings. *Clin J Pain* 2001; 17(1):11–19.

Arendt-Nielsen L, Andersen OK, Jensen TS. Brief, prolonged and repeated stimuli applied to hyperalgesic skin areas: a psychophysical study. *Brain Res* 1996; 712(1):165–167.

Ashina M, Stallknecht B, Bendtsen L, et al. In vivo evidence of altered skeletal muscle blood flow in chronic tension-type headache. *Brain* 2002; 125(Pt 2):320–326.

Asmundsen GJG, Vlaeyen JWS, Crombez G (Eds). *Understanding and Treating Fear of Pain.* Oxford University Press, 2004.

Audette JF, Wang F, Smith H. Bilateral activation of motor unit potentials with unilateral needle stimulation of active myofascial trigger points. *Am J Phys Med Rehabil* 2004; 83(5):368–374.

Babenko V, Svensson P, Graven-Nielsen T, et al. Duration and distribution of experimental muscle hyperalgesia in humans following combined infusions of serotonin and bradykinin. *Brain Res* 2000; 853(2):275–281.

Bartoli V, Dorigo B, Grisillo D, Beconi D. Fibrositic myofascial pain in intermittent claudication: significance of trigger areas in the calf. *Angiology* 1980; 31(1):11–20.

Bergman S, Herrstrom P, Hogstrom K, et al. Chronic musculoskeletal pain, prevalence rates, and sociodemographic associations in a Swedish population study. *J Rheumatol* 2001; 28(6):1369–1377.

Blangsted AK, Sogaard K, Christensen H, Sjogaard G. The effect of physical and psychosocial loads on the trapezius muscle activity during computer keying tasks and rest periods. *Eur J Appl Physiol* 2004; 91(2–3):253–258.

Borg-Stein J, Simons DG. Focused review: myofascial pain. *Arch Phys Med Rehabil* 2002; 83(3 Suppl 2):S40–S47.

Bowsher D, Rigge M, Sopp L. Prevalence of chronic pain in the British population: a telephone survey of 1037 households. *The Pain Clinic* 1991; 4:223–230.

Brulin C, Winkvist A, Langendoen S. Stress from working conditions among home care personnel with musculoskeletal symptoms. *J Adv Nurs* 2000; 31(01):181–189.

Buskila D, Neumann L, Odes LR, et al. The prevalence of musculoskeletal pain and fibromyalgia in patients hospitalized on internal medicine wards. *Semin Arthritis Rheum* 2001; 30(6):411–417.

Carlson CR, Reid KI, Curran SL, et al. Psychological and physiological parameters of masticatory muscle pain. *Pain* 1998; 76(3):297–307.

Chelimsky TC, Mcneeley KM, Comfort B, Piantadosi CA, LaManna JC. Effect of exercise and ischemia on tissue oximetry and cytochrome in normal subjects, patients with chronic limb pain, and patients with mitochondrial mitopathies. *Adv Exp Med Biol* 1997; 411:445–451.

Chen JT, Chung KC, Hou CR, et al. Inhibitory effect of dry needling on the spontaneous electrical activity recorded from myofascial trigger spots of rabbit skeletal muscle. *Am J Phys Med Rehabil* 2001; 80(10):729–735.

Chesterton LS, Barlas P, Foster NE, Baxter GD, Wright CC. Gender differences in pressure pain threshold in healthy humans. *Pain* 2003; 101(3):259–266.

Davidoff RA. Trigger points and myofascial pain: toward understanding how they affect headaches. *Cephalalgia* 1998; 18(7):436–448.

De Stefano R, Selvi E, Villanova M, et al. Image analysis quantification of substance P immunoreactivity in the trapezius muscle of patients with fibromyalgia and myofascial pain syndrome. *J Rheumatol* 2000; 27(12):2906–2910.

Elovic E. Principles of pharmaceutical management of spastic hypertonia. *Phys Med Rehabil Clin N Am* 2001; 12(4):793–816.

Fishbain DA, Goldberg M, Steele R, Rosomoff H. DSM-III diagnoses of patients with myofascial pain syndrome (fibrositis). *Arch Phys Med Rehabil* 1989; 70(6):433–438.

Francis K, Bach JR, DeLisa JA. Evaluation and rehabilitation of patients with adult motor neuron disease. *Arch Phys Med Rehabil* 1999; 80(8):951–963.

Frenette J. Accumulation of PDGF+ cells and internalisation of the PDGF receptor at myotendinous junction following modified hindlimb muscle use in the rat. *J Anat* 2000; 196(Pt 2):211–216.

Frenette J, Cai B, Tidball JG. Complement activation promotes muscle inflammation during modified muscle use. *Am J Pathol* 2000; 156(6):2103–2110.

Frenette J, St Pierre M, Cote CH, Mylona E, Pizza FX. Muscle impairment occurs rapidly and precedes inflammatory cell accumulation after mechanical loading. *Am J Physiol Regul Integr Comp Physiol* 2002; 282(2):R351–R357.

Fricton JR, Kroening R, Haley D, Siegert R. Myofascial pain syndrome of the head and neck: a review of clinical characteristics of 164 patients. *Oral Surg, Oral Med, Oral Pathol* 1985; 60(6):615–623.

Furlan AD, van Tulder MW, Cherkin DC, et al. Acupuncture and dry-needling for low back pain. *Cochrane Database Syst Rev* 2005; 1:CD001351.

Ge HY, Madeleine P, Arendt-Nielsen L. Sex differences in temporal characteristics of descending inhibitory control: an evaluation using repeated bilateral experimental induction of muscle pain. *Pain* 2004; 110(1–2):72–78.

Ge HY, Madeleine P, Arendt-Nielsen L. Gender differences in pain modulation evoked by repeated injections of glutamate into the human trapezius muscle. *Pain* 2005; 113(1–2):134–140.

Geisser ME, Haig AJ, Theisen ME. Activity avoidance and function in persons with chronic back pain. *J Occup Rehabil* 2000; 10:215–227.

Gerwin RD. Neurobiology of the myofascial trigger point. *Baillieres Clin Rheumatol* 1994; 8(4):747–762.

Gerwin RD, Shannon S, Hong CZ, Hubbard D, Gevirtz R. Interrater reliability in myofascial trigger point examination. *Pain* 1997; 69(1–2):65–73.

Goubert L, Crombez G, Van Damme S, et al. Confirmatory factor analysis of the Tampa Scale for Kinesiophobia: invariant two-factor model across low back pain patients and fibromyalgia patients. *Clin J Pain* 2004; 20:103–110.

Graven-Nielsen T. Thermosensitivity of muscle: high-intensity thermal stimulation of muscle tissue induces muscle pain in humans. *J Physiol* 2002; 540(Pt 2):647–656.

Graven-Nielsen T, Mense S. The peripheral apparatus of muscle pain: evidence from animal and human studies. *Clin J Pain* 2001; 17(1):2–10.

Graven-Nielsen T, Svensson P, Arendt-Nielsen L. Effects of experimental muscle pain on muscle activity and co-ordination during static and dynamic motor function. *Electroencephalogr Clin Neurophysiol* 1997; 105(2):156–164.

Graven-Nielsen T, Aspegren Kendall S, Henriksson KG, et al. Ketamine reduces muscle pain, temporal summation, and referred pain in fibromyalgia patients. *Pain* 2000a; 85(3):483–491.

Graven-Nielsen T, Svensson P, Arendt-Nielsen L. Effect of muscle pain on motor control—a human experimental approach. *Adv Physiother* 2000b; 2:26–38.

Graven-Nielsen T, Segerdahl M, Svensson P, Arendt-Nielsen L. Methods for induction and assessment of pain in humans with clinical and pharmacological examples. In: Kruger LR (Ed). *Methods in Pain Research.* CRC Press, 2001, pp 263–304.

Griggs RC, Karpati G. Muscle pain, fatigue, and mitochondriopathies. *N Engl J Med* 1999; 341(14):1077–1078.

Hanten WP, Olson SL, Butts NL, Nowicki AL. Effectiveness of a home program of ischemic pressure followed by sustained stretch for treatment of myofascial trigger points. *Phys Ther* 2000; 80(10):997–1003.

Harden RN, Bruehl SP, Gass S, Niemiec C, Barbick B. Signs and symptoms of the myofascial pain syndrome: a national survey of pain management providers. *Clin J Pain* 2000; 16(1):64–72.

Henriksson KG. Hypersensitivity in muscle pain syndromes. *Curr Pain Headache Rep* 2003; 7(6):426–432.

Hinderer SR, Dixon K. Physiologic and clinical monitoring of spastic hypertonia. *Phys Med Rehabil Clin N Am* 2001; 12(4):733–746.

Hoheisel U, Mense S, Simons DG, Yu XM. Appearance of new receptive fields in rat dorsal horn neurons following noxious stimulation of skeletal muscle: a model for referral of muscle pain? *Neurosci Lett* 1993; 153(1):9–12.

Hong CZ, Simons DG. Pathophysiologic and electrophysiologic mechanisms of myofascial trigger points. *Arch Phys Med Rehabil* 1998; 79(7):863–872.

Hsieh CY, Hong CZ, Adams AH, et al. Interexaminer reliability of the palpation of trigger points in the trunk and lower limb muscles. *Arch Phys Med Rehabil* 2000; 81(3):258–264.

Kaergaard A, Andersen JH. Musculoskeletal disorders of the neck and shoulders in female sewing machine operators: prevalence, incidence, and prognosis. *Occup Environ Med* 2000; 57(8):528–534.

Kaufman MP, Longhurst JC, Rybicki KJ, Wallach JH, Mitchell JH. Effects of static muscular contraction on impulse activity of groups III and IV afferents in cats. *J Appl Physiol* 1983; 55(1 Pt 1):105–112.

Kellgren JH. Observations on referred pain arising from muscle. *Clin Sci* 1938; 3:175–190.

Kendall FP, McCreary EK, Provance PG. Muscles. *Testing and Function*, 4th ed. Baltimore, MD: Williams and Wilkins, 1993.

Kniffki K, Mense S, Schmidt R. Muscle receptors with fine afferent fibers which may evoke circulatory reflexes. *Circ Res* 1981; 48(Suppl 1):125–131.

Koelbaek J, Graven-Nielsen T, Schou O, Arendt-Nielsen L. Generalised muscular hyperalgesia in chronic whiplash syndrome. *Pain* 1999; 83(2):229–234.

Koh H, Robinson PG. Occlusal adjustment for treating and preventing temporomandibular joint disorders. *J Oral Rehabil* 2004; 31(4):287–292.

Kumar S. Disability, injury and ergonomics intervention. *Disabil Rehabil* 2001; 23(18):805–814.

Kupers RC, Svensson P, Jensen TS. Central representation of muscle pain and mechanical hyperesthesia in the orofacial region: a positron emission tomography study. *Pain* 2004; 108(3):284–293.

Li G, Buckle P. Current techniques for assessing physical exposure to work-related musculoskeletal risks, with emphasis on posture-based methods. *Ergonomics* 1999; 42(5):674–695.

Linton SJ, van Tulder MW. Preventive interventions for back and neck pain problems: what is the evidence? *Spine* 2001; 26(7):778–787.

Lundberg U. Stress responses in low-status jobs and their relationship to health risks: musculoskeletal disorders. *Ann New York Acad Sci* 1999; 896:162–172.

Lundberg U, Dohns IE, Melin B, et al. Psychophysiological stress responses, muscle tension, and neck and shoulder pain among supermarket cashiers. *J Occup Health Psychol* 1999; 4(3):245–255.

Madeleine P, Lundager B. Sensory manifestations in experimental and work-related chronic neck-shoulder pain. *Eur J Pain* 1998; 2(2):251–260.

Madeleine P, Lundager B, Voigt M, Arendt-Nielsen L. Shoulder muscle co-ordination during chronic and acute experimental neck-shoulder pain. An occupational pain study. *Eur J Appl Physiol Occup Physiol* 1999; 79(2):127–140.

Marchettini P. Muscle pain: animal and human experimental and clinical studies. *Muscle Nerve* 1993; 16(10):1033–1039.

Matre DA, Sinkjaer T, Svensson P, Arendt-Nielsen L. Experimental muscle pain increases the human stretch reflex. *Pain* 1998; 75(2–3):331–339.

McCracken LM, Zayfert C, Gross RT. The Pain Anxiety Symptoms Scale: development and validation of a scale to measure fear of pain. *Pain* 1992; 50:67–73.

McCracken LM, Faber SD, Janeck AS. Pain-related anxiety predicts non-specific physical complaints in persons with chronic pain. *Behav Res Ther* 1998; 36(6):621–630.

Mense S. Nociception from skeletal muscle in relation to clinical muscle pain. *Pain* 1993; 54(3):241–289.

Mense S. Group III and IV receptors in skeletal muscle: are they specific or polymodal? *Prog Brain Res* 1996; 113:83–100.

Mense S, Simons DG, Russell IJ. *Muscle Pain. Understanding its Nature, Diagnosis and Treatment,* 1st ed. Philadelphia: Lippincott Williams and Wilkins, 2001.

Mense S, Stahnke M. Responses in muscle afferent fibres of slow conduction velocity to contractions and ischaemia in the cat. *J Physiol* 1983; 342:383–397.

Moxley RT. Proximal myotonic myopathy: mini-review of a recently delineated clinical disorder. *Neuromuscul Disord* 1996; 6(2):87–93.

Muggleton JM, Allen R, Chappell PH. Hand and arm injuries associated with repetitive manual work in industry: a review of disorders, risk factors and preventive measures. *Ergonomics* 1999; 42(5):714–739.

Nahit ES, Hunt IM, Lunt M, et al. Effects of psychosocial and individual psychological factors on the onset of musculoskeletal pain: common and site-specific effects. *Ann Rheum Dis* 2003; 62(8):755–760.

Nelson DV, Novy DM. Psychological characteristics of reflex sympathetic dystrophy versus myofascial pain syndromes. *Reg Anesth* 1996; 21(3):202–208.

Nice DA, Riddle DL, Lamb RL, Mayhew TP, Rucker K. Intertester reliability of judgments of the presence of trigger points in patients with low back pain. *Arch Phys Med Rehabil* 1992; 73(10):893–898.

Njoo KH, Van der Does E. The occurrence and inter-rater reliability of myofascial trigger points in the quadratus lumborum and gluteus medius: a prospective study in non-specific low back pain patients and controls in general practice. *Pain* 1994; 58(3):317–323.

Preedy VR, Adachi J, Ueno Y, et al. Alcoholic skeletal muscle myopathy: definitions, features, contribution of neuropathy, impact and diagnosis. *Eur J Neurol* 2001; 8(6):677–687.

Putz-Anderson V, Bernard B, Burt S, et al. Musculoskeletal disorders and workplace factors: a critical review of epidemiologic evidence for work related musculoskeletal disorders of the neck, upper extremity and low back. Bernard B (Ed). 2001. Public Health Service, Centers for Disease Control and Prevention, National Institute for Occupational Safety and Health.

Rosendal L, Larsson B, Kristiansen J, et al. Increase in muscle nociceptive substances and anaerobic metabolism in patients with trapezius myalgia: microdialysis in rest and during exercise. *Pain* 2004; 112(3):324–334.

Rosenstiel AK, Keefe FJ. The use of coping strategies in chronic low back pain patients. Relationship to patient characteristics and current adjustments. *Pain* 1983; 17:33–44.

Rosomoff HL, Fishbain DA, Goldberg M, Santana R, Rosomoff RS. Physical findings in patients with chronic intractable benign pain of the neck and/or back. *Pain* 1989; 37(3):279–287.

Ruch TC. Visceral sensation and referred pain. In: Fulton JF (Ed). *Howell's Textbook of Physiology.* Philadelphia: Saunders, 1949, pp 385–401.

Sahrmann SA. *Diagnosis and Treatment of Movement Impairment Syndromes.* St. Louis: Mosby, 2002.

Schapiro RT. Management of spasticity, pain, and paroxysmal phenomena in multiple sclerosis. *Curr Neurol Neurosci Rep* 2001; 1(3):299–302.

Schroeder BS. Musculoskeletal pelvic pain in a pediatric and adolescent gynecology practice. *J Pediatr Adolesc Gynecol* 2000; 13(2):90.

Sessle BJ, Hu JW, Amano N, Zhong G. Convergence of cutaneous, tooth pulp, visceral, neck and muscle afferents onto nociceptive and non-nociceptive neurones in trigeminal subnucleus caudalis (medullary dorsal horn) and its implications for referred pain. *Pain* 1986; 27(2):219–235.

Severeijns R, Vlaeyen JWS, van der Hout MA, Weber WE. Pain catastrophising predicts pain intensity, disability and psychological distress independent of the level of physical impairment. *Clin J Pain* 2001; 17:165–172.

Simons DG. Clinical and etiological update of myofascial pain from trigger points. *J Musculoskel Pain* 1996; 4(1–2):93–121.

Simons DG. Endplate potentials are common to midfiber myofascial trigger points. *Am J Physical Med Rehabil* 2002; 81(3):212–222.

Simons DG. Review of enigmatic MTrPs as a common cause of enigmatic musculoskeletal pain and dysfunction. *J Electromyogr Kinesiol* 2004; 14(1):95–107.

Simons DG, Mense S. Understanding and measurement of muscle tone as related to clinical muscle pain. *Pain* 1998; 75(1):1–17.

Simons DG, Travell JG. Myofascial origins of low back pain. 2. Torso muscles. *Postgrad Med* 1983a; 73(2):81–92.

Simons DG, Travell JG. Myofascial origins of low back pain. 3. Pelvic and lower extremity muscles. *Postgrad Med* 1983b; 73(2):99–105.

Simons DG, Travell JG, Simons LS. *Travell & Simons' Myofascial Pain and Dysfunction: The Trigger Point Manual,* Vol. 1, 2nd ed. Baltimore: Williams and Wilkins, 1999.

Skootsky SA, Jaeger B, Oye RK. Prevalence of myofascial pain in general internal medicine practice. *West J Med* 1989; 151(2):157–160.

Slater H, Arendt-Nielsen L, Wright A, Graven-Nielsen T. Sensory and motor effects of experimental muscle pain in patients with lateral epicondylalgia and controls with delayed onset muscle soreness. *Pain* 2005; 114(1–2):118–130.

Slocumb JC. Neurological factors in chronic pelvic pain: trigger points and the abdominal pelvic pain syndrome. *Am J Obstet Gynecol* 1984; 149(5):536–543.

Sorensen J, Graven-Nielsen T, Henriksson KG, Bengtsson M, Arendt-Nielsen L. Hyperexcitability in fibromyalgia. *J Rheumatol* 1998; 25(1):152–155.

Stubbs DA. Ergonomics and occupational medicine: future challenges. *Occup Med (London)* 2000; 50:277–282.

Sullivan MJI, Bishop SR, Pivot J. *The Pain Catastrophising Scale: Development and Validation, Psychological Assessment,* 1995; 7:155–163.

Sullivan MJ, Stanish W, Waite H, Sullivan M, Tripp DA. Catastrophising, pain and disability in patients with soft-tissue injuries. *Pain* 1998; 77:253–260.

Svensson P, Graven-Nielsen T. Craniofacial muscle pain: review of mechanisms and clinical manifestations. *J Orofac Pain* 2001; 15(2):117–145.

Szabo RM, King KJ. Repetitive stress injury: diagnosis or self-fulfilling prophecy? *J Bone Joint Surg* 2000; 82(American):1314–1322.

Thomae MK, Porteous JE, Brock JR, et al. Back pain in Australian military helicopter pilots: a preliminary study. *Aviat Space Environ Med* 1998; 69(5):468–473.

Travell JG, Simons DG. *Myofascial Pain and Dysfunction: The Trigger Point Manual.* Baltimore: Williams and Wilkins, 1992.

Tunks E, Crook J. Regional soft tissue pains: alias myofascial pain? *Best Pract Res Clin Rheumatol* 1999; 13(2):345–369.

Vasseljen OJ, Westgaard RH. Can stress-related shoulder and neck pain develop independently of muscle activity? *Pain* 1996; 64(2):221–230.

Vasseljen O, Holte KA, Westgaard RH. Shoulder and neck complaints in customer relations: individual risk factors and perceived exposures at work. *Ergonomics* 2001; 44(4):355–372.

Vecchiet L, Vecchiet J. Referred muscle pain: clinical and pathophysiologic aspects. *Curr Rev Pain* 1999; 3(6):489–498.

Vowles KE, Gross RT. Work-related beliefs about injury and physical capability for work in individuals with chronic pain. *Pain* 2003; 101:291–298.

Vlaeyen JWS, Linton SJ. Fear-avoidance and its consequences in chronic musculoskeletal pain: a state of the art. *Pain* 2000; 85:317–332.

Waddell G, Newton M, Henderson I, Somerville D, Main CA. Fear-Avoidance Beliefs Questionnaire (FABQ) and the role of fear-avoidance in chronic low back pain and disability. *Pain* 1993; 52:157–168.

Wahlstrom J, Lindegard A, Ahlborg G Jr, Ekman A, Hagberg M. Perceived muscular tension, emotional stress, psychological demands and physical load during VDU work. *Int Arch Occup Environ Health* 2003; 76(8):584–590.

Wang K, Svensson P, Arendt-Nielsen L. Effect of tonic muscle pain on short-latency jaw-stretch reflexes in humans. *Pain* 2000; 88(2):189–197.

Weiss JM. Pelvic floor myofascial trigger points: manual therapy for interstitial cystitis and the urgency-frequency syndrome. *J Urol* 2001; 166(6):2226–2231.

Westgaard RH. Effects of physical and mental stressors on muscle pain. *Scand J Work Environ Health* 1999a; 25(Suppl 4):19–24.

Westgaard RH. Muscle activity as a releasing factor for pain in the shoulder and neck. *Cephalalgia* 1999b; 19(Suppl 25):1–8.

Westgaard RH. Work-related musculoskeletal complaints: some ergonomics challenges upon the start of a new century. *Appl Ergon* 2000; 31(6):569–580.

Wolfe F, Simons DG, Fricton J, et al. The fibromyalgia and myofascial pain syndromes: a preliminary study of tender points and trigger points in persons with fibromyalgia, myofascial pain syndrome and no disease. *J Rheumatol* 1992; 19(6):944–951.

Core Curriculum for Professional Education in Pain, edited by J. Edmond Charlton, IASP Press, Seattle, © 2005.

34

Visceral Pain

I. Characteristics of visceral pain

   A. Know the distinct clinical features of visceral pain (Vecchiet et al 1993; Mayer and Gebhart 1994; Gebhart 1995; Cervero and Laird 1999).

      1. Be aware of the diffuse localization of visceral pain and referral to somatic sites.
      2. Be aware of mechanistic differences between somatic and visceral pain.
      3. Be aware of the relationship between the clinical features of visceral pain and the underlying neurobiology.

   B. Know the general organization of the visceral pain system.

II. Peripheral mechanisms (Cervero 1994; Gebhart 2000)

   A. Know the anatomical organization of visceral innervation.

      1. Be aware of differences in innervation between visceral and somatic structures.
      2. Be aware of differences in density of innervation between visceral and somatic structures.

   B. Know the properties of visceral nociceptors (Ness and Gebhart 1990).

      1. Be aware that stimuli adequate for activation of visceral nociceptors differ from stimuli adequate for activation of somatic nociceptors.
      2. Be aware of location in tissue of visceral nociceptors.
      3. Be aware that visceral nociceptors are polymodal.
      4. Be aware of the neurochemistry of visceral sensory neuron cell bodies.

   C. Know mechanisms of visceral nociceptor sensitization.

      1. Be aware of contributions of amine, peptide, and other mediators to sensitization of visceral nociceptors.
      2. Be aware of contributions of ligand-gated ion channels to sensitization of visceral nociceptors.

III. Central mechanisms (Ness and Gebhart 1990; Cervero and Laird 1999)

   A. Know pattern of termination of visceral afferent fibers in the spinal cord.

      1. Be aware of differences in the areas of spinal cord projection between visceral and somatic nociceptors.
      2. Be aware of differences in segmental distribution and spread between visceral and somatic nociceptors.

   B. Know properties of spinal neurons that receive visceral input.

      1. Be aware of viscerosomatic and viscero-visceral convergence onto spinal neurons.
      2. Be aware of convergent cutaneous receptive fields of visceroreceptive spinal neurons.

   C. Know mechanisms of central sensitization of visceroreceptive spinal neurons.

      1. Be aware of the role of neuroactive peptide transmitters (e.g., substance P and calcitonin gene-related peptide) and excitatory amino acids in central sensitization of visceroreceptive spinal neurons.

2. Be aware of second-messenger pathways in visceroreceptive spinal neurons (e.g., nitric oxide, MAP kinase, etc.) in central sensitization of visceroreceptive spinal neurons.

D. Know ascending pathways in the spinal cord that convey visceral nociceptive information to supraspinal sites.

    1. Be aware of the spinothalamic pathway.
    2. Be aware of the dorsal column pathway.

E. Know the differences in supraspinal sites that receive visceral and cutaneous nociceptive input.

IV. Visceral pain modulation

A. Know descending modulatory influences on visceroreceptive spinal neurons.

B. Know peripheral and central mechanisms of visceral pain modulation.

REFERENCES

Cervero F. Sensory innervation of the viscera: peripheral basis of visceral pain. *Physiol Rev* 1994; 74:95–138.

Cervero F, Laird JMA. Visceral pain. *Lancet* 1999; 353:2145–2148.

Gebhart GF (Ed). *Visceral Pain,* Progress in Pain Research and Management, Vol. 5. Seattle: IASP Press, 1995.

Gebhart GF. Peripheral contributions to the pathobiology of visceral pain. *Am J Physiol* 2000; 278:G834–G838.

Mayer EM, Gebhart GF. Basic and clinical aspects of visceral hyperalgesia. *Gastroenterology* 1994; 107:207–293.

Ness TJ, Gebhart GF. Visceral pain: a review of experimental studies. *Pain* 1990; 41:167–234.

Vecchiet L, Albe-Fessard D, Lindblom U, Giamberardino MA (Eds). *New Trends in Referred Pain and Hyperalgesia,* Vol. 7. Amsterdam: Elsevier, 1993.

Core Curriculum for Professional Education in Pain, edited by J. Edmond Charlton, IASP Press, Seattle, © 2005.

35

Chronic Urogenital Pain

Following self-directed learning and/or instruction, attainment of the following general (I, II, III, etc.) and specific (A, B, C, etc.) learning outcomes relating to knowledge and skills can be tested.

I. Can apply the neuroscience understanding of visceral, somatic, and neuropathic pain in the context of urogenital pain.

   A. Can describe the anatomy of urogenital structures, bony pelvis and associated musculature, and autonomic and sensory nerves, with special reference to the hypogastric plexus and pudendal nerve (Wesselmann et al. 1997).

   B. Can explain concepts of visceral hyperalgesia, viscerosomatic convergence/hyperalgesia, and viscero-visceral hyperalgesia (Giamberardino 2000).

   C. Can describe the influence of sex and gender (Fillingim et al. 1998, 1999) and hormones (Bradshaw et al. 1999) on pain experience.

II. Can outline the epidemiology of urogenital pain (Mathias et al. 1996; Zondervan et al. 1998; Kreiger et al. 2002; Parsons et al. 2002; Diokno et al. 2003).

III. Can apply the clinical distinction between gastrointestinal, urological, gynecological, and musculoskeletal pain (see www.pelvicpain.org/pdf/FRM_Pain_Questionnaire.pdf).

   A. Can obtain a focused history.

   B. Can undertake a relevant physical examination.

   C. Can identify any features suspicious of malignancy.

   D. Can identify pathological conditions of the pelvis that cause pain.

IV. Can apply psychological principles to clinical assessment, explanation, and treatment (Elcombe et al. 1997).

   A. Can identify and manage distress and concerns, for example fertility, sexuality, and sexual functioning (Berghuis et al. 1996).

   B. Can identify patients in whom sexual and physical abuse may be an unresolved issue and can discuss appropriate referral (Collett et al. 1998; Raphael et al. 2001).

V. Can explain the importance of the doctor-patient relationship in influencing outcome (Selfe et al. 1998).

   A. Can demonstrate good consultation skills.

   B. Can demonstrate nondiscriminatory and empathic attitudes and practice.

   C. Can outline the components of a multidisciplinary care model (Collett et al. 2000).

VI. Can identify in men the features of the following *nonspecific* clinical conditions and symptoms, investigations, and management options:

   A. Prostatitis/prostatodynia (Kreiger et al. 2002; Moldwin 2002; Sant et al. 2003).

   B. Type III chronic prostatitis/chronic pelvic pain syndrome (CP/CPPS).

179

C. Interstitial cystitis (Berger et al. 1998; Mann 1998; Warren and Keay 2002).

D. Testicular/scrotal pain (Ness 2001).

E. Penile pain.

F. Perineal pain (Nickel et al. 2001).

G. Musculoskeletal pain (Clauw et al. 1997; Weiss 2001).

VII. Can identify in men the features of the following *specific* clinical conditions and symptoms, investigations, and management options:

A. Bacterial prostatitis (Potts 2001).

B. Epididymitis (Berger 1991; Nickel et al. 2002).

C. Orchitis (Berger 1994).

D. Hernia pain (Karlsson et al. 1994).

E. Nerve entrapment pain (Robert et al. 1998; Shafik and Doss 1999).

F. Cancer pain (Gerstenbluth et al. 2002).

G. Miscellaneous.

VIII. Can identify in women features of the following clinical conditions, investigations (Howard 1993, 2000; Cody and Ascher 2000), and management options (Prentice 2000; Stones 2003):

A. Endometriosis (Vercellini 2000).

B. Adhesions.

C. Chronic pelvic inflammatory disease.

D. Ovarian cycle dependent/functional (Stones 2003b).

E. Dysmenorrhea.

F. Interstitial cystitis/urethral syndrome (Parsons et al. 2002).

G. Musculoskeletal pain (King Baker 1998; Weiss 2001).

H. Vestibulitis (Glazer et al. 1995; Zolnoun et al. 2003).

I. Vulvodynia (Smart and Maclean 2003).

K. Postsurgical pain (Perry 2003).

L. Nerve entrapment pain (Robert et al. 1998; Shafik and Doss 1999).

REFERENCES

Bradshaw HB, Temple JL, Wood E, Berkley KJ. Estrous variations in behavioral responses to vaginal and uterine distention in the rat. *Pain* 1999; 82:187–197.

Berger RE. Acute epididymitis: etiology and therapy. *Semin Urol* 1991; 9(1):28–31.

Berger RE. Infection of the male reproductive tract. *Curr Ther Endocrinol Metab* 1994; 5:305–309.

Berger RE, Miller JE, Rothman I, Krieger JN, Muller CH. Bladder petechiae after cystoscopy and hydrodistension in men diagnosed with prostate pain. *J Urol* 1998; 159(1):83–85.

Berghuis JP, Heiman JR, Rothman I, Berger RE. Psychological and physical factors involved in chronic idiopathic prostatitis. *J Psychosom Res* 1996; 41(4):313–325.

Clauw DJ, Schmidt M, Radulovic D, et al. The relationship between fibromyalgia and interstitial cystitis. *J Psychiatr Res* 1997; 31(1):125–131.

Diokno AC, Homma Y, Sekiguchi Y, Suzuki Y. Interstitial cystitis, gynecologic pelvic pain, prostatitis, and their epidemiology. *Int J Urol* 2003;10(1):S1–6.

Cody RF, Ascher SM. Diagnostic value of radiological tests in chronic pelvic pain. *Bailliere's Clin Obstet Gynaecol* 2000; 14:433–466.

Collett BJ, Cordle CJ, Stewart CR, Jagger C. A comparative study of women with chronic pelvic pain, chronic nonpelvic pain and those with no history of pain attending general practitioners. *Br J Obstet Gynaecol* 1998; 105:87–92.

Collett BJ, Cordle C, Stewart C. Setting up a multidisciplinary clinic. *Bailliere's Clin Obstet Gynaecol* 2000; 14:541–556.

Elcombe S, Gath D, Day A. The psychological effects of laparoscopy on women with chronic pelvic pain. *Psychol Med* 1997; 27(5):1041–1050.

Fillingim RB, Maixner W, Kincaid S, Silva S. Sex differences in temporal summation but not sensory-discriminative processing of thermal pain. *Pain* 1998; 75:121–127.

Fillingim RB, Edwards RR, Powell T. The relationship of sex and clinical pain to experimental pain responses. *Pain* 1999; 83:419–425.

Gerstenbluth RE, Seftel AD, MacLennan GT, et al. Distribution of chronic prostatitis in radical prostatectomy specimens with up-regulation of bcl-2 in areas of inflammation. *J Urol* 2002; 167(5):2267–2270.

Giamberardino MA. Visceral hyperalgesia. In: Devor M, Rowbotham MC, Wiesenfeld-Hallin Z (Eds). *Proceedings of the 9th World Congress on Pain,* Progress in Pain Research and Management, Vol. 16. Seattle: IASP Press, 2000, pp 523–550.

Glazer H, Rodke G, Swencions C, Hertz R, Young AW. Treatment of vulvar vestibulitis with electromyographic biofeedback of pelvic floor musculature. *J Repro Med* 1995; 40:283–290.

Howard F. The role of laparoscopy in chronic pelvic pain: promise and pitfalls. *Obstet Gynecol Survey* 1993; 48:357–387.

Howard FM. The role of laparoscopy as a diagnostic tool in chronic pelvic pain. *Bailliere's Clin Obstet Gynaecol* 2000; 14:467–494.

Karlsson JL, Sward, Kalebo P, Thomee R. Chronic groin injuries in athletes: recommendations for treatment and rehabilitation. *Sports Med* 1994; 17(2):141–148.

King Baker P. Musculoskeletal problems. In: Steege JF, Metzger DA, Levy BS (Eds). *Chronic Pelvic Pain: An Integrated Approach.* Philadelphia: Saunders, 1998, pp 215–240.

Kreiger JN, Ross SO, Riley DE. Chronic prostatitis: epidemiology and role of infection. *Urology* 2002; 60:8–12.

Mann O. Pelvic joint dysfunctions, lifting injuries, and testicular pain. *J Occup Environ Med* 1998; 40(5):419–421.

Mathias SD, Kupperman M, Liberman RF, Lipschutz RC, Steege JF. Chronic pelvic pain: prevalence, health-related quality of life, and economic correlates. *Obstet Gynecol* 1996; 87:321–327.

Moldwin RM. Similarities between interstitial cystitis and male chronic pelvic pain syndrome. *Curr Urol Rep* 2002; 3(4):313–318.

Ness TJ. Chronic urologic pain syndromes. *Curr Pain Headache Rep* 2001; 5(1):27–34.

Nickel JC, Downey J, Hunter D, Clark J. Prevalence of prostatitis-like symptoms in a population based study using the National Institutes of Health chronic prostatitis symptom index. *J Urol* 2001; 165(3):842–845.

Nickel JC, Siemens DR, Nickel KR, Downey J. The patient with chronic epididymitis: characterization of an enigmatic syndrome. *J Urol* 2002; 167(4):1701–1704.

Parsons CL, Dell J, Stanford EJ, et al. Increased prevalence of interstitial cystitis: previously unrecognized urologic and gynecologic cases identified using new symptoms questionnaire and intravesical potassium sensitivity. *Urology* 2002; 60:573–578.

Potts JM. The four categories of prostatitis: a practical approach to treatment. *Cleve Clin J Med* 2001; 68(5):389–90, 392–393, 397.

Prentice A. Medical management of chronic pelvic pain. *Bailliere's Clin Obstet Gynaecol* 2000; 14:495–499.

Raphael KG, Widom CS, Lange C. Childhood victimization and pain in adulthood: a prospective investigation. *Pain* 2001; 92:283–293.

Robert R, Prat-Pradal D, Labat JJ, et al. Anatomic basis of chronic perineal pain: role of the pudendal nerve. *Surg Radiol Anat* 1998; 20:93–98.

Sant GR, Propert KJ, Hanno PM, et al. A pilot clinical trial of oral pentosan polysulfate and oral hydroxyzine in patients with interstitial cystitis. *J Urol* 2003; 170:810–815.

Selfe SA, Matthews Z, Stones RW. Factors influencing outcome in consultations for chronic pelvic pain. *J Womens Health* 1998; 7:1041–1048.

Shafik A, Doss SH. Pudendal canal: surgical anatomy and clinical implications. *Am Surg* 1999; 65:176–180.

Smart O, Maclean AB. Vulvodynia. *Curr Opin Obstet Gynecol* 2003, 15:497–500.

Stones RW. Chronic pelvic pain. In: Shaw RW, Soutter WP, Stanton SL (Eds). *Gynaecology,* 3rd ed. Edinburgh: Churchill Livingstone; 2003, pp 879–890.

Stones RW. Pelvic vascular congestion-half a century later. *Clin Obstet Gynecol* 2003; 46:831–836.

Stones RW, Mountfield J. *Interventions for Treating Chronic Pelvic Pain in Women.* Cochrane Library. Oxford: Update Software, 2000, Issue 4.

Vercellini P, De Giorgi O, Pisacreta A, et al. Surgical management of endometriosis. *Bailliere's Clin Obstet Gynaecol* 2000; 14:501–523.

Warren JW, Keay SK. Interstitial cystitis. *Curr Opin Urol* 2002; 12(1):69–74.

Weiss JM. Pelvic floor myofascial trigger points: manual therapy for interstitial cystitis and the urgency-frequency syndrome. *J Urol* 2001; 166(6):2226–2231.

Wesselmann U, Brunett AL, Heinberg LJ. The urogenital and rectal pain syndromes. *Pain* 1997; 73:269–294.

Zolnoun DA, Hartmann KE, Steege JF. Overnight 5% lidocaine ointment for treatment of vulvar vestibulitis. *Obstet Gynecol* 2003; 102:84–87.

Zondervan KT, Yudkin PL, Vessey MP, et al. The prevalence of chronic pelvic pain in women in the United Kingdom: a systematic review. *Br J Obstet Gynaecol* 1998; 105:93–99.

Core Curriculum for Professional Education in Pain, edited by J. Edmond Charlton, IASP Press, Seattle, © 2005.

36

Pain and Pregnancy and Labor

I. Perception of pain in pregnancy

Know the factors that can influence the perception of pain in pregnancy compared with the nonpregnant state:

A. Fear of pain (Saisto and Halmesmaki 2003): may be primary (usually in nulliparous women, and may be associated with pre-existing psychological morbidity and/or ignorance), or secondary (e.g., as a result of a previous bad experience).

B. Increased susceptibility to pain due to generalized anxiety (related to the pregnancy, its outcome, its implications for the woman, or other concerns).

C. Positive attitudes to pregnancy and its social implications: may increase tolerance to pain, especially in labor (pain is seen as a "positive" force rather than a destructive one).

D. Level of education: poor knowledge and/or misinformation may exacerbate the above.

E. Age/parity: younger women may have increased tolerance to pain, but older multiparae may be more relaxed and therefore less fearful.

F. Neuroendocrine system (Whipple et al. 1990; Shapira et al. 1995): sex steroids, e.g., 17 beta-estradiol and progesterone, can modulate the opioid system during pregnancy (e.g., via spinal dynorphin pathways), increasing pain tolerance.

II. Causes of pain in pregnancy

Be familiar with the spectrum of conditions that can present with pain during pregnancy:

A. Not specific to, but common during, pregnancy.

1. Headache: most commonly tension headache or migraine; both have similar triggers and treatment. Recurrence may be due to reluctance to take analgesics in pregnancy, but the usual pattern is improvement over time, usually in the first trimester. It is important to exclude depression, sleep deprivation, pre-eclampsia, subarachnoid hemorrhage, cerebral tumors, and other focal lesions. Management is with simple measures, nondrug treatments, analgesics, and beta-blockers if headache is recurrent and severe.

2. Back pain: occurs in approximately 50% of pregnant women (Rathmell et al. 1997). Pain is increased by preexisting problems, multiparity, and increased age. Its early presentation (commonly the first trimester) suggests that weight gain is not the only factor; neuronal and endocrine mechanisms have been implicated (the polypeptide relaxin, secreted by the corpus luteum, softens the pelvic ligaments to allow accommodation of the developing fetus and facilitate vaginal delivery, and is thought to contribute to back problems during and after pregnancy). The pain is typically described as dull (lumbar), stabbing (gluteal), burning (thoracic), and/or accompanied by paresthesia (root compression). Management includes normal daily activity where possible, physiotherapy and analgesics. Sacroiliitis is common and may respond to manipulation. Epidural steroid injections are usually avoided in pregnancy if possible.

3. Nerve entrapment: carpal tunnel syndrome is the most common; approximately 50% of sufferers experience pain. Although common in normal pregnancy, it may be associated with excessive fluid retention, e.g., pre-eclampsia, heart failure. Treatment is with elevation and splints, or surgery. Entrapment of the lateral cutaneous nerve of the thigh (meralgia paraesthetica) may also cause pain/paresthesia. Nerve entrapment may cause abdominal pain (see below).

4. Abdominal pain: nonspecific pain is common in pregnancy and may occasionally be severe; it is thought to be related to the physical presence of the enlarging uterus and stretching/displacement of abdominal structures. Softening and stretching of the ligaments of the symphysis pubis may cause suprapubic pain that can be severe, especially if there is distraction of the symphysis. Nerve entrapment may also occur.

5. Other potentially dangerous conditions that may present with pain should also be considered, e.g., sickle crisis, pulmonary embolism. Trauma is also an important cause of pain, and pregnant women are often victims of domestic violence.

B. Specific to pregnancy: obstetric causes of abdominal pain include torsion/rupture of ovarian cysts, ectopic pregnancy, amnionitis/pelvic infection, labor, placental abruption, and uterine rupture.

III. Management of pain in pregnancy

Be familiar with the principles of management:

A. Nonpharmacological methods are used where possible. The risk of harm to both mother and fetus should always be considered.

B. The neuroendocrine changes of pregnancy mean that parturients are more susceptible to anesthetics (both local and general) and analgesics.

C. Placental transfer of drugs depends on protein binding, lipid solubility, maternal metabolism, and molecular weight. With the exception of large polar molecules, e.g., insulin/heparin, all drugs are transferred to a degree. Drugs may also have indirect fetal effects via maternal effects (e.g., by affecting the mother's blood pressure).

D. Be aware that the pharmacokinetics and pharmacodynamics of analgesics are altered in pregnancy.

IV. Mechanisms and characteristics of labor pain

Understand the causes, pathways, and features of labor pain:

A. Causes

1. First stage: uterine contractions and dilatation of the lower uterine segment and cervix to allow passage of the fetus.
2. Second stage: greater pressure of the presenting part on pain-sensitive pelvic structures and distension of surrounding structures.

B. Pathways

1. Uterus and cervix: mainly via A-delta and C fibers passing in the sympathetic nerves to the sympathetic chain; referred to the T10–L1 dermatomes.
2. Vagina and pelvic outlet: via A-delta and C fibers passing in the parasympathetic bundle in the pudendal nerves; referred to the S2–S4 dermatomes.
3. Other: contributions from the ilioinguinal, genitofemoral, and perforating branch of the posterior cutaneous nerve of the thigh; somatic pain experienced in the L2–S5 dermatomes.

C. Features

1. Over 90% of women experience severe/unbearable labor pain, although recollection fades with time.

2. Typically, pain is similar to other types of visceral pain, i.e., intermittent, severe, and colicky; it starts in the lower abdomen and back, spreading to the perineum and thighs (Lowe 2000).

3. Pain may be influenced by the factors already listed above, in particular by social, societal, and cultural aspects. Certain cultures are more emotive and expressive than other, more stoic ones, leading possibly to differences in pain *behavior* rather than in the extent of pain felt. Fatigue and general debility, common in late pregnancy, may also contribute to the experience of labor pain.

V. Consequences of labor pain

A. Understand that labor pain may have adverse physiological and psychological consequences:

1. Respiratory: causes hyperventilation, leading to hypocapnia and respiratory acidosis.
2. Cardiovascular: increases cardiac output and blood pressure via sympathetic activity; this may be problematic in cardiac disease and pre-eclampsia. Increased venous return associated with uterine contractions may also contribute.
3. Neuroendocrine: increases maternal catecholamine secretion with risk of uteroplacental constriction.
4. Gastrointestinal: effect of labor on gastric emptying and acidity is unclear, although delayed emptying and increased acid secretion have been suggested. Opioids are well known to induce gastric stasis.
5. Psychological: severe labor pain has been implicated in contributing to long-term emotional stress, with potential adverse consequences on maternal mental health and family relationships.

B. Understand also that pain during labor may have benefits:

1. Indicates to the mother and those assisting labor/delivery that contractions are occurring.
2. May have positive connotations regarding childbirth, related to societal/cultural influences.
3. May indicate problems (e.g. uterine rupture, placental abruption).

VI. Management of labor pain

Be familiar with methods of management of labor pain (available techniques will vary according to local resources and customs):

A. Nonpharmacological:

1. Psychological preparation/support, e.g., sympathetic partner, relatives and care-givers; appropriate relaxing environment; psychoprophylaxis, i.e., positive conditioning, distraction, and relaxation techniques (Simkin and O'Hara 2002).
2. Hypnosis: needs appropriately trained hypnotist; 10–20% women are not susceptible to hypnosis, and side effects include anxiety states.
3. Aromatherapy, reflexology, and acupuncture: labor-intensive, and their role is thought to be limited.
4. Transcutaneous electrical nerve stimulation (TENS): often used in early labor and for low levels of pain, but its efficacy in labor is not supported by a systematic review (Carroll et al. 1997).
5. Others: include abdominal decompression and distraction techniques.

B. Systemic analgesia:

1. Parenteral:
   a. "Pure" opioids, e.g., pethidine (meperidine), morphine, diamorphine; more recently fentanyl and remifentanil. Many of the apparent "analgesic" effects may be due to sedation (Olofsson et al. 1996). All cross the placenta easily, and both mother and baby need monitoring during and after labor.
   b. Mixed agents, e.g., meptazinol, tramadol: show no evidence of greater efficacy or safety than traditional opioids.

2. Inhalational:
   a. Nitrous oxide: available premixed 50:50 with oxygen in many countries, where it is widely used but of limited efficacy. May cause nausea, drowsiness, or euphoria and may interact with opioids to cause maternal desaturation.
   b. Volatile agents: most have been studied and found to be helpful, though limited by difficulties in delivery (e.g. draw-over vaporizers and scavenging required) and side effects, particularly sedation.

C. Regional analgesia:

1. Local infiltration/nerve blocks:
   a. Paracervical block: rarely used because of the high risk of intravascular injection and fetal bradycardia.
   b. Pudendal block: used for vaginal deliveries (including instrumental). Blocks the pudendal nerve (S2–S4) arising from the sacral plexus, supplying the lower vagina, vulva and perineum. Ineffective for procedures requiring extensive manipulation e.g. mid-cavity forceps/rotations.

2. Neuraxial techniques:
   a. Caudal: rarely used in developed countries because lumbar epidurals are easier to manage and more flexible.
   b. Spinal: useful for single procedures, e.g., instrumental delivery, but less commonly used for labor, because the effect of a single-shot spinal may not last long enough, even if opioids and local anesthetic are used together.
   c. Lumbar epidural: widely used in developed countries. Has the following advantages:
      i.   Thought to be the most effective form of analgesia in labor.
      ii.   Provides analgesia for instrumental/assisted delivery.
      iii. Avoids the need for general anesthesia with its attendant risks, since the epidural can be topped up for cesarean section or other procedures.
      iv.   Improves the management of pre-eclampsia and thought to be of benefit in multiple pregnancy and prematurity.
      v.   Reduces cardiovascular, respiratory, and neurological stress in systemic disease.
      vi.   May improve neonatal acid-base status in maternal exhaustion.

3. Contra-indications are similar to those in non-obstetric practice; hypovolemia and coagulopathy are the most common. Thrombocytopenia, e.g., associated with pre-eclampsia, may contraindicate neuraxial techniques, although the benefits must be weighed against the risks, and the "safe" cut-off for platelet count is unknown (most authorities using a cut-off of 70–100 x 10^9/l).

4. Brief summary of techniques:
   a. An epidural catheter is usually placed at L3–L4 or L4–L5. In combined spinal-epidural (CSE) techniques, intrathecal local anesthetic and opioid (e.g., bupivacaine 2–4 mg with fentanyl 10–20 µg) are injected first, using either a needle-through-needle or separate-space method. More rapid onset and better analgesia have been claimed for CSE, but these are disputed.
   b. Epidural analgesia is commonly achieved using low-dose mixtures (e.g., bupivacaine 0.1% with fentanyl 2 µg/mL) by infusion (8–15 mL/h) or bolus (10–15 mL as required). Patient-controlled analgesia is also used, but it requires more complex delivery systems, and its advantages and disadvantages are still disputed.
   c. Bupivacaine is still widely used; ropivacaine and levobupivacaine have been introduced more recently. Fentanyl is the most commonly used opioid; in the United States sufentanil is popular.

5. Complications are as for nonpregnant patients. If accidental dural puncture occurs during epidural analgesia, postdural puncture headache occurs in ~50% of cases; the risk of headache after spinal anesthesia with 25–27 G pencil-point needles is <2% (Choi et al. 2003). Neurological lesions are common after childbirth, so women should be warned of the small extra risk from regional analgesia (Loo et al. 2000).

REFERENCES

Carroll D, Tramer M, McQuay H, Nye B, Moore A. Transcutaneous electrical nerve stimulation in labour pain: a systematic review. *Br J Obstet Gynaecol* 1997; 104:169–175.

Choi PT, Galinski SE, Takeuchi L, et al. PDPH is a common complication of neuraxial blockade in parturients: a meta-analysis of obstetrical studies. *Can J Anaesth* 2003; 50:460–469.

Loo CC, Dahlgren G, Irestedt L. Neurological complications in obstetric regional anaesthesia. *Int J Obstet Anesth* 2000; 9:99–124.

Lowe N. The nature of labor pain. *Am J Obstet Gynecol* 2000; 186:S16–24.

Olofsson C, Ekblom A, Ekman-Ordeberg G, Hjelm A Irestedt L. Lack of analgesic effect of systemically administered morphine or pethidine on labour pain. *Br J Obstet Gynaecol* 1996; 103:968–972.

Rathmell J, Viscomi C, Ashburn M. Management of nonobstetric pain during pregnancy and lactation. *Anesth Analg* 1997; 85:1074–1087.

Saisto T, Halmesmaki E. Fear of childbirth: a neglected dilemma. *Acta Obstet Gynecol Scand* 2003; 82:201–208.

Shapira SC, Magora F, Chrubasik S, et al. Assessment of pain threshold and pain tolerance in women in labour and in the early post-partum period by pressure algometry. *Eur J Anaesthesiol* 1995; 12:495–499.

Simkin P, O'Hara M. Nonpharmacologic relief of pain during labor: systematic reviews of five methods. *Am J Obstet Gynaecol* 2002; 186:S131–159.

Whipple B, Josimovich JB, Komisaruk BR. Sensory thresholds during the antepartum, intrapartum and postpartum periods. *Int J Nursing Stud* 1990; 27:213–221.

Core Curriculum for Professional Education in Pain, edited by J. Edmond Charlton, IASP Press, Seattle, © 2005.

37

Headache

I. Know the anatomy and physiology relevant to headache (Lance 1998; Olesen et al. 2000; Silberstein et al. 2002).

    A. Pain-sensitive structures of the head

    B. Physiology of trigeminal nociception

    C. Cephalic vascular system and its innervation

II. Be aware of major hypotheses about mechanisms of headache.

    A. Peripheral nociception, including the concepts of perivascular neuroinflammation and dilatation of cerebral arteries

    B. Central dysmodulation

    C. 5-hydroxytryptamine, calcitonin gene-related peptide, and nitric oxide involvement

    D. Myofascial mechanisms

III. Be able to record a systematic case history of headache and to use a headache diary. Be able to differentiate multiple headache disorders in a single patient. Be able to elicit and understand the clinical significance of the following:

    A. Duration and frequency of attacks

    B. Severity, quality, location, and aggravation by physical activity

    C. Duration and mode of onset

    D. Aura symptoms (immediately preceding headache)

    E. Associated symptoms (e.g., nausea, phonophobia, photophobia)

    F. Precipitating and aggravating factors

    G. Relieving factors

    H. Psychosocial stress

    I. Present or previous traumas and diseases that may cause headache.

    J. Family history

IV. Know how to select and carry out an appropriate examination on the basis of the case history.

    A. General physical examination.

    B. Neurological examination

    C. Pericranial palpation

V. Be aware of the International Classification of Headache Disorders, second edition (ICHD-2; Headache Classification Subcommittee of the International Headache Society 2004). Be aware of the internationally accepted diagnostic criteria for the following headache disorders:

A. Migraine with and without aura.

B. Tension-type headache

C. Cluster headache

D. Chronic post-traumatic headache

E. Medication overuse headache

F. Trigeminal neuralgia

VI. Know the indications for further investigation of headache.

VII. Understand the physical, psychological, and social factors that may contribute to headache, and know the importance of counseling and other nonpharmacological means of treatment (Lance 1998; Olesen et al. 2000; Silberstein et al. 2002).

VIII. Know how to explain about medication overuse headache and how to stop the overuse before intensifying prophylactic drug treatment.

IX. Be able to use the following pharmacological agents appropriately, and be aware of possible alternatives (Lance 1998; Olesen et al. 2000; Silberstein et al. 2002).

A. Acetaminophen, acetylsalicylic acid, and other nonsteroidal anti-inflammatory drugs (NSAIDs) for acute headaches (and migraine attacks), and their possible combination with antiemetics and sedatives

B. Ergotamine and triptans for acute attacks of migraine

C. Oxygen inhalation and sumatriptan injections for acute attacks of cluster headache

D. Beta-blockers for prophylaxis of migraine

E. Verapamil for prophylaxis of cluster headache

X. Know, for the above-mentioned pharmacological agents:

A. Rationale for use

B. Appropriate dosage and route of administration

C. Effects and side effects

D. Degree of documentation by controlled clinical trials

E. Risk of inappropriate use in daily or near-daily headache

REFERENCES

Headache Classification Subcommittee of the International Head-ache Society. The International Classification of Headache Disorders, 2nd ed. *Cephalalgia* 2004, 24 (Suppl 1):1–160.

Lance JW. *Mechanism and Management of Headache,* 6th ed. London: Butterworth-Heinemann, 1998.

Olesen J, Tfelt-Hansen P, Welch KMA. *The Headaches,* 2nd ed. Philadelphia: Lippincott, Williams and Wilkins, 2000.

Silberstein SD, Lipton RB, Goadsby PJ. *Headache in Clinical Practice,* 2nd ed. London: Martin Dunitz, 2002.

Core Curriculum for Professional Education in Pain, edited by J. Edmond Charlton, IASP Press, Seattle, © 2005.

38

Orofacial Pain

I. Anatomical, physiological, and psychological aspects of orofacial pain (Dubner et al. 1978; Dworkin and LeResche 1992; Zarb et al. 1994; Fricton and Dubner 1995; Sessle et al. 1995; Sessle 2000; Lund et al. 2001; Svensson and Graven-Nielsen 2001). Have a broad general knowledge of the anatomy and physiology of the orofacial structures, particularly of the peripheral nerve distribution of the major trigeminal nerve trunks and other cranial nerves, the anatomical relations of the structures they innervate, and their primary central connections.

   A. Be able to recognize the commonalties between the trigeminal system and the spinal and lemniscal systems that make current concepts of nociceptive transmission and its control applicable to the trigeminal system.

   B. Recognize the features that distinguish these systems, e.g., in the trigeminal system, the proportion of myelinated to unmyelinated fibers and the properties of some of these fibers are different from those in spinal nerves; the occurrence of sites (e.g., tooth pulp, cornea) in the orofacial region that are predominantly or exclusively innervated by nociceptive afferents; the bilateral and disproportionately large representation of the orofacial region in higher levels of the somatosensory system; the exquisite sensibility of orofacial tissues.

   C. Be familiar with psychological and psychosocial factors associated with orofacial pain and other pain conditions.

II. Diagnosis of orofacial pain (Attanasio and Mohl 1992; Dworkin and LeResche 1992; Zarb et al. 1994; Fricton and Dubner 1995; Okeson 1995; Sessle et al. 1995; Sharav 1999; Zakrzewska and Harrison 2002; Lund et al. 2001).

   A. Have a broad general knowledge of the major diagnostic features and possible etiological, epidemiological, and pathophysiological aspects of pain associated with:

      1. Specific sites: tooth and surrounding structures, temporomandibular joint, muscle, mucosa, sinus, bone, salivary glands
      2. Orofacial pain conditions including neuralgias, neuropathic pain, painful temporomandibular disorders, and neurovascular and other headaches.

   B. Pain history and clinical examination.

      1. Know the general principles of taking a structured orofacial pain history and carrying out a clinical examination of the orofacial region and adjacent structures.
      2. Be aware that there are objective and validated tests and procedures used for differential diagnosis of many of the above but that some diagnostic approaches still lack reliability, validity, specificity, or sensitivity. Tests and procedures include tooth pulp vitality and tooth percussion tests, muscle palpation tests, salivary tests, quantitative sensory and neurophysiological tests, and other physical exams; behavioral and psychosocial assessments; radiographs and other imaging techniques; microbiological and serological tests; biopsies; and controlled nerve blocks.
      3. Know the common orofacial patterns of pain referral. Be aware that orofacial pain may sometimes be referred from remote sites (e.g., earache, cardiac pain, intracranial lesions).

III.   Treatment of orofacial pain (Attanasio and Mohl 1992; Zarb et al. 1994; Fricton and Dubner 1995; Okeson 1995; Sessle et al. 1995; Sharav 1999; Zakrzewska 1999; Lund et al. 2001; Mohl et al. 2002).

    A.   Be informed of the current evidence-based management approaches, and their indications and contra-indications, for the different types of orofacial pain noted in section II. Some of the commonly used therapeutic approaches include pharmacological agents, surgery, physical medicine, and multidisciplinary approaches, as well as the use of support groups. Be able to inform the patient on these topics.

REFERENCES

Attanasio R, Mohl N. Educational guidelines of temporomandibular disorders. *J Craniomandib Disord Facial Oral Pain* 1992; 6:123–134.

Dubner R, Sessle BJ, Storey AT. *The Neural Basis of Oral and Facial Function.* New York: Plenum, 1978.

Dworkin SF, LeResche L. Research diagnostic criteria for temporomandibular disorders: review, criteria, examinations and specifications, critique. *J Craniomandib Disord Facial Oral Pain* 1992; 6:301–355.

Fricton J, Dubner R. *Advances in Temporomandibular Disorders and Orofacial Pain.* New York: Raven Press, 1995.

Lund JP, Lavigne G, Dubner R, Sessle BJ. *Orofacial Pain: From Basic Science to Clinical Management.* Chicago: Quintessence, 2001.

Mohl ND, Attanasio R, Sessle BJ, Truelove E, Fricton JR. Third Educational Conference to Develop the Curriculum in Temporomandibular Disorders and Orofacial Pain. *J Orofac Pain* 2002; 16:173–199.

Okeson JP. *Bell's Orofacial Pains,* 5th ed. Chicago: Quintessence, 1995.

Sessle BJ. Acute and chronic craniofacial pain: brainstem mechanisms of nociceptive transmission and neuroplasticity, and their clinical correlates. *Crit Rev Oral Biol Med* 2000; 11:57–91.

Sessle BJ, Bryant PS, Dionne RD. *Temporomandibular Disorders and Related Pain Conditions,* Progress in Pain Research and Management, Vol. 4. Seattle: IASP Press, 1995.

Sharav Y. Orofacial pain. In: Wall PD, Melzack R (Eds). *Textbook of Pain,* 4th ed. Edinburgh: Churchill Livingstone, 1999, pp 711–737.

Svensson P, Graven-Nielsen T. Craniofacial muscle pain: review of mechanisms and clinical manifestations. *J Orofac Pain* 2001; 15:117–145.

Zakrzewska JM, Harrison SD. *Assessment and Management of Orofacial Pain.* Amsterdam: Elsevier, 2002.

Zarb GA, Carlsson GE, Sessle BJ, Mohl ND. *Temporomandibular Joint and Masticatory Muscle Disorders.* Copenhagen: Munksgaard, 1994.

Core Curriculum for Professional Education in Pain, edited by J. Edmond Charlton, IASP Press, Seattle, © 2005.

39

Neuropathic Pain

I. Definition

    A. Know the current definition of neuropathic pain (Merskey and Bogduk 1994) and reasons for growing criticism against it (Hansson 2002; Backonja 2003).

        1. Recognize that neuropathic pain is a consequence of injury or disease affecting the somatosensory system.

        2. Know that the patient with neuropathic pain may have concomitant non-neuropathic pain.

II. Epidemiology of common neuropathic pain syndromes (MacDonald et al. 2000)

    A. Know that painful peripheral neuropathy is a common complication in HIV/AIDS, diabetes, alcoholism, and vasculitis (Ziegler et al. 1992; Schmader 2002; Schiffito et al. 2002; Koike et al. 2003; Daousi et al. 2004; Wolfe and Trivedi 2004).

    B. Know that 4 out of 5 patients with idiopathic polyneuropathy and 1 in 3 patients with Guillain Barré syndrome have neuropathic pain (Moulin et al. 1997; Forsberg et al. 2004; Wolfe and Trivedi 2004).

    C. Know that peripheral neuropathic pain is common after surgical procedures (MacRae 2001), including herniorrhaphy (Poobalan et al. 2001; Neumeyer et al. 2004), thoracotomy (Perttunen et al. 1999, Gotoda et al. 2001), and mastectomy (Wallace et al. 1996; Smith et al. 1999), as well as during treatment with chemotherapeutic agents (Quasthoff and Hartung 2002).

    D. Know that patients with stroke, spinal cord injury, multiple sclerosis, and syringomyelia frequently develop neuropathic pain, whereas patients with central nervous system tumors or infection rarely do so (Österberg et al. 1994; Andersen et al. 1995; Cohodarevic et al. 2000; Siddall et al. 2003).

    E. Know that population studies show carpal tunnel syndrome to be very common in certain occupations and in people engaged in repetitive manual work (Atroshi et al. 2003).

    F. Know that the annual incidence of herpes zoster is around 2–4 cases per 1000 population and that the risk of contracting it increases with age (Schmader 2002).

III. Etiology

    A. Know the common causes for neural damage and subsequent pain, i.e., metabolic disease, infection, ischemia, injury, entrapment, connective tissue disease, acquired immunodeficiency, malignancy, drugs, and toxins (Woolf and Mannion 1999; Dworkin 2002; Gonzales et al. 2003; Sommer 2003).

    B. Know that neuropathic pain may develop without any identifiable cause (e.g., intercostal neuralgia, idiopathic polyneuropathy).

    C. Know that painful neuropathy may be the first manifestation of a systemic disease.

IV. Clinical characteristics of neuropathic pain (Jensen et al. 2001; Dworkin 2002; Hansson 2002)

    A. Know the common symptoms associated with neuropathic pain, e.g., burning pain, electric shock-like pain, pain paroxysms, dysesthesia, and paresthesia (Jensen et al. 2001; Dworkin 2002; Hansson 2002; Sommer 2003). Be aware that aching pain is common in polyneuropathy (Otto et al. 2003) and central pain (Hansson 2002).

B. Know that questionnaires have been developed to differentiate neuropathic pain from non-neuropathic pain, e.g., the LANSS Pain Scale (Bennett 2001) and the Neuropathic Pain Questionnaire (Krause and Backonja 2003) or to measure various characteristics, e.g., the Neuropathic Pain Scale (Galer and Jensen 1997) and the Neuropathic Pain Inventory (Bouhassira et al. 2004).

C. Know the common signs associated with neuropathic pain, including positive (mechanical and thermal allodynia and hyperalgesia, temporal and spatial summation), negative (sensory loss, weakness, and muscle atrophy), and other signs (neuroma signs, referred sensation, swelling, skin flare and discoloration, hyperhidrosis, hypohidrosis, and trophic changes) (Bowsher 1996; Baron 2000; Jensen et al. 2001; Jänig and Baron 2003).

D. Know that simple bedside tests alone have low power of distinguishing neuropathic pain from non-neuropathic pain (Rasmussen et al. 2004).

V. Pathological changes in the nervous system

A. Know the pathological changes that occur in the affected nerve(s), e.g., Wallerian degeneration, sprouting, formation of end-neuromas and neuromas-in-continuity, and compression-induced atrophy (Devor and Seltzer 1999; Burnett and Zager 2004).

B. Know the pathological changes that occur in the central nervous system following disease or injury, such as necrosis, apoptosis, gliosis, demyelination, and cavitation, and know that late effects may occur, e.g., syrinx formation following spinal cord injury (Profyris et al. 2004).

VI. Pathophysiological mechanisms in the peripheral nerve fibers for neuropathic pain (Devor and Seltzer 1999; Woolf and Mannion 1999; Woolf 2004)

A. Changes in the peripheral afferents.

1. Know that injury causes ectopic discharges at the site of injury, at the neuroma, and at the dorsal root ganglion.
2. Know that increased activity is also seen in neighboring uninjured C fibers (Wu et al. 2001).
3. Know that upregulation of several sodium channels, downregulation of potassium channels, and reduction in threshold in TRP transducer ion channels have a major role in the generation and maintenance of increased activity.
4. Know that sensitization of a subgroup of mechanoinsensitive C fibers may contribute to hyperalgesia (Orstavik et al. 2003).
5. Know that A fibers may undergo phenotype switch, and start expressing brain-derived neurotrophic factor (BDNF) and substance P.
6. Be familiar with the role of inflammatory mediators, e.g., cytokines, prostaglandins, and serotonin, in the maintenance of peripheral sensitization.
7. Know that hypersensitivity of adrenergic receptors in injured terminals may make them excessively sensitive to the effects of circulating norepinephrine.

B. Central changes following peripheral nerve injury or disease (Woolf and Mannion 1999; Ji et al. 2003).

1. Understand the concept of central sensitization and know that several forms of central sensitization occur (both dependent on and independent of nociceptor activity).
2. Appreciate that increased and prolonged ectopic activity in peripheral nociceptors (and in non-nociceptors following phenotype switch) promotes increased synaptic efficacy in the dorsal horn and increased responsiveness of dorsal horn neurons and expansion of their receptive fields.
3. Appreciate that central sensitization explains many features of neuropathic pain, including referral outside the injured nerve's territory and touch-evoked pain.
4. Be aware that central sensitization-like phenomena occur in the rostroventral medulla, amygdala, anterior cingulate cortex, and trigeminal brainstem complex.

5. Be aware of reports of increased sprouting of central terminals of injured fibers within the dorsal horn, and know that conclusive evidence is still lacking.

C. Be familiar with the significance of activation in spinal astrocytes and microglia in chronic neuropathic pain (Watkins et al. 2001).

D. Be aware of increased spontaneous activity in the thalamus as the result of injury to the peripheral and central nervous systems, and understand its relation to pain (Lenz et al. 2000; Nandi et al. 2003).

E. Be aware of the structural and functional neuroplastic changes that occur at the subcortical and cortical level following injury to the peripheral or central nervous system and contribute to perception of pain (Flor 2002, 2003; Wall et al. 2002).

F. Be aware of the evidence suggesting disruption of spinal inhibition involving, e.g., GABAergic and cannabinoid mechanisms (Drew et al. 2004).

G. Be aware of the mechanisms of descending modulation of spinal nociceptive processing, and know that this phenomenon has both inhibitory and facilitatory components (Porreca et al. 2002).

VII. Investigations (Cruccu et al. 2004)

A. Know the common bedside tests used to assess positive and negative signs (Cruccu et al. 2004).

B. Know the advantages and limitations of conventional neurophysiological tests, e.g., that nerve conduction studies will show level of pathology but cannot detect abnormal C-fiber or A-delta-fiber function (Treede 2003).

C. Know the advantages and limitations of quantitative sensory testing (Shy et al. 2003; Chong and Cros 2004).

D. Know the advantages and limitations of laser-evoked potentials (Treede 2003; Truini et al. 2004).

E. Be aware of the use of structural magnetic resonance imaging and know that it has diagnostic value in sciatica and trigeminal neuralgia and may be useful in selected cases of nerve injury or entrapment (Meaney 1995; Akimoto et al. 2002; Koltzenburg and Bendzsus 2004).

F. Be aware of the potential of functional brain imaging in assessment of neuropathic pain.

G. Be aware that skin punch biopsies are useful in the diagnosis of small-fiber neuropathies (Griffin et al. 2001).

VIII. Know the following common neuropathic pain syndromes, including their clinical features, supporting laboratory and radiographic findings, differential diagnosis, natural course, and proposed pathology.

A. Painful focal neuropathies (including mononeuropathies, plexopathies, and radiculopathies).

1. Syndromes related to compression of peripheral nerves or nerve roots, e.g., lumbar and cervical radiculopathies, carpal and tarsal tunnel syndrome, and meralgia paresthetica (Stewart 2000).
2. Syndromes related to inflammation of peripheral nerves (e.g., acute herpes zoster and Guillain-Barré syndrome (Moulin et al. 1997; Haanpää et al. 1999).
3. Syndromes related to ischemia/infarction of peripheral nerves, e.g., diabetic or vasculitic mononeuropathies (Griffin 2001; Dyck and Vindebank 2002).
4. Syndromes associated with nerve injury, with or without neuroma formation, e.g., stump pain, postmastectomy pain, postherniorrhaphy pain (Macrae 2001).
5. Common syndromes with unknown etiology (e.g., intercostal neuralgia).

B. Painful polyneuropathies (including acute-onset and slow-onset distal symmetrical polyneuropathies)

1. HIV (Schiffito et al. 2002; Luciano et al. 2003).

2. Mixed small- and large-diameter-fiber polyneuropathies, e.g., diabetic, vasculitic, toxic, inflammatory, and paraneoplastic (Otto et al. 2003; Sommer 2003; Wolfe and Trivedi 2004).
3. Small-fiber neuropathies, e.g., idiopathic, Fabry's disease, amyloid, acute-onset diabetic neuropathy (Luciano et al. 2002; Lacomis 2003).

C. Postherpetic neuralgia (Watson 2003).

D. Trigeminal neuralgia and other cranial neuralgias (Nurmikko and Eldridge 2001).

E. Phantom limb pain (Flor 2002).

F. Brachial plexus avulsion (Wynn Parry 1980).

G. Central post-stroke pain (Bowsher 1996; Gonzales and Casey 2003).

H. Other common central pain syndromes, e.g., spinal cord injury, spinal cord tumor, tethered cord syndrome, multiple sclerosis, syringomyelia (Gonzales and Casey 2003; Finnerup and Jensen 2004).

I. Cancer-associated neuropathic pain, e.g., tumor invasion of nerve and plexus, epidural metastases, post-radiation syndromes, and drug-induced neuropathies.

J. Complex regional pain syndrome (CRPS) type II (Jänig and Baron 2003).

IX. Therapeutic interventions applied in neuropathic pain

A. Know the common pharmacological approaches used for neuropathic pain of all types.

1. Be aware of the multiple coexisting mechanisms in many neuropathic pain conditions and the advantages and disadvantages of combination therapy.
2. Be aware of the limitations of controlled clinical trials, and familiar with methods for assessing the quality of publications (Jadad and McQuay 1993).
3. Know specific agents and syndromes where data from controlled clinical trials have established efficacy (Sindrup and Jensen 1999; Dworkin et al. 2003a).

   a. Tricyclic antidepressants (McQuay et al. 1996).
   b. Serotonin-norepinephrine reuptake inhibitors (SNRIs), e.g., venlafaxine and duloxetine (Sindrup et al. 2003; Rowbotham et al. 2004).
   c. Gabapentin and pregabalin (Mellegers et al. 2001, Dworkin et al. 2003b).
   d. Other antiepileptic drugs, e.g., carbamazepine in trigeminal neuralgia and lamotrigine in diabetic and HIV neuropathy (Eisenberg et al. 2001; Simpson et al. 2003).
   e. Opioids (Kalso et al. 2004).
   f. Topical treatments, e.g., capsaicin, lidocaine patch (Meier et al. 2003; Mason et al. 2005).
   g. Tramadol (Dühmke et al. 2004).
   h. Cannabinoids in multiple sclerosis (Svendsen et al. 2004, Rog et al. 2005).
   i. Bupropion (Schemenuck et al. 2001).
   j. Dextromethorphan (Sang et al. 2002).

4. Know agents which may have efficacy but data are insufficient or conflicting (e.g., selective serotonin reuptake inhibitors [SSRIs], adenosine, i.v. ketamine).
5. Be aware of data suggesting lack of effect of drugs in certain neuropathic pains, e.g., amitriptyline in HIV neuropathy (Kieburtz et al. 1998), dextromethorphan in postherpetic neuralgia (Sang et al. 2002), topiramate in diabetic neuropathy (Thienel et al. 2005), riluzole in peripheral neuropathic pain (Galer et al. 2000), and sodium valproate in spinal cord injury (Drewes et al. 1994).
6. Be aware of the lack of evidence supporting the use of nonsteroidal anti-inflammatory drugs in neuropathic pain.
7. Know the contraindications, side effects, and interactions of drugs commonly used in neuropathic pain, and how to minimize the risk of adverse effects.
8. Know the indications and contraindications for prescribing strong opioids in neuropathic pain.

9. Know the drugs traditionally used in the treatment of sympathetically mediated pain and be aware of the limited data in support of their use (e.g., corticosteroids. phenoxybenzamine, prazosin, guanethidine, and clonidine).

B. Know the data supporting intrathecal and epidural administration of drugs (ziconotide, morphine, clonidine, and bupivacaine) in selected cases (Bennett et al. 2000).

1. Be aware of the indications and contraindications for drug delivery systems.
2. Be aware of risks and complications (e.g., infection, overdosing, granuloma formation, catheter migration).

C. Know the limited role of regional approaches in the management of chronic neuropathic pain other than in syndromes in which pain is thought to be primarily sympathetically mediated (Abram 2000). Know that published evidence supporting the use of chemical sympathectomy in neuropathic pain is virtually absent (Mailis and Furlan 2001). Be aware of the indications, techniques, and potential complications of sympathetic blockade.

D. Know the role of surgical approaches to pain management in patients with neuropathic pain.

1. Be aware of the role of peripheral procedures in selected patients with specific pain syndromes, e.g., decompression of entrapped peripheral nerves, microvascular decompression in trigeminal neuralgia, or controlled gangliolysis in trigeminal neuralgia (Stewart 2000; Nurmikko and Eldridge 2001).
2. Be aware of the conflicting reports regarding surgical procedures in the treatment of post-injury neuromas.
3. Be aware of extremely limited data supporting the use of neurolytic procedures in peripheral neuropathic pain (e.g., cryosurgery, phenol).
4. Be aware of the data suggesting efficacy of dorsal root entry zone lesions in selected patients with specific pain syndromes, e.g., avulsion of the brachial plexus, or pain following spinal cord injury (Sindou et al. 2001).

E. Be familiar with neurostimulation in the management of neuropathic pain.

1. Be aware of the limited data published on the efficacy of transcutaneous electrical nerve stimulation and other similar electric stimulation methods.
2. Be aware that there are insufficient data supporting the efficacy of acupuncture in the management of neuropathic pain to warrant any conclusions.
3. Be aware of the data supporting the use of peripheral nerve stimulation in selected neuropathic syndromes (Eisenberg et al. 2004; Johnson and Burchiel 2004).
4. Be aware of the emerging data supporting the use of spinal cord stimulation in the management of selected neuropathic pain conditions (Quigley et al. 2003; Mailis-Gagnon et al. 2004).
5. Be aware of the data suggesting benefit from motor cortex stimulation in selected neuropathic pains.
6. Be aware of the data suggesting benefit from deep brain stimulation in selected patients with neuropathic pain.

F. Know the utility of rehabilitation to neuropathic pain management.
1. Understand the fundamental importance of physical therapy in treatment for some neuropathic disorders (e.g., CRPS).
2. Know the analgesic potential of orthoses and prostheses in selected patients with particular pain syndromes (e.g., a prosthesis for a patient with stump pain and phantom pain).
3. Have knowledge of a multidisciplinary approach to the patient with pain and related disabilities secondary to neuropathic lesion, and understand the importance of maintained function as a goal equal in importance to the goal of pain relief.

G. Recognize the need for behavioral and psychological approaches to neuropathic pain.

1. Know that depression and anxiety are commonly associated with neuropathic pain and may need specific therapy.
2. Know that sleep disturbance is common in neuropathic pain.
3. Know that quality of life is severely reduced in chronic neuropathic pain.
4. Be aware of the efficacy of cognitive-behavioral pain management programs in neuropathic pain.

REFERENCES

Abram SE. Neural blockade for neuropathic pain. *Clin J Pain* 2000; 16(2 Suppl):S56–61.

Akimoto H, Nagaoka T, Nariai T, et al. Preoperative evaluation of neurovascular compression in patients with trigeminal neuralgia by use of three-dimensional reconstruction from two types of high-resolution magnetic resonance imaging. *Neurosurgery* 2002; 51:956–961.

Andersen G, Vestergaard K, Ingeman-Nielsen M, Jensen TS. Incidence of post-stroke pain. *Pain* 1995; 61:187–193.

Atroshi I, Gummesson C, Johnsson R, McCabe SJ, Ornstein E. Severe carpal tunnel syndrome potentially needing surgical treatment in a general population. *J Hand Surg [Am]* 2003; 28:639–644.

Backonja M-M. Defining neuropathic pain. *Anesth Analg* 2003; 97:785–790.

Baron R. Peripheral neuropathic pain: from mechanisms to symptoms. *Clin J Pain* 2000; 16(2 Suppl):S12–20.

Bennett G, Deer T, Du Pen S, et al. Future directions in the management of pain by intraspinal drug delivery. *J Pain Symptom Manage* 2000; 20:S44–50.

Bennett M. The LANSS Pain Scale: the Leeds assessment of neuropathic symptoms and signs. *Pain* 2001; 92:147–157.

Bouhassira D, Attal N, Fermanian J, et al. Development and validation of the Neuropathic Pain Symptom Inventory. *Pain* 2004; 108:248–257.

Bowsher D. Central pain: clinical and physiological characteristics. *J Neurol Neurosurg Psychiatry* 1996; 61:62–69.

Burnett MG, Zager EL. Pathophysiology of peripheral nerve injury: a brief review. *Neurosurg Focus* 2004; 16(5):E1.

Chong PST, Cros DP. Technology literature review: quantitative sensory testing. *Muscle Nerve* 2004; 29:734–747.

Cohodarevic T, Mailis A, Montanera W. Syringomyelia: pain, sensory abnormalities and neuroimaging. *J Pain* 2000; 1:54–66.

Cruccu G, Anand P, Attal N, et al. EFNS Guidelines on neuropathic pain assessment. *Eur J Neurol* 2004; 11:153–162.

Daousi C, MacFarlane IA, Woodward A, et al. Chronic painful peripheral neuropathy in an urban community: a controlled comparison of people with and without diabetes. *Diabet Med* 2004; 21:976–982.

Devor M, Seltzer Z. Pathophysiology of damaged nerves in relation to chronic pain. In: Wall PD, Melzack R (Eds). *Textbook of Pain*. Edinburgh: Churchill Livingstone, 1999, pp 129–144.

Dyck PJ, Vindebank AJ. Diabetic and nondiabetic lumbosacral radiculoplexus neuropathies: new insights into pathophysiology and treatment. *Muscle Nerve* 2002; 25:477–491.

Dworkin RH. An overview of neuropathic pain: syndromes, symptoms, signs and several mechanisms. *Clin J Pain* 2002; 18:343–349.

Dworkin RH, Backonja M, Rowbotham MC, et al. Advances in neuropathic pain. Diagnosis, mechanisms, and treatment recommendations. *Arch Neurol* 2003a; 60:1524–1534.

Dworkin RH, Corbin AE, Young JP Jr, et al. Pregabalin for the treatment of postherpetic neuralgia: a randomized, placebo-controlled trial. *Neurology* 2003b; 60:1274–1283.

Eisenberg E, Lurie Y, Braker C, Daoud D, Ishay A. Lamotrigine reduces painful diabetic neuropathy: a randomized, controlled study. *Neurology* 2001; 57:505–509.

Eisenberg E, Waisbrod H, Gerbershagen HU. Long-term peripheral nerve stimulation for painful nerve injuries. *Clin J Pain* 2004; 20:143–146.

Finnerup NB, Jensen TS. Spinal cord injury pain—mechanisms and treatment. *Eur J Neurology* 2004; 11:73–82.

Flor H. Phantom-limb pain. Characteristics, causes and treatment. *Lancet Neurol* 2002; 1:182–189.

Flor H. Remapping somatosensory cortex after injury. *Adv Neurol* 2003; 93:195–204.

Forsberg A, Press R, Einarsson U. Impairment in Guillain-Barré syndrome during first two years after onset: a prospective study. *J Neurol Sci* 2004; 227:131–138.

Galer BS, Jensen MP. Development and preliminary validation of a pain measure specific to neuropathic pain: the Neuropathic Pain Scale. *Neurology* 1997; 48:332–338.

Galer BS, Twilling U, Harle J, et al. Lack of efficacy of riluzole in the treatment of peripheral neuropathic pain conditions. *Neurology* 2000; 55:971–975.

Gonzales GR, Casey KL. Central pain syndromes. In: Jensen TS, Wilson PR, Rice ACR (Eds). *Clinical Pain Management: Chronic Pain*. London: Arnold, 2003, pp 403–416.

Griffin JW. Vasculitic neuropathies. *Rheum Dis Clin North Am* 2001; 27:751–760.

Griffin JW, McArthur JC, Polydefkis M. Assessment of cutaneous innervation by skin biopsies. *Curr Opin Neurol* 2001; 14:655–659.

Gotoda Y, Kambara N, Sakai T, et al. The morbidity, time course, and predictive factors for persistent post-thoracotomy pain. *Eur J Pain* 2001; 5:89–96.

Haanpää M, Laippala P, Nurmikko T. Pain and somatosensory dysfunction in acute herpes zoster. *Clin J Pain* 1999; 15:78–84.

Hansson P. Neuropathic pain: clinical characteristics and diagnostic workup. *Eur J Pain* 2002; 6(Suppl A):47–50.

Jänig W, Baron R. Complex regional pain syndrome: mystery explained? *Lancet Neurol* 2003; 2:687–695.

Jensen TS, Gottrup H, Sindrup SH, Bach FW. The clinical picture of neuropatic pain. *Eur J Pharmacol* 2001; 429:1–11.

Ji R-R, Kohno T, Moore KA, Woolf CJ. Central sensitization and LTP. Do pain and memory share similar mechanisms? *Trends Neurosci* 2003; 26:696–705.

Johnson MD, Burchiel KJ. Peripheral stimulation for treatment of trigeminal postherpetic neuralgia and trigeminal posttraumatic neuropathic pain: a pilot study. *Neurosurgery* 2004; 55:135–141.

Kalso E, Edwards JE, Moore RA, McQuay HJ. Opioids in chronic non-cancer pain: systematic review of efficacy and safety. *Pain* 2004; 112:372–380.

Kieburtz K, Simpson D, Yiannoutsos C, et al. A randomized trial of amitriptyline and mexiletine for painful neuropathy in HIV infection. *Neurology* 1998; 51(6):1682–1688.

Koike H, Iijima M, Sgiura M, et al. Alcoholic neuropathy is clinicopathologically distinct from thiamine-deficiency neuropathy. *Ann Neurol* 2003; 54:19–29.

Koltzenburg M, Bendszus M. Imaging of peripheral nerve lesions. *Curr Opin Neurol* 2004; 17:621–626.

Krause SJ, Backonja MM. Development of a neuropathic pain questionnaire. *Clin J Pain* 2003; 19:306–314.

Lenz FA, Lee JI, Garonsik IM, et al. Plasticity of pain-related neuronal activity in the human thalamus. *Prog Brain Res* 2000; 129:259–273.

Luciano CA, Russell JW, Banerjee TK. Physiological characterization of neuropathy in Fabry's disease. *Muscle Nerve* 2002; 26:622–629.

Luciano CA, Pardo CA, McArthur JC. Recent developments in the HIV neuropathies. *Curr Opin Neurol* 2003; 16:403–409.

MacDonald BK, Cockerell OC, Sander JW, Shorvon SD. The incidence and lifetime prevalence of neurological disorders in a prospective community-based study in the UK. *Brain* 2000; 123:665–676.

Macrae WA. Chronic pain after surgery. *Br J Anaesth* 2001; 87:88–98.

Mailis A, Furlan A. Sympathectomy for neuropathic pain. *Cochrane Database Syst Rev* 2002; 1:CD002918.

Mailis-Gagnon A, Furlan AD, Sandoval JA, Taylor R. Spinal cord stimulation for chronic pain. *Cochrane Database Syst Rev* 2004; 3:CD003783.

Meaney JF, Eldridge PR, Dunn LT, et al. Demonstration of neurovascular compression in trigeminal neuralgia with magnetic resonance imaging. Comparison of surgical findings in 52 consecutive operative cases. *J Neurosurg* 1995; 83:799–805.

Merskey H, Bogduk N (Eds). *Classification of Chronic Pain: Descriptions of Chronic Pain Syndromes and Definitions of Pain Terms,* 2nd ed. Seattle: IASP Press, 1994.

Moulin DE, Hagen N, Feasley TE, Amiseh R, Hahn R. Pain in Guillain-Barré syndrome. *Neurology* 1997; 48:328–331.

Nandi D, Aziz T, Carter H, Stein J. Thalamic field potentials in chronic central pain treated by periventricular gray stimulation: a series of eight cases. *Pain* 2003; 101:97–107.

Neumayer L, Giobbie-Hunder A, Jonasson O, et al. Open mesh versus laparoscopic mesh repair of inguinal hernia. *N Engl J Med* 2004; 350:1819–1827.

Nurmikko TJ, Eldridge PR. Trigeminal neuralgia. *Br J Anaesth* 2001; 87:117–132.

Orstavik K, Weidner C, Schmidt et al. Pathological C-fibers in patients with a chronic painful condition. *Brain* 2003; 126:567–578.

Österberg A, Boivie J, Holmgren H, Thuomas K-A, Johansson I. The clinical characteristics and sensory abnormalities of patients with central pain caused by multiple sclerosis. In: Gebhart GF, Hammond DL, Jensen TS (Eds). *Proceedings of the 7th World Congress on Pain,* Progress in Pain Research and Management, Vol. 2. Seattle: IASP Press, 1994, pp 789–796.

Otto M, Bak S, Bach FW, Jensen TS, Sindrup SH. Pain phenomena and possible pain mechanisms in patients with painful polyneuropathy. *Pain* 2003; 101:187–192.

Perttunen K, Tasmuth T, Kalso E. Chronic pain after thoracic surgery: a follow-up study. *Acta Anaesthesiol Scand* 1999; 43:563–567.

Poobalan AS, Bruce J, King PM, et al. Chronic pain and quality of life following open inguinal hernia repair. *Br J Surg* 2001; 88:1122–1126.

Porreca F, Ossipov MH, Gebhart GF. Chronic pain and medullary descending facilitation. *Trends Neurosci* 2002; 25:319–325.

Profyris C, Cheema SS, Zang D, et al. Degenerative and regenerative mechanisms governing spinal cord injury. *Neurobiol Dis* 2004; 15:415–436.

Quasthoff S, Hartung P. Chemotherapy-induced peripheral neuropathy. *J Neurol* 2002; 249:9–17.

Quigley DG, Arnold J, Eldridge PR, et al. Long-term outcome of spinal cord stimulation and hardware complications. *Sterotact Funct Neurourg* 2003; 81:50–56.

Rasmussen PV, Sindrup SH, Jensen TS, Bach FW. Symptoms and signs in patients with suspected neuropathic pain. *Pain* 2004; 110(1–2):461–469.

Rowbotham MC, Goli V, Kunz NR, Lei D. Venlafaxine extended release in the treatment of painful diabetic neuropathy. *Pain* 2004; 110:697–706.

Sang CN, Booher S, Gilron I, Parada S, Max MB. Dextromethorphan and memantine in painful diabetic neuropathy and postherpetic neuralgia: efficacy and dose-response trials. *Anesthesiology* 2002; 96:1053–1061.

Schiffito G, McDermott M, McArthur JC, et al. Incidence of and risk factors for HIV associated distal sensory polyneuropathy. *Neurology* 2002; 58:1764–1768.

Schmader KE. Epidemiology and impact on quality of life of postherpetic neuralgia and painful diabetic neuropathy. *Clin J Pain* 2002; 18:350–354.

Schemenuck MR, Sherman S, Davis B. Double-blind, randomized trial of bupropion SR for the treatment of neuropathic pain. *Neurology* 2001; 57:1583–1588.

Shy ME, Frohmann EM, So YT, et al. Quantitative sensory testing: report of the Therapeutics and Technology Assessment Subcommittee of the American Academy of Neurology. *Neurology* 2003; 60:898–904.

Siddall PJ, McClelland JM, Rutkowski SB, Cousins MJ. A longitudinal study of the prevalence and characteristics of pain in the first 5 years following spinal cord injury. *Pain* 2003; 103:249–257.

Simpson DM, McArthur JC, Olney M, et al. Lamotrigine for HIV-associated painful sensory neuropathies: a placebo-controlled trial. *Neurology* 2003; 60:1508–1514.

Sindrup SH, Jensen TS. Efficacy of pharmacological treatments of neuropathic pain: an update and effect related to mechanism of drug action. *Pain* 1999; 83:389–400.

Sindrup SH, Bach FW, Madsen C, Gran LE, Jensen TS. Venlafaxine versus imipramine in painful polyneuropathy: a randomized, controlled trial. *Neurology* 2003; 60:1284–1249.

Sindou M, Martens P, Wael M. Microsurgical DREZotomy for pain due to spinal cord and/or cauda equina injuries: long-term results in a series of 44 patients. *Pain* 2001; 92:159–171.

Smith WCS, Bourne D, Squair J, Phillips DO, Chamber AW. A retrospective study of post mastectomy pain syndrome. *Pain* 1999; 83:91–95.

Sommer C. Painful neuropathies. *Curr Opin Neurol* 2003; 16:623–628.

Stewart JD. *Focal Peripheral Neuropathies,* 3rd ed. Philadelphia: Lippincott William & Wilkins, 2000.

Svendsen KB, Jensen TS, Bach FW. Does the cannabinoid dronabinol reduce central pain in multiple sclerosis? Randomised double blind placebo controlled crossover trial. *BMJ* 2004; 329:253.

Thienel U, Neto W, Schwabe SK, Vijapurkar U. Topiramate in painful diabetic polyneuropathy: findings from three double-blind, placebo-controlled trials. *Acta Neurol Scand* 2005; in press.

Treede RD. Neurophysiological studies of pain pathways in peripheral and central nervous system disorders. *J Neurol* 2003; 250:1152–1161.

Truini A, Romanelli A, Galeotti F, Iannetti GD, Cruccu G. Laser evoked potentials for assessing sensory neuropathy in human patients. *Neurosci Lett* 2004; 361:25–28.

Wallace MS, Wallace AM, Lee J, Dobke MK. Pain after breast surgery: a survey of 282 women. *Pain* 1996; 66:195–205.

Watkins LR, Milligan ED, Maier SF. Spinal cord glia: new players in pain. *Pain* 2001; 93:201–205.

Watson CPN. Postherpetic neuralgia. In: Jensen TS, Wilson PR, Rice ASC (Eds). *Chronic Pain: Clinical Pain Management.* London: Arnold, 2003, pp 451–458.

Wolfe GI, Trivedi JA. Painful neuropathy and its nonsurgical treatment. *Muscle Nerve* 2004; 30:3–19.

Woolf CJ. Dissecting out mechanisms responsible for peripheral neuropathic pain: implications for diagnosis and therapy. *Life Sci* 2004; 74:2605–2610.

Woolf CJ, Mannion RJ. Neuropathic pain: aetiology, symptoms, mechanisms and management. *Lancet* 1999; 353:1959–1964.

Wu G, Ringkamp M, Hartke TV, et al. Early onset of spontaneous activity in uninjured C-fiber nociceptors after injury to neighboring nerve fibers. *J Neurosci* 2001; 21:RC140(1–5).

Wynn Parry CB. Pain in avulsion lesions of the brachial plexus. *Pain* 1980; 9:41–53.

Ziegler D, Gries FA, Spuler M, Lessmann F. The epidemiology of diabetic neuropathy. *J Diabet Complications* 1992; 6:49–57.

Core Curriculum for Professional Education in Pain, edited by J. Edmond Charlton, IASP Press, Seattle, © 2005.

40

Complex Regional Pain Syndromes

I.   Know the definition of complex regional pain syndrome (CRPS) and be aware of the inciting traumatologic events (Stanton-Hicks et al. 1995).

  A. CRPS type I (reflex sympathetic dystrophy). Minor injuries or fracture of a limb precede the onset of symptoms.

  B. CRPS type II (causalgia) develops after injury to a major peripheral nerve.

II. Know the common clinical characteristics of CRPS (Veldman et al. 1993; Birklein et al. 2000; Baron and Wasner 2001; Wasner et al. 2003, Fördereuther et al. 2004).

  A. Know the common sensory signs and symptoms associated with CRPS:

    1. Continuous burning pain in the distal part of the affected extremity.
    2. Pain is disproportionate in intensity to the inciting event and usually increases when the extremity is in a dependent position.
    3. Stimulus-evoked pains include mechanical and thermal allodynia and/or hyperalgesia, and deep somatic allodynia (pain due to touching the joints and movement of joints).
    4. Sensory abnormalities are most pronounced distally, and have no consistent spatial relationship to individual nerve territories or to the site of the inciting lesion.

  B. Know the common autonomic abnormalities associated with CRPS:

    1. Swelling of the distal extremity especially in the acute phase
    2. Hyper- or hypohidrosis
    3. Vasodilatation or vasoconstriction
    4. Changes in skin temperature

  C. Know the common trophic changes associated with CRPS:

    1. Abnormal nail growth
    2. Increased or decreased hair growth
    3. Fibrosis
    4. Thin, glossy skin
    5. Osteoporosis

  D. Know the common motor abnormalities associated with CRPS:

    1. Weakness
    2. Coordination deficits
    3. Tremor
    4. Dystonia
    5. Neglect-like symptoms or symptoms of disturbed body perception of the affected extremity

  E. Know that sympathetically maintained pain (SMP) may occur in CRPS (Baron et al. 1999; Ali et al. 2000; Baron et al. 2002).

    1. Be aware that this pain component may be relieved by specific sympatholytic procedures (e.g., sympathetic blocks).

2. Know that SMP is defined to be a symptom or the underlying mechanism in a subset of patients with CRPS and not a clinical entity. The positive effect of a sympathetic blockade is not essential for the diagnosis of CRPS.

F. Understand that CRPS evolves through different stages, although the duration of each stage may be variable.

III. Know the proposed pathophysiological mechanisms of CRPS (Baron et al. 1999; Birklein et al. 2001; Huygen et al. 2002; Juottonen et al. 2002; Jänig and Baron 2003; Maihofner et al. 2003).

A. In the periphery:

1. Know the abnormal characteristics of primary afferents after lesion in CRPS-II (e.g., spontaneous discharge, sensitization, ectopic mechanosensitivity, or acquired responsiveness to norepinephrine).
2. Understand the proposed role in spontaneous discharge of sodium channel accumulation in the terminal membrane.
3. Understand the proposed role of acquired norepinephrine responsiveness in intact C nociceptor terminals whose axons travel in a damaged nerve.
4. Be aware of the potential role of an inflammatory reaction and neurogenic inflammation in the acute phase of CRPS.

B. For the central nervous system:

1. Understand the proposed role of N-methyl-D-aspartate (NMDA)-receptor mediated hyperexcitability in the spinal cord dorsal horn.
2. Understand how spinal cord neuron hyperexcitability can account for pain that shows a distally generalized distribution.
3. Understand that a persistent source of nociceptor drive may dynamically maintain hyperexcitability in central neurons.
4. Realize that the somatosensory cortical maps are changed in S1.
5. Understand that an unilateral inhibition of central sympathetic vasoconstrictor activity is involved in vascular abnormalities.
6. Realize that motor abnormalities must be generated in the central nervous system.

IV. Know the proposed diagnostic procedures in CRPS (Galer et al. 1998; Allen et al. 1999; Bruehl et al. 1999; Harden et al. 1999; Oerlemans et al. 1999; Sieweke et al. 1999; van de Beek et al. 2002; Wasner et al. 2002, 2003).

A. Realize that CRPS diagnosis is based upon clinical criteria and that there is so far no gold standard nor any objective diagnostic tool.

B. Be aware that CRPS may be potentially overdiagnosed.

C. Know the categories of clinical signs and symptoms that are important for diagnosis, know the interpretation of these diagnostic criteria for clinical use and the sensitivity and specificity (sensitivity 0.85, specificity 0.60).

1. Positive sensory abnormalities: spontaneous pain, mechanical hyperalgesia, thermal hyperalgesia, deep somatic hyperalgesia.
2. Vascular abnormalities: vasodilation, vasoconstriction, skin temperature asymmetries, skin color changes.
3. Edema, sweating abnormalities: swelling, hyperhidrosis, hypohidrosis.
4. Motor, trophic changes: motor weakness, tremor, dystonia, coordination deficits, nail changes, hair changes, skin atrophy, joint stiffness, soft tissue changes.
5. Interpretation. One or more symptoms of three or more categories each AND one or more signs of two or more categories each.

E. Know the diagnostic tests which may aid the diagnosis of CRPS.

    1. Understand the roles that X-ray, three-phase bone scan, quantitative sensory testing (QST), autonomic testing, and thermography play in CRPS diagnosis.

V. Know the therapeutic interventions applied in CRPS (Kingery 1997; Price et al. 1998; Stanton-Hicks et al. 1998, 2002; Kemler et al. 2000; van Hilten et al. 2000; Perez et al. 2001; Forouzanfar et al. 2002; Moseley 2004).

A. Know the basic guidelines in the treatment of CRPS.

    1. Realize that treatment should be immediate after diagnosis.
    2. Realize that even a suspected CRPS should be evaluated by a pain specialists to start adequate therapy immediately.
    3. Have knowledge of a multidisciplinary approach to the patient with CRPS, and understand that the treatment is most importantly directed toward restoration of full function of the affected area.
    4. Know that severity of the disease determines the therapeutic regime and that reduction of pain is the precondition with which all other interventions must comply.
    5. Realize that the intensity of therapy (in particular physiotherapy) should be adapted to the severity of the disease. It should be gentle and below pain threshold and must not exacerbate the pain since every painful stimulus may worsen the syndrome.

B. Know pharmacological approaches typically used for neuropathic pain of all types.

    1. Know specific agents for which data from controlled clinical trials have established efficacy in CRPS (e.g., gabapentin, corticosteroids, Ca-modulating drugs, free radical scavengers).
    2. Know agents for which substantial anecdotal evidence exists for efficacy in CRPS (e.g., antidepressants, anticonvulsants, opioids, capsaicin, lidocaine).
    3. Know drugs typically used in the treatment of sympathetically mediated pain and be aware of the limited data in support of their use (e.g., phenoxybenzamine, prazosin, guanethidine, reserpine, and clonidine).

C. Know the role of interventional approaches in the management of CRPS.

    1. Be aware of the indications, techniques, and potential complications of sympathetic blockade in CRPS.
    2. Know the different types of local sympathetic blocks.
    3. Know the indications, advantages and disadvantages, and drugs and techniques employed in regional intravenous blockade.
    4. Understand the limited role of surgical sympathectomy in patients who respond to temporary sympathetic blocks.
    5. Be aware of the methods employed to document effective regional sympathetic block (e.g., thermography and laser Doppler).
    6. Be aware of the existence, possible causes, and treatment of post-sympathectomy pain.

D. Be aware of neurostimulatory approaches to the management of CRPS.

    1. Be aware of the variability in response to transcutaneous electrical nerve stimulation and the multiple methods that can be employed.
    2. Understand the limited role played by percutaneous electrical nerve stimulation.
    3. Be aware of the data supporting the value of dorsal column stimulation.
    4. Be aware of the data supporting motor cortex stimulation.
    5. Be aware of the data supporting and refuting the value of deep brain stimulation.

E. Be aware of the response of pain to clonidine and refractory dystonia to intrathecal baclofen.

F. Be aware of the data supporting and the data refuting the value of acupuncture.

G. Understand the fundamental importance of physical and occupational therapy in treatment for CRPS.

H. Know the utility of psychiatric and psychological approaches to management of CRPS.

REFERENCES

Ali Z, Raja SN, Wesselmann U, et al. Intradermal injection of norepinephrine evokes pain in patients with sympathetically maintained pain. *Pain* 2000; 88:161–168.

Allen G, Galer BS, Schwartz L. Epidemiology of complex regional pain syndrome: a retrospective chart review of 134 patients. *Pain* 1999; 80:539–544.

Baron R, Wasner G. Complex regional pain syndromes. *Curr Pain Headache Rep* 2001; 5:114–123.

Baron R, Levine JD, Fields HL. Causalgia and reflex sympathetic dystrophy: does the sympathetic nervous system contribute to the generation of pain? *Muscle Nerve* 1999; 22:678–695.

Baron R, Schattschneider J, Binder A, Siebrecht D, Wasner G. Relation between sympathetic vasoconstrictor activity and pain and hyperalgesia in complex regional pain syndromes: a case-control study. *Lancet* 2002; 359:1655–1660.

Birklein F, Riedl B, Sieweke N, Weber M, Neundorfer B. Neurological findings in complex regional pain syndromes—analysis of 145 cases. *Acta Neurol Scand* 2000; 101:262–269.

Birklein F, Schmelz M, Schifter S, Weber M. The important role of neuropeptides in complex regional pain syndrome. *Neurology* 2001; 57:2179–2184.

Bruehl S, Harden RN, Galer BS, et al. External validation of IASP diagnostic criteria for Complex Regional Pain Syndrome and proposed research diagnostic criteria. *Pain* 1999; 81:147–154.

Fördereuther S, Sailer U, Staube A. Impaired self-perception of the hand in complex regional pain syndrome (CRPS). *Pain* 2004; 110:756–761.

Forouzanfar T, Koke AJ, van Kleef M, Weber WE. Treatment of complex regional pain syndrome type I. *Eur J Pain* 2002; 6:105–122.

Galer BS, Bruehl S, Harden RN. IASP diagnostic criteria for complex regional pain syndrome: a preliminary empirical validation study. *Clin J Pain* 1998; 14:48–54.

Harden RN, Bruehl S, Galer BS, et al. Complex regional pain syndrome: are the IASP diagnostic criteria valid and sufficiently comprehensive? *Pain* 1999; 83:211–219.

Huygen FJ, De Bruijn AG, De Bruin MT, et al. Evidence for local inflammation in complex regional pain syndrome type 1. *Mediators Inflamm* 2002; 11:47–51.

Jänig W, Baron R. Complex regional pain syndrome: mystery explained? *Lancet Neurol* 2003; 2:687–697.

Juottonen K, Gockel M, Silen T, et al. Altered central sensorimotor processing in patients with complex regional pain syndrome. *Pain* 2002; 98:315–323.

Kemler MA, Barendse GA, van Kleef M, et al. Spinal cord stimulation in patients with chronic reflex sympathetic dystrophy. *N Engl J Med* 2000; 343:618–624.

Kingery WS. A critical review of controlled clinical trials for peripheral neuropathic pain and complex regional pain syndromes. *Pain* 1997; 73:123–139.

Maihofner C, Handwerker HO, Neundorfer B, Birklein F. Patterns of cortical reorganization in complex regional pain syndrome. *Neurology* 2003; 61:1707–1715.

Moseley GL. Graded motor imagery is effective for long-standing complex regional pain syndrome: a randomised controlled trial. *Pain* 2004; 108:192–198.

Oerlemans HM, Oostendorp RA, de Boo T, Perez RS, Goris RJ. Signs and symptoms in complex regional pain syndrome type I/reflex sympathetic dystrophy: judgment of the physician versus objective measurement. *Clin J Pain* 1999; 15:224–232.

Perez RS, Kwakkel G, Zuurmond WW, de Lange JJ. Treatment of reflex sympathetic dystrophy (CRPS type 1): a research synthesis of 21 randomized clinical trials. *J Pain Symptom Manage* 2001; 21:511–526.

Price DD, Long S, Wilsey B, Rafii A. Analysis of peak magnitude and duration of analgesia produced by local anesthetics injected into sympathetic ganglia of complex regional pain syndrome patients. *Clin J Pain* 1998; 14:216–226.

Sieweke N, Birklein F, Riedl B, Neundorfer B, Handwerker HO. Patterns of hyperalgesia in complex regional pain syndrome. *Pain* 1999; 80:171–177.

Stanton-Hicks M, Jänig W, Hassenbusch S, et al. Reflex sympathetic dystrophy: changing concepts and taxonomy. *Pain* 1995; 63:127–133.

Stanton-Hicks M, Baron R, Boas R, et al. Complex Regional Pain Syndromes: guidelines for therapy. *Clin J Pain* 1998; 14:155–166.

Stanton-Hicks M, Burton AW, Bruehl SP, et al. An updated interdisciplinary clinical pathway for CRPS: report of an expert panel. *Pain Practice* 2002; 2:1–16.

van de Beek WJ, Schwartzman RJ, van Nes SI, Delhaas EM, van Hilten JJ. Diagnostic criteria used in studies of reflex sympathetic dystrophy. *Neurology* 2002; 58:522–526.

van Hilten BJ, van de Beek WJ, Hoff JI, Voormolen JH, Delhaas EM. Intrathecal baclofen for the treatment of dystonia in patients with reflex sympathetic dystrophy. *N Engl J Med* 2000; 343:625–630.

Veldman PH, Reynen HM, Arntz IE, Goris RJ. Signs and symptoms of reflex sympathetic dystrophy: prospective study of 829 patients. *Lancet* 1993; 342:1012–1016.

Wasner G, Schattschneider J, Baron R. Skin temperature side differences—a diagnostic tool for CRPS? *Pain* 2002; 98:19–26.

Wasner G, Schattschneider J, Binder A, Baron R. Complex regional pain syndrome—diagnostic, mechanisms, CNS involvement and therapy. *Spinal Cord* 2003; 41:61–75.

Core Curriculum for Professional Education in Pain, edited by J. Edmond Charlton, IASP Press, Seattle, © 2005.

41

Pain in Infants, Children, and Adolescents

I.   Pain in infants

A.   Know that the postnatal period is a time of considerable synaptic growth and reorganization in the dorsal horn of the spinal cord (Fitzgerald 2000; Fitzgerald and Howard 2003) and that the developing nociceptive system responds differently to injury (i.e., increased excitability and sensitization) when compared to the mature adult system (see Chapter 3).

B.   Understand that some inhibitory mechanisms in the dorsal horn are immature at birth and descending inhibition is delayed (Fitzgerald and Koltzenburg 1986; Boucher et al. 1998; Jennings and Fitzgerald 1998).

C.   Know that behavioral studies on human infants have revealed comparable findings of plasticity and increased excitability in the developing nervous system and that in comparison to adults, young infants have exaggerated reflex responses (i.e., lower thresholds and longer-lasting muscle contractions) in response to certain types of trauma, such as needle insertion (Andrews and Fitzgerald 1994, 1999).

D.   Recognize that repeated mechanical stimulation at strong (but not pain-inducing) intensities can cause sensitization in very young infants (Fitzgerald et al. 1988) and that preliminary studies have noted a striking hypersensitivity (to touch as well as pain) in infants after surgery (Andrews and Fitzgerald 2002).

E.   Recognize the differing immediate, short-term, and long-term effects of pain exposure on the developing nervous system (Anand 2000; Anand et al. 2000; Grunau 2000, 2002, 2003; Bhutta and Anand 2002; Goldschneider and Anand 2003). Appreciate that pain experienced by neonates has both immediate and longer-term effects on their pain reactivity (Johnston and Stevens 1996; Porter et al. 1998; Grunau et al. 2001a,b; Johnston et al. 2003).

F.   Know that circumcised infants displayed a stronger pain response to subsequent routine immunizations at 4 and 6 months than uncircumcised infants (Taddio et al. 1995) and that studies of former premature infants who required intensive care have shown behavioral differences related to early pain experiences (Grunau et al. 2001a,b).

G.   Appreciate the complexities in effects of pain and opiate exposure in vulnerable infants (Abbott and Guy 1995; Anand et al. 1999; Bhutta et al. 2001; Lidow et al. 2001; Rahman et al. 1998).

H.   Recognize that the differences in pharmacokinetics and pharmacodynamics among neonates, preterm infants, and full-term infants warrant special dosing considerations for infants and close monitoring when they receive opioids. Know the guidelines for neonatal and child analgesia administration and appreciate the pharmacokinetics and pharmacodynamics specific to the major opioids, nonsteroidal anti-inflammatory drugs (NSAIDs), and adjunctive analgesics (Clinical Practice Guideline 1992; Olkkola et al. 1995; Kart et al. 1997; Krane et al. 2003; Maunuksela and Olkkola 2003; McGrath and Brown 2003; Yaster 2003; Yaster et al. 2003a).

I.   Know practical interventions for managing pain and distress in infants such as developmental care, containment, sucrose, feeding, and kangaroo care (Franck and Lawhon 2000; Stevens et al. 2004).

II.   Children's pain perception

A.   Know that children can experience many different types of acute, recurrent, and chronic pain (Goodman and McGrath 1991; McGrath et al. 2000; Perquin et al. 2000) and that the lifetime prevalence for most types of recurrent and chronic pain increases with age (McGrath 1999).

B.   Know that children's age and developmental level influence their perception of pain (McGrath and Unruh 1987; Ross and Ross 1988; McGrath 1990) and that children's understanding of pain, pain coping strategies, and the impact of pain increase with age (Ross and Ross 1984; Gaffney and Dunne 1987; Harbeck and Peterson 1992; Gaffney 1993).

C.   Know that most studies of children's acute pain caused by invasive medical procedures reveal that pain intensity and overt distress generally decrease with age (Jay et al. 1983; Fradet et al. 1990; Jacobsen et al. 1990; Lander and Fowler-Kerry 1991; Humphrey et al. 1992; Fanurik et al. 1993; Bournaki 1997; Goodenough et al. 1997).

D.   However, appreciate that the effect of age probably varies depending on the type of pain and the nature of children's previous pain experiences—that is, positive experiences with similar painful situations (Dahlquist et al. 1986; Bijttebier and Vertommen 1998; Thastum et al. 2001; McGrath and Hillier 2003). Some studies of postoperative pain show increasing pain with age (Bennett-Branson and Craig 1993), while others show age-related decreases (Palermo and Drotar 1996) or no differences (Gidron et al. 1995).

E.   Recognize that children's memories of past pain experiences and pain-coping efficacy also shape responses to present pain situations; prior difficulties can undermine active efforts to cope and heighten anxiety and rumination (Chen et al. 1999, 2000a,b). Thus, effective early intervention for children at risk is critical because it not only influences the child's present pain experience but also expectations of, and strategies for, coping with future pain situations.

F.   Know that the results of studies evaluating sex- and gender-related trends in children's pain perception yield equivocal results (Ross and Ross 1984; Grunau and Craig 1987; Fradet et al. 1990; Jacobsen et al. 1990; Fowler-Kerry and Lander 1991; Schechter et al. 1991; Humphrey et al. 1992; Manne et al. 1992; Bennett-Branson and Craig 1993; Tesler et al. 1998).

G.   Appreciate that in addition to experiential and maturational factors, temperament and children's reactivity are likely to play a substantial role in shaping children's response to pain (Peterson and Toler 1986; Field et al. 1988; Blount et al. 1989; Wallace 1989; Schechter et al. 1991; Siegel and Smith 1991; Peterson et al. 1999; Zeltzer et al. 1999; Chen et al. 2000a,b). Child development theorists have proposed that consistent, inherent predispositions underlie and modulate the expression of activity, reactivity, emotionality, and sociability.

H.   Appreciate that biopsychosocial, as well as developmental, factors modify all children's pain perceptions and pain behaviors. Situational factors, particularly cognitive, behavioral, and emotional factors, vary with the circumstances in which a child experiences pain and can profoundly affect a child's pain level and distress (Ross and Ross 1988; McGrath and Hillier 2003).

I.   Understand that family beliefs, attitudes, and parental pain history influence how children learn about pain, its impact, and how to cope with different types of pain (Edwards et al. 1985a,b; Bush et al. 1986; Gil et al. 1991; Walker et al. 1994; Schanberg et al. 1998). In particular, children's chronic pain problems should be viewed within the broader context of their family (Covelman et al. 1990; Ehde et al. 1991; Gil et al. 1991; Walker 1999; McGrath and Hillier 2001).

J.   Know that only a few studies have focused on the specific impact of culture on children's pain (Abu-Saad 1984; Zeltzer and LeBaron 1985; Pfefferbaum et al. 1990; Harrison 1991; Lewis et al. 1993; Rosmus et al. 2000), and empiric data on specific cultural differences in pain experience and responses are lacking (Bernstein and Pachter 2003).

III. Treating children's pain problems: drug therapies

   A. Understand that managing a child's pain requires a dual focus on addressing the primary cause, usually through pharmacological or physical interventions, and the contributing factors or secondary causes, usually through a cognitive-behavioral approach or specific psychological interventions (McGrath 1990).

   B. Know that analgesics include acetaminophen, NSAIDs, and opioids and that adjuvant analgesics include a variety of drugs with analgesic properties that were initially developed to treat other health problems, such as anticonvulsants and antidepressants. Appreciate the unique aspects of using these agents in infants and children (Morselli et al. 1980; Andersen et al. 1997; Finley 2001) and know the guidelines for analgesic administration in infants and children (Wolf 2001; Krane et al. 2003).

   C. Understand that neonates and infants require the same three categories of analgesic drugs as older children. However, premature and term newborns show reduced clearance of most opioids. The differences in pharmacokinetics and pharmacodynamics among neonates, preterm infants, and full-term infants warrant special dosing considerations for infants and close monitoring when they receive opioids (Wong et al. 2003).

   D. Understand that children should receive analgesics at regular times, "by the clock," to provide consistent pain relief and prevent breakthrough pain. The specific drug schedule (e.g., every 4 or 6 hours) is based on the drug's duration of action and the child's pain severity (Clinical Practice Guideline 1992).

   E. Recognize that the management of acute procedural pain requires appropriate pharmacological management (Liossi 2002; Schechter 2003). Understand that children who receive multiple invasive procedures throughout a prolonged time period, are at risk for developing increasing anxiety about these procedures, but that many brief cognitive-behavioral interventions can effectively lessen children's anxiety and pain (Ellis and Spanos 1994; Jay et al. 1995; Kazak et al. 1998; Barrera 2000; Kazak and Kunin-Batson 2001).

   F. Know that regional techniques for the administration of local anesthetics and analgesics are an integral part of pain control for children. Be aware of the central and peripheral nerve blocks available and the indications for their use in children of all ages (Brown et al. 1999; Peng and Chan 1999; Dalens 2003; Desparmet et al. 2003; Wilder 2003; Yaster et al. 2003b).

   G. Understand that children with severe pain may require progressively higher and more frequent opioid doses due to drug tolerance and that they should receive the doses they need to relieve their pain (Collins and Weisman 2003; McGrath and Brown 2003). Appreciate that the fear of opioid addiction in children has been greatly exaggerated.

   H. Understand that active participation of children and parents is important in pain management (Schechter 1985; Romsing and Walther-Larsen 1996).

IV. Treating children's pain: nondrug therapies

   A. Appreciate that an extensive array of nondrug therapies is available to treat children's pain, including counseling, guided imagery, hypnosis, biofeedback, behavioral management, acupuncture, massage, homeopathic remedies, naturopathic approaches, and herbal medicines (Kemper and Gardiner 2003; Lin 2003; McCarthy et al. 2003; McGrath et al. 2003).

   B. Know how to use basic psychological and behavioral approaches to pain in children (Broome et al. 1998; Kazak and Kunin-Batson 2001; Kuttner and Solomon 2003; McGrath and Hillier 2003). Understand that the evidence base supporting the efficacy of cognitive and behavioral approaches is strong (Zeltzer and LeBaron 1982; Kellerman et al. 1983; Katz et al. 1987; Blount et al. 1990; Jay and Elliott 1990; Routh and Sanfilippo 1991; Powers et al. 1993; Ellis and Spanos 1994; Janicke and

Finney 1999; Walco et al. 1999; Anie and Green 2000; McGrath and Hollahan 2003). These methods can mitigate some of the factors that intensify pain, distress, and disability for children.

C. Be aware that providing age-appropriate information, some simple pain-coping methods like attention and distraction, and giving children as much choice as possible can effectively lessen children's pain and distress during invasive procedures (McGrath and Hillier 2003). These cognitive approaches can be easily incorporated into routine clinical practice.

D. Understand how to use a consistent cognitive-behavioral approach to target the multiple factors that typically contribute to children's recurrent and chronic pain (McGrath and Finley 1999; Walker 1999; McGrath and Hillier 2001).

E. Recognize that specialized multidisciplinary programs have been developed to treat certain pain problems for children including sickle cell pain (Dampier and Shapiro 2003), musculoskeletal pain (Varni et al. 1989; Kulas and Schanberg 2003), complex regional pain syndromes (Berde and Solodiuk 2003; Berde et al. 2003), chronic headache (Hillier and McGrath 2001; Hämäläinen and Masek 2003), abdominal pain (Apley 1975; Sanders et al. 1994; Scharff et al. 2003), burn pain (Kahana 2003), and cancer pain (Collins and Weisman 2003).

F. Understand that increasing attention is focusing on the special problem of pain for children with developmental disabilities; realize that pain assessment techniques are available (McGrath et al. 1998; Hunt et al. 1999; Oberlander 2001; Breau et al. 2002; Hadden and von Baeyer 2002; Stallard et al. 2002; Terstegen et al. 2003) and that practical guidelines for pain management have been detailed (Oberlander and Craig 2003).

G. Appreciate that children are increasingly using complementary and alternative therapies (Spigelblatt et al. 1994; Kemper and Gardiner 2003; Lin 2003), but that pediatric research is just beginning on many of the therapies regarded as complementary to traditional medical approaches such as acupuncture (Zeltzer et al. 2002). Thus, the efficacy of complementary therapies for treating children's pain is unknown.

H. Know that physical therapies are a major component of many pain management programs for children (McCarthy et al. 2003), especially for children with neuropathic pain (Lee et al. 2002).

I.   Recognize that the neurosurgical approaches for treating pain in children are comparable to those used for adults' pain, but understand that there have been no studies documenting the effectiveness of particular procedures for children (Smith and Madsen 2003).

V.   Assessing pain in infants and children

A. Know that pain onset, location, intensity, quality, duration (or frequency, if recurring), spatial extent, temporal pattern, and accompanying physical symptoms are the key pain characteristics for assessment (McGrath and Brown 2003). These characteristics are obtained from a child and parental report during the diagnostic interview and clinical examination. When possible, clinicians should obtain a quantitative rating of pain intensity.

B. Recognize that many physiological parameters have been monitored in infants and children as potential pain measures including heart rate, respiration rate, blood pressure, palmar sweating, cortisol and cortisone levels, O_2 levels, vagal tone, and endorphin concentrations (Harpin and Rutter 1982; Jay et al. 1983; Owens and Todt 1984; Johnston and Strada 1986; Gunnar et al. 1987; Szyfelbein et al. 1987). Understand how behavioral and biological measures may be used to assess pain (Sweet and McGrath 1998; McGrath and Gillespie 2001; Oberlander and Saul 2002).

C. Recognize that from birth, infants exhibit an array of distress behaviors and physiological changes in response to tissue damage (Craig and Grunau 1993) and that many behavioral pain measures have been developed and validated for use with infants (Stevens et al. 2000). Know the unique challenges of assessing pain in infants and preverbal children (Stevens et al. 2000; Craig et al. 2002; Peters et al., in press).

D. Know that children can use many analogue, facial, and verbal rating scales for assessing pain intensity and that many behavioral and self-report measures have been developed and validated for use with children and adolescents (Beyer and Wells 1989; Champion et al. 1998; Finley and McGrath 1998; McGrath 1998; RCN Institute 1999; McGrath and Gillespie 2001; Gaffney et al. 2003).

E. Appreciate that different measures are required depending on the age and developmental level of children and recognize the impact of any developmental disability or neurological impairment on assessing pain in children (Stevens et al. 2000; Chambers and Johnston 2002; Craig et al. 2002; Gaffney et al. 2003; Johnston et al. 2003; Oberlander and Craig 2003).

F. Know that a child's pain level should be routinely documented to ensure that health care providers assume appropriate responsibility for controlling pain.

VI.   Special considerations for acute pain management

A. Know the clinical guidelines for the management of acute procedural and postoperative pain in infants and children, including injuries, postoperative pain, burns, common pediatric diseases, and repeated invasive procedures (Finley 2001; Morton 2001; Bouwmeester et al. 2003; Schechter 2003).

B. Know the primary approaches to pain management in the neonatal and pediatric intensive care unit (Tobias and Rasmussen 1994; Chambliss and Anand 1997; Macfadyen and Buckmaster 1999; Franck and Lawhon 2000; Stevens 2001; Tobias 2003; Wong et al. 2003).

C. Know the primary approaches for pain control and sedation guidelines for treating children in the emergency department and the appropriate monitoring for respiratory, cardiovascular and neurological status (Selbst and Zempsky 2003).

D. Appreciate the role of combined analgesic, anxiolytic, and amnesiac agents in the management of children's acute pain (Joseph et al. 1999; Krauss 1999).

VII. Special considerations for chronic pain management

A. Understand that chronic pain causes significant suffering, disability, anxiety, and emotional distress for many children and adolescents (McGrath 1999; Perquin et al. 2000). Appreciate that chronic pain often has nociceptive and neuropathic components and is affected by environmental and psychological factors, so a multimodal therapeutic regimen is usually required. Understand that independent of initial etiology, children may continue to experience long-term pain and disability (Bursch et al. 1998, 2003).

B. Although psychological interventions are an integral component of treatment programs for chronic pain, be aware that the evidence base supporting the use of cognitive and behavioral interventions for relieving chronic pain other than headache is weak, as assessed by the number of controlled trials that have been conducted in children and by the few types of chronic pain that have been formally studied (McGrath and Holahan 2003).

C. Appreciate that significant gaps exist within our evidence base for multidisciplinary treatment programs and psychological therapies for treating chronic pain in children. Reviews of psychological therapies for childhood headache (Holden et al. 1999; Janicke and Finney 1999; McGrath et al. 2001; Hermann and Blanchard 2003), recurrent abdominal pain (Blanchard and Scharff 2002; Weydert et al. 2003), disease-related pain (Walco et al. 1999), sickle cell disease (Anie and Green 2000), and chronic pain including headache (Eccleston et al. 2002; McGrath and Holahan 2003) have stressed the need for well-designed studies to obtain much-needed information on treatment efficacy for particular pain conditions.

D.   Understand that most of the pharmacological management of neuropathic pain in children and adolescents is based on extrapolation from adult studies. While tricyclic antidepressants and gabapentin are well-established analgesics for these conditions in adults, evidence for efficacy in children is confined to case reports or very small series (McGraw and Kosek 1997; Rusy et al. 2001).

E.   Be aware that certain children with chronic pain may also have long-standing emotional problems suggestive of mood disorders, anxiety disorders, and somatoform disorders (Ernst et al. 1984; Egger et al. 1998; Zwaigenbaum et al. 1999; Holden et al. 2001).

VIII. Palliative care for children

A.   Understand that pain control is an integral component of pediatric palliative care because children may experience many different types of pain from invasive procedures, the cumulative effects of toxic therapies, progressive disease, or psychological factors (World Health Organization 1998).

B.   Know that pain control should include regular pain assessments, appropriate analgesics administered at regular dosing intervals, adjunctive drug therapy for symptom and side-effect control, and non-drug interventions to modify the situational factors that can exacerbate pain and suffering (World Health Organization 1998; Goldman et al. 2003; McGrath and Brown 2003).

C.   Although specific drugs and doses are determined by the needs of each child, general guidelines for drug therapies to control pain for children in palliative care have been developed (Pichard-Leandri and Gauvain-Piquard 1989; Galloway and Yaster 2000; McGrath and Brown 2003). Recognize that children may not report all side effects (i.e., constipation, dysphoria) voluntarily, so they should be asked specifically about these problems.

D.   Appreciate that special problems in pain control may arise when children die at home, unless parents and medical and nursing teams communicate openly (Howell and Martinson 1993; Goldman 1994; Sourkes 1996; Davies and Howell 1998; Stevens 1998).

IX. Ethical considerations for children

A.   Understand the primary ethical concerns related to the undertreatment of pain in infants and children, end-of-life care, and the use of placebo controls in treatment trials (Kenny 2001; Walco et al. 2003).

B.   Know that experimental pains induced by electrical stimuli, pressure, and cold water immersion have been used to study pain and tolerance thresholds, pain intensity ratings, coping strategies, and cognitive-behavioral interventions in children (Zeltzer et al. 1989; Fanurik et al. 1993; Miller et al. 1994; Hogeweg et al. 1996; McGrath et al. 2003). However, appreciate that the use of experimental pain in children continues to be a controversial issue, and that ethical guidelines have been recommended for its use (McGrath 1993).

REFERENCES

Abbott FV, Guy ER. Effects of morphine, pentobarbital and amphetamine on formalin-induced behaviours in infant rats: sedation versus specific suppression of pain. *Pain* 1995; 62(3):303–312.

Abu-Saad H. Cultural components of pain: the Arab-American child. *Issues Compr Pediatr Nurs* 1984; 7(2-3):91–99.

Anand KJS. Effects of perinatal pain and stress. In: Mayer EA, Saper CB (Eds). *Progress in Brain Research*. Amsterdam: Elsevier Science, 2000, pp 117–129.

Anand KJ, Coskun V, Thrivikraman KV, Nemeroff CB, Plotsky PM. Long-term behavioral effects of repetitive pain in neonatal rat pups. *Physiol Behav* 1999; 66(4):627–637.

Anand KJS, Stevens BJ, McGrath PJ (Eds). *Pain in Neonates,* 2nd ed. Amsterdam: Elsevier, 2000.

Andersen BJ, McKee AS, Holford NH. Size, myths and clinical pharmacokinetics of analgesia in paediatric patients. *Clin Pharmacokinet* 1997; 33:313–327.

Andrews K, Fitzgerald M. The cutaneous withdrawal reflex in human neonates: sensitization, receptive fields, and the effects of contralateral stimulation. *Pain* 1994; 56(1):95-101.

Andrews K, Fitzgerald M. Cutaneous flexion reflex in human neonates: a quantitative study of threshold and stimulus-response characteristics after single and repeated stimuli. *Dev Med Child Neurol* 1999; 41(10):696–703.

Andrews K, Fitzgerald M. Wound sensitivity as a measure of analgesic effects following surgery in human neonates and infants. *Pain* 2002; 99(1-2):185–195.

Anie KA, Green J. Psychological therapies for sickle cell disease and pain. *Cochrane Database Syst Rev* 2000; (3):CD001916.

Apley J. *The Child with Abdominal Pains*. Oxford: Blackwell Scientific, 1975.

Barrera M. Brief clinical report: procedural pain and anxiety management with mother and sibling as co-therapists. *J Pediatr Psychol* 2000; 25(2):117–121.

Bennett-Branson SM, Craig KD. Post-operative pain in children: developmental and family influences on spontaneous coping strategies. *Can J Behav Sci* 1993; 25:355–383.

Berde CB, Solodiuk J. Multidisciplinary programs for management of acute and chronic pain in children. In: Schechter N, Berde C, Yaster M (Eds). *Pain in Infants, Children and Adolescents,* 2nd ed. Philadelphia: Lippincott, Williams and Wilkins, 2003, pp 471–486.

Berde CB, Lebel AA, Olsson G. Neuropathic pain in children. In: Schechter N, Berde C, Yaster Y. *Pain in Infants, Children and Adolescents,* 2nd ed. Philadelphia: Lippincott, Williams and Wilkins, 2003, pp 620–641.

Bernstein BA, Pachter LM. Cultural considerations in children's pain. In: Schechter N, Berde C, Yaster M (Eds). *Pain in Infants, Children and Adolescents,* 2nd ed. Philadelphia: Lippincott, Williams and Wilkins, 2003, pp 142–156.

Beyer JE, Wells N. The assessment of pain in children. *Pediatr Clin N Am* 1989; 36:837–854.

Bhutta AT, Anand KJ. Vulnerability of the developing brain: neuronal mechanisms. *Clin Perinatol* 2002; 29(3):357–372.

Bhutta AT, Rovnaghi C, Simpson PM, et al. Interactions of inflammatory pain and morphine in infant rats: long-term behavioral effects. *Physiol Behav* 2001; 273(1-2):51–58.

Bijttebier P, Vertommen H. The impact of previous experience on children's reactions to venepunctures. *J Health Psychol* 1998; 3:39–46.

Blanchard EB, Scharff L. Psychosocial aspects of assessment and treatment of irritable bowel syndrome in adults and recurrent abdominal pain in children. *J Consult Clin Psychol* 2002; 70:725–738.

Blount RL, Sturges JW, Powers SW. Analysis of child and adult behavioral variations by phase of medical procedure. *Behav Ther* 1990; 21:33–48.

Boucher T, Jennings E, Fitzgerald M. The onset of diffuse noxious inhibitory controls in postnatal rat pups: a C-Fos study. *Neurosci Lett* 1998; 257(1):9–12.

Bournaki MC. Correlates of pain-related responses to venipunctures in school-age children. *Nurs Res* 1997; 46:147–154.

Bouwmeester NJ, van den Anker JN, Hop WC, Anand KJ, Tibboel D. Age- and therapy-related effects on morphine requirements and plasma concentrations of morphine and its metabolites in post-operative infants. *Br J Anaesth* 2003; 90(5):642–652.

Breau LM, McGrath PJ, Camfield CS, Finley GA. Psychometric properties of the non-communicating children's pain checklist-revised. *Pain* 2002; 99(1–2):349–357.

Broome M, Rehwaldt M, Fogg L. Relationships between cognitive-behavioral techniques, temperament, observed distress and pain reports in children and adolescents during lumbar puncture. *J Pediatr Nurs* 1998; 1:48–54.

Brown TC, Eyres RL, McDougall RJ. Local and regional anaesthesia in children. *Br J Anaesth* 1999; 83:65–77.

Bursch B, Walco GA, Zeltzer L. Clinical assessment and management of chronic pain and pain-associated disability syndrome. *J Dev Behav Pediatr* 1998; 19:45–53.

Bursch B, Joseph MH, Zeltzer LK. Pain-associated disability syndrome. In: Schechter N, Berde C, Yaster M (Eds). *Pain in Infants, Children and Adolescents,* 2nd ed. Philadelphia: Lippincott, Williams and Wilkins, 2003, pp 841–848.

Bush JP, Melamed BG, Sheras PL, et al. Mother-child patterns of coping with anticipatory medical stress. *Health Psychol* 1986; 5:137–157.

Chambers CT, Johnston C. Developmental differences in children's use of rating scales. *J Pediatr Psychol* 2002; 27(1):27–36.

Chambliss CR, Anand KJ. Pain management in the pediatric intensive care unit. *Curr Opin Pediatr* 1997; 9(3):246–253.

Champion GD, Goodenough B, von Baeyer CL, Thomas W. Measurement of pain by self-report. In: Finley GA, McGrath PJ (Eds). *Measurement of Pain in Infants and Children*, Progress in Pain Research and Management, Vol. 10. Seattle: IASP Press, 1998, pp 123–160.

Chen E, Zeltzer LK, Craske MG, Katz ER. Alteration of memory in the reduction of children's distress during repeated aversive medical procedures. *J Clin Consult Psychol* 1999; 67:481–490.

Chen E, Craske MG, Katz ER, Schwartz E, Zeltzer LK. Pain-Sensitive temperament: does it predict procedural distress and response to psychological treatment among children with cancer? *J Pediatr Psychol* 2000a; 25:269–278

Chen E, Zeltzer LK, Craske MG, Katz ER. Children's memories for painful cancer treatment procedures: implications for distress. *Child Dev* 2000b; 71:933–947.

Clinical Practice Guideline. *Acute Pain Management in Infants, Children, and Adolescents: Operative and Medical Procedures.* Rockville, MD: Agency for Health Care Policy and Research, 1992.

Collins JJ, Weisman SJ. Management of pain in childhood cancer. In: Schechter N, Berde C, Yaster M (Eds). *Pain in Infants, Children and Adolescents,* 2nd ed. Philadelphia: Lippincott, Williams and Wilkins, 2003, pp 517–538.

Covelman K, Scott S, Buchanan B, et al. Pediatric pain control: a family systems model. In: Tyler DC, Krane EJ (Eds). *Pediatric Pain: Advances in Pain Research Therapy.* New York: Raven Press, 1990, pp 225–236.

Craig KD, Grunau RVE. Neonatal pain perception and behavioral measurement. In: Anand KJS, McGrath PJ (Eds). *Pain in Neonates.* Amsterdam: Elsevier, 1993, pp 67–105.

Craig KD, Korol CT, Pillai R. Challenges of judging pain in vulnerable infants. Stevens B, Grunau RE (Eds). *Clin Perinatol* 2002; 29(3):445–458.

Dahlquist LM, Gil KM, Armstrong D, et al. Preparing children for medical examinations: the importance of previous medical experience. *Health Psychol* 1986; 5:249–259.

Dalens B. Peripheral nerve blockade in the management of postoperative pain in children. In: Schechter N, Berde C, Yaster M. *Pain in Infants, Children and Adolescents*, 2nd ed. Philadelphia: Lippincott, Williams and Wilkins, 2003, pp 363–395.

Dampier C, Shapiro BS. Management of pain in sickle cell disease. In: Schechter N, Berde C, Yaster Y. *Pain in Infants, Children and Adolescents,* 2nd ed. Philadelphia: Lippincott, Williams and Wilkins, 2003, pp 489–516.

Davies B, Howell D. Special services for children. In: Doyle D, Hanks GWC, MacDonald N (Eds). *Oxford Textbook of Palliative Medicine, 2nd* ed. Oxford: Oxford University Press, 1998, pp 1078–1084.

Desparmet JF, Hardart RA, Yaster M. Central blocks in children and adolescents. In: Schechter N, Berde C, Yaster M (Eds). *Pain in Infants, Children and Adolescents,* 2nd ed. Philadelphia: Lippincott, Williams and Wilkins, 2003, pp 339–362.

Eccleston C, Morley S, Williams A, Yorke L, Mastroyannopoulou K. Systematic review of randomised controlled trials of psychological therapy for chronic pain in children and adolescents, with a subset meta-analysis of pain relief. *Pain* 2002; 99(1–2):157–165.

Edwards PW, O'Neill GW, Zeichner A, Kuczmierczyk AR. Effects of familial pain models on pain complaints and coping strategies. *Percept Mot Skills* 1985a; 61:1053–1054.

Edwards PW, Zeichner A, Kuczmierczyk AR, Boczkowski J. Familial pain models: the relationship between family history of pain and current pain experience. *Pain* 1985b; 21:379–384.

Egger HL, Angold A, Costello EJ. Headaches and psychopathology in children and adolescents. *J Am Acad Child Adolesc Psychiatry* 1998; 37:951–958.

Ehde DM, Holm JE, Metzger DL. The role of family structure, functioning, and pain modeling in headache. *Headache* 1991; 31:35–40.

Ellis JA, Spanos NP. Cognitive-behavioral interventions for children's distress during bone marrow aspirations and lumbar punctures: a critical review. *J Pain Symptom Manage* 1994; 9(2):96–108.

Ernst AR, Routh DK, Harper DC. Abdominal pain in children and symptoms of somatization disorder. *J Pediatr Psychol* 1984; 9:77–86.

Fanurik D, Zeltzer LK, Roberts MC, Blount RL. The relationship between children's coping styles and psychological interventions for cold pressor pain. *Pain* 1993; 53(2):213-222.

Field T, Alpert B, Vega-Lahr N, Goldstein S, Perry S. Hospitalization stress in children: sensitizer and repressor coping styles. *Health Psychol* 1988; 7:433–445.

Finley GA. Pharmacological management of procedure pain. In: Finley GA, McGrath PJ (Eds). *Acute and Procedural Pain in Infants and Children*, Progress in Pain Research and Management, Vol. 20. Seattle: IASP Press, 2001.

Finley GA, McGrath P (Eds). *Measurement of Pain in Infants and Children*, Progress in Pain Research and Management, Vol. 20. Seattle: IASP Press, 1998.

Fitzgerald M. Development of the peripheral and spinal pain system. In: Anand KJS, Stevens BJ, McGrath PJ (Eds). *Pain in Neonates*, 2nd ed. Amsterdam: Elsevier, 2000.

Fitzgerald M, Howard RF. The neurobiologic basis of pediatric pain. In: Schechter NL, Berde CB, Yaster M (Eds). *Pain in Infants, Children, and Adolescents*, 2nd ed. Baltimore: Lippincott Williams and Wilkins, 2003, pp 19–42.

Fitzgerald M, Koltzenburg M. The functional development of descending inhibitory pathways in the dorsolateral funiculus of the newborn rat spinal cord. *Brain Res* 1986; 389(1-2):261–270.

Fitzgerald M, Shaw A, MacIntosh N. Postnatal development of the cutaneous flexor reflex: comparative study of preterm infants and newborn rat pups. *Dev Med Child Neurol* 1988; 30(4):520–526.

Fowler-Kerry S, Lander J. Assessment of sex differences in children's and adolescents' self-reported pain from venipuncture. *J Pediatr Psychol* 1991; 16:783–793.

Fradet C, McGrath PJ, Kay J, Adams S, Luke B. A prospective survey of reactions to blood tests by children and adolescents. *Pain* 1990; 40:53–60.

Franck LS, Lawhon G. Environmental and behavioral strategies to prevent and manage neonatal pain. In: Anand KJS, Stevens BJ, McGrath PJ (Eds). *Pain in Neonates*, 2nd ed. Amsterdam: Elsevier, 2000, pp 203–216.

Gaffney A. Cognitive developmental aspects of pain in school-age children. In: Schechter NL, Berde C, Yaster M (Eds). *Pain in Infants, Children and Adolescents*. Baltimore: Williams and Wilkins, 1993, pp 75–85.

Gaffney A, Dunne EA. Children's understanding of the causality of pain. *Pain* 1987; 29:91–104.

Gaffney A, McGrath P, Dick B. Measuring pain in children: developmental and instrument issues. In: Schechter N, Berde C, Yaster M (Eds). *Pain in Infants, Children and Adolescents*, 2nd ed. Philadelphia: Lippincott, Williams and Wilkins, 2003, pp 128–141.

Galloway KS, Yaster M. Pain and symptom control in terminally ill children. *Pediatr Clin North Am* 2000; 47:711–747.

Gidron Y, McGrath PJ, Goodday R. The physical and psychosocial predictors of adolescents' recovery from oral surgery. *J Behav Med* 1995; 18:385–399.

Gil KM, Williams DA, Thompson RJ Jr, Kinney TR. Sickle cell disease in children and adolescents: the relation of child and parent pain coping strategies to adjustment. *Pediatr Psychol* 1991; 16:643–663.

Goldman A (Ed). *Care of the Dying Child.* New York: Oxford University Press, 1994.

Goldman A, Frager G, Pomietto M. Pain and palliative care. In: Schechter N, Berde C, Yaster M (Eds). *Pain in Infants, Children and Adolescents,* 2nd ed. Philadelphia: Lippincott, Williams and Wilkins, 2003, pp 539–562.

Goldschneider K, Anand KJS. Long-term consequences of pain in neonates. In: Schechter N, Berde C, Yaster M (Eds). *Pain in Infants, Children and Adolescents,* 2nd ed. Philadelphia: Lippincott, Williams and Wilkins, 2003, pp 58–70.

Goodenough B, Kampel L, Champion GD, et al. An investigation of the placebo effect and age-related factors in the report of needle pain from venipuncture in children. *Pain* 1997; 72(3):383–391.

Goodman JE, McGrath PJ. The epidemiology of pain in children and adolescents: a review. *Pain* 1991; 46(3):247–264.

Grunau RE. Long-term consequences of pain in human neonates. In: Anand KJS, Stevens BJ, McGrath PJ. *Pain in Neonates,* 2nd ed. Amsterdam: Elsevier, 2000, pp 55–76.

Grunau RE. Early pain in preterm infants: a model of long term effects. *Clin Perinatol* 2002; 29:373–394.

Grunau RE. Self-regulation and behavior in preterm children: effects of early pain. In: McGrath PJ, Finley A (Eds). *Pediatric Pain: Biological and Social Context,* Progress in Pain Research and Management, Vol. 26. Seattle: IASP Press, 2003.

Grunau RVE, Craig KD. Pain expression in neonates: facial action and cry. *Pain* 1987; 28:395–410.

Grunau RE, Oberlander TF, Whitfield MF, Fitzgerald C, Lee SK. Demographic and therapeutic determinants of pain reactivity in very low birth weight neonates at 32 weeks post-conceptional age. *Pediatrics* 2001a; 107:105–112.

Grunau RE, Oberlander TF, Whitfield MF, et al. Pain reactivity in former extremely low birth weight infants at corrected age 8 months compared with term born controls. *Infant Behav Develop* 2001b; 24:41–55.

Gunnar MR, Isensee J, Fust LS. Adrenocortical activity and the Brazelton Neonatal Assessment Scale: moderating effects of the newborn's biobehavioral status. *Child Dev* 1987; 58:1448–1458.

Hadden KL, von Baeyer CL. Pain in children with cerebral palsy: common triggers and expressive behaviors. *Pain* 2002; 99(1–2):281–288.

Hämäläinen M, Masek BJ. Diagnosis, classification, and medical management of headache in children and adolescents. In: Schechter N, Berde C, Yaster M (Eds). *Pain in Infants, Children and Adolescents,* 2nd ed. Philadelphia: Lippincott, Williams and Wilkins, 2003, pp 707–718.

Harbeck C, Peterson L. Elephants dancing in my head: a developmental approach to children's concepts of specific pains. *Child Dev* 1992; 63:138–149.

Harpin VA, Rutter N. Development of emotional sweating in the newborn infant. *Arch Disease Childhood* 1982; 57:691–695.

Harrison A, Badran S, Ghalib R, Rida S. Arabic children's pain descriptions. *Pediatr Emerg Care* 1991; 7(4):199–203.

Hermann C, Blanchard EB. Biofeedback in the treatment of headache and other childhood pain. *Appl Psychophysiol Biofeedback* 2002; 27(2):143–162.

Hillier LM, McGrath PA. A cognitive-behavioral program for treating recurrent headache. In: McGrath PA, Hillier LM (Eds). *The Child with Headache: Diagnosis and Treatment,* Progress in Pain Research and Management, Vol. 19. Seattle: IASP Press, 2001, pp 183–220.

Hogeweg JA, Kuis W, Oostendorp RA, Helders PJ. The influence of site of stimulation, age, and gender on pain threshold in healthy children. *Phys Ther* 1996; 76(12):1331–1339.

Holden EW, Deichmann MM, Levy JD. Empirically supported treatments in pediatric psychology: recurrent pediatric headache. *J Pediatr Psychol* 1999; 24(2):91–109.

Holden EW, Bachanas P, Kullgren K, Gladstein J. Chronic daily headache in children and adolescents. In: McGrath PA, Hillier LM (Eds). *The Child with Headache: Diagnosis and Treatment,* Progress in Pain Research and Management, Vol. 19. Seattle: IASP Press, 2001, pp 221–241.

Howell DA, Martinson IM. Management of the dying child. In: Pizzo PA, Poplack DG (Eds). *Principles and Practice of Pediatric Oncology,* 2nd ed. Philadelphia: J.B. Lippincott, 1993, pp 1115–1124.

Humphrey GB, Boon CM, van Linden van den Heuvell GF, van de Wiel HB. The occurrence of high levels of acute behavioral distress in children and adolescents undergoing routine venipunctures. *Pediatrics* 1992; 90:87–91.

Hunt AM, Goldman A, Mastroyannopoulou K, Seers K. Identification of pain cues of children with severe neurological impairment. *Pain* 1999.

Jacobsen PB, Manne SL, Gorfinkle K, Schorr O. Analysis of child and parent behavior during painful medical procedures. *Health Psychol* 1990; 9:559–576.

Janicke DM, Finney JW. Empirically supported treatments in pediatric psychology: recurrent abdominal pain. *J Pediatr Psychol* 1999; 24(2):115–127.

Jay SM, Elliot CH. A stress inoculation program for parents whose children are undergoing painful medical procedures. *J Consult Clin Psychol* 1990; 58(6):799–804.

Jay SM, Ozolins M, Elliott CH, Caldwell S. Assessment of children's distress during painful medical procedures. *Health Psychol* 1983; 2:133–147.

Jay S, Elliott CH, Fitzgibbons I, Woody P, Siegel S. A comparative study of cognitive behavior therapy versus general anesthesia for painful medical procedures in children. *Pain* 1995; 62(1):3–9.

Johnston CC, Stevens BJ. Experience in a neonatal intensive care unit affects pain response. *Pediatrics* 1996; 98:925–930.

Johnston CC, Strada ME. Acute pain response in infants: a multidimensional description. *Pain* 1986; 24:373–382.

Johnston CC, Stevens B, Boyer K, Porter F. Development of psychologic responses to pain and assessment of pain in infants and toddlers. In: Schechter N, Berde C, Yaster M (Eds). *Pain in Infants, Children and Adolescents,* 2nd ed. Philadelphia: Lippincott, Williams and Wilkins, 2003, pp 105–127.

Joseph MH, Brill J, Zeltzer LK. Pediatric pain relief in trauma. *Pediatr Rev* 1999; 20:75–83.

Kahana MD. Burn pain management: avoiding the "private nightmare." In: Schechter N, Berde C, Yaster M (Eds). *Pain in Infants, Children and Adolescents,* 2nd ed. Philadelphia: Lippincott, Williams and Wilkins, 2003, pp 642–650.

Kart T, Christup LL, Rasmussen M. Recommended use of morphine in neonates, infants and children based on a literature review: Part 1. Pharmacokinetics. *Paediatr Anaesth* 1997; 7:5–11.

Katz ER, Kellerman J, Ellenberg L. Hypnosis in the reduction of acute pain and distress in children with cancer. *J Pediatr Psychol* 1987; 12(3):379–394.

Kazak AE, Kunin-Batson A. Psychological and integrative interventions in pediatric procedure pain. In: Finley GA, McGrath PJ (Eds). *Acute and Procedural Pain in Infants and Children,* Progress in Pain Research and Management, Vol. 20. Seattle: IASP Press, 2001.

Kazak AE, Penati B, Brophy P, Himelstein B. Pharmacologic and psychologic interventions for procedural pain. *Pediatrics* 1998; 102(1)Pt 1:59–66.

Kellerman J, Zeltzer L, Ellenberg L, Dash J. Adolescents with cancer. Hypnosis for the reduction of the acute pain and anxiety associated with medical procedures. *J Adolesc Health Care* 1983; 4(2):85–90.

Kemper KJ, Gardiner P. Complementary and alternative medical therapies in pediatric pain treatment. In: Schechter N, Berde C, Yaster M (Eds). *Pain in Infants, Children and Adolescents,* 2nd ed. Philadelphia: Lippincott, Williams and Wilkins, 2003, pp 449–461.

Kenny NP. The politics of pediatric pain. In: Finley GA, McGrath PJ (Eds). *Acute and Procedural Pain in Infants and Children,* Progress in Pain Research and Management, Vol. 20. Seattle: IASP Press, 2001.

Krane EJ, Leong MS, Golianu B, Leong YY. Treatment of pediatric pain with nonconventional analgesics. In: Schechter N, Berde C, Yaster M (Eds). *Pain in Infants, Children and Adolescents,* 2nd ed. Philadelphia: Lippincott, Williams and Wilkins, 2003, pp 225–240.

Krauss B. Practical aspects of procedural sedation and analgesia. In: Krauss B, Brustowicz RM (Eds). *Pediatric Procedural Sedation and Analgesia.* Philadelphia: Lippincott Williams & Williams, 1999, pp 223–236.

Kulas D, Schanberg L. Musculoskeletal pain in children. In: Schechter N, Berde C, Yaster M (Eds). *Pain in Infants, Children and Adolescents,* 2nd ed. Philadelphia: Lippincott, Williams and Wilkins, 2003, pp 578–598.

Kuttner L, Solomon R. Hypnotherapy and imagery for managing children's pain. In: Schechter N, Berde C, Yaster M (Eds). *Pain in Infants, Children and Adolescents,* 2nd ed. Philadelphia: Lippincott, Williams and Wilkins, 2003, pp 317–328.

Lander J, Fowler-Kerry S. Age differences in children's pain. *Percept Mot Skills* 1991; 73:415–418.

Lee BH, Scharff L, Sethna NF, et al. Physical therapy and cognitive-behavioral treatment for complex regional pain syndromes. *J Pediatr* 2002; 141(1):135–140.

Lewis M, Ramsay D, Kawakami K. Differences between Japanese infants and Caucasian American infants in behavioral and cortisone response to inoculation. *Child Dev* 1993; 64:1722–1731.

Lidow MS, Song ZM, Ren K. Long-term effects of short-lasting early local inflammatory insult. *Neuroreport* 2001; 12(2):399–403.

Lin YC. Acupuncture. In: Schechter N, Berde C, Yaster M (Eds). *Pain in Infants, Children and Adolescents,* 2nd ed. Philadelphia: Lippincott, Williams and Wilkins, 2003, pp 462–470.

Liossi C. *Procedure-Related Cancer Pain in Children.* Oxford: Radcliffe Medical Press, 2002.

Macfadyen AJ, Buckmaster MA. Pain management in the pediatric intensive care unit. *Crit Care Clin* 1999; 15(1):185–200.

Manne SL, Jacobsen PB, Redd WH. Assessment of acute pediatric pain: do child self-report, parent ratings, and nurse ratings measure the same phenomenon? *Pain* 1992; 48:45–52.

Maunuksela EL, Olkkola KT. Nonsteroidal anti-inflammatory drugs in pediatric pain management. In: Schechter N, Berde C, Yaster M. *Pain in Infants, Children and Adolescents,* 2nd ed. Philadelphia: Lippincott, Williams and Wilkins, 2003, pp 171–180.

McCarthy CF, Shea AM, Sullivan P. Physical therapy management of pain in children. In: Schechter N, Berde C, Yaster M (Eds). *Pain in Infants, Children and Adolescents,* 2nd ed. Philadelphia: Lippincott, Williams and Wilkins, 2003, pp 434–448.

McGrath PA. *Pain in Children: Nature, Assessment and Treatment.* New York: Guilford Publications, 1990.

McGrath PA. Inducing pain in children—a controversial issue. *Pain* 1993; 52(3):255–257.

McGrath PA. Chronic pain in children. In: Crombie I, Croft P, Linton S, LeResche L, Von Korff M (Eds). *Epidemiology of Pain*. Seattle: IASP Press, 1999, pp 81–101.

McGrath PA, Brown SC. Pain control in children. In: Doyle D, Hanks GWC, NM (Eds). *Oxford Textbook of Palliative Medicine*. Oxford: Oxford University Press, 2003, pp 1–35.

McGrath PA, Gillespie J. Pain assessment in children and adolescents. In: Turk DC, Melzack R (Eds). *Handbook of Pain Assessment*, 2nd ed. New York: Guilford Press, 2001, pp 97–118.

McGrath PA, Hillier LM. Recurrent headache: triggers, causes and contributing factors. In: McGrath PA, Hillier LM (Eds). *The Child with Headache: Diagnosis and Treatment*, Progress in Pain Research and Management, Vol. 19. Seattle: IASP Press, 2001, pp 77–107.

McGrath PA, Hillier LM. Modifying the psychologic factors that intensify children's pain and prolong disability. In: Schechter N, Berde C, Yaster M (Eds). *Pain in Infants, Children and Adolescents*, 2nd ed. Philadelphia: Lippincott, Williams and Wilkins, 2003, pp 85–104.

McGrath PA, Holahan AL. Psychological Interventions with children and adolescents: evidence for their effectiveness in treating chronic pain. *Semin Pain Med* 2003; 1(2):1–11.

McGrath PA, Speechley KN, Siefert CE, et al. A survey of children's acute, recurrent, and chronic pain: validation of the Pain Experience Interview. *Pain* 2000; 87:59–73.

McGrath PA, Stewart D, Koster AL. Nondrug therapies for childhood headache. In: McGrath PA, Hillier LM (Eds). *The Child with Headache: Diagnosis and Treatment*, Progress in Pain Research and Management, Vol. 19. Seattle: IASP Press, 2001, pp 129–158.

McGrath PJ. Behavioral measures of pain. In: Finley GA, McGrath PJ (Eds). *Measurement of Pain in Infants and Children*, Progress in Pain Research and Management, Vol. 10. Seattle: IASP Press, 1998, pp 83–102.

McGrath PJ, Finley GA (Eds). *Chronic and Recurrent Pain in Children and Adolescents*, Progress in Pain Research and Management, Vol. 13. Seattle: IASP Press, 1999.

McGrath PJ, Unruh A. *Pain in Children and Adolescents*. Amsterdam: Elsevier, 1987.

McGrath PJ, Rosmus C, Canfield C, Campbell MA, Hennigar A. Behaviours caregivers use to determine pain in non-verbal, cognitively impaired individuals. *Dev Med Child Neurol* 1998; 40(5):340–343.

McGrath PJ, Dick B, Unruh AM. Psychologic and behavioral treatment of pain in children and adolescents. In: Schechter N, Berde C, Yaster M (Eds). *Pain in Infants, Children and Adolescents*, 2nd ed. Philadelphia: Lippincott, Williams and Wilkins, 2003, pp 303–316.

McGraw T, Kosek P. Erythromelalgia pain managed with gabapentin. *Anesthesiology* 1997; 86:988–990.

Miller A, Barr RG, Young SN. The cold pressor test in children: methodological aspects and the analgesic effect of intraoral sucrose. *Pain* 1994; 56(2):175–183.

Morselli PL, Franco-Morselli R, Bossi L. Clinical pharmacokinetics in newborns and infants: age-related differences and therapeutic implications. *Clin Pharmacokinet* 1980; 5:485–527.

Morton NS. Simple and systemic management of postoperative pain. In: Finley GA, McGrath PJ (Eds). *Acute and Procedural Pain in Infants and Children*, Progress in Pain Research and Management, Vol. 20. Seattle: IASP Press, 2001.

Oberlander TF. Understanding pain in infants with developmental disabilities. *J Infants Young Child* 2001; 14(2):33–47.

Oberlander TF, Craig KD. Pain and children with developmental disabilities. In: Schechter N, Berde C, Yaster M (Eds). *Pain in Infants, Children and Adolescents*, 2nd ed. Philadelphia: Lippincott, Williams and Wilkins, 2003, pp 599–619.

Oberlander T, Saul JP. Methodological considerations for the use of heart rate variability as a measure of pain reactivity in vulnerable infants. Stevens B, Grunau RE (Eds). *Clin Perinatol* 2002; 29(3):427–444.

Olkkola KT, Hamunen K, Maunuksela EL. Clinical pharmacokinetics and pharmacodynamics of opioid analgesics in infants and children. *Clin Pharmacokinet* 1995; 28:383–404.

Owens ME, Todt EH. Pain in infancy: neonatal reaction to a heel lance. *Pain* 1984; 20:77–86.

Palermo TM, Drotar D. Prediction of children's postoperative pain: the role of presurgical expectations and anticipatory emotions. *J Pediatr Psychol* 1996; 21:683–698.

Peng PW, Chan VW. Local and regional block in post-operative pain control. *Surg Clin North Am* 1999; 79:345–370.

Perquin CW, Hazebroek-Kampschreur AA, Hunfeld JA, et al. Pain in children and adolescents: a common experience. *Pain* 2000; 87(1):51–58.

Peters JWB, Duivenvoorden HJ, Grunau RE, et al. The value of the Neonatal Facial Coding System to assess postoperative pain in infants. *Clin J Pain;* in press.

Peterson L, Toler SM. An information seeking disposition in child surgery patients. *Health Psychol* 1986; 5:343–358.

Peterson L, Crowson J, Saldana L, Holdridge S. Of needles and skinned knees: children's coping with medical procedures and minor injuries for self and other. *Health Psychol* 1999; 18:197–200.

Pfefferbaum B, Admas J, Aceves J. The influence of culture on pain in Anglo and Hispanic children with cancer. *J Am Acad Child Adolesc Psychiatry* 1990; 29:642–647.

Pichard-Leandri E, Gauvain-Piquard A (Eds). *La Douleur chez l'enfant*. Paris: Medsi/McGraw Hill, 1989.

Porter FL, Wolf CM, Miller JP. The effect of handling and immobilization on the response to acute pain in newborn infants. *Pediatrics* 1998; 102(6):1383–1389.

Powers SW, Blount RL, Bachanas PJ, Cotter MW, Swan SC. Helping preschool leukemia patients and their parents cope during injections. *J Pediatr Psychol* 1993; 18:681–695.

Rahman W, Dashwood MR, Fitzgerald M, Aynsley-Green A, Dickenson AH. Postnatal development of multiple opioid receptors in the spinal cord and development of spinal morphine analgesia. *Brain Res Dev Brain Res* 1998; 108(1–2):239–254.

RCN Institute. *Clinical Guideline for the Recognition and Assessment of Acute Pain in Children: Recommendations*. London: RCN Publishing, 1999.

Romsing J, Walther-Larsen S. Postoperative pain in children: a survey of parents' expectations and perceptions of their children's experiences. *Paediatr Anaesth* 1996 6(3): 215–218.

Rosmus C, Johnston CC, Chan-Yip A, Yang F. Pain response in Chinese and non-Chinese Canadian infants: is there a difference? *Soc Sci Med* 2000; 51(2):175–184.

Ross DM, Ross SA. Childhood pain: the school-aged child's viewpoint. *Pain* 1984; 20:179–191.

Ross DM, Ross SA. *Childhood Pain: Current Issues, Research, and Management*. Baltimore: Urban & Schwarzenberg, 1988.

Routh DK, Sanfilippo MD. Helping children cope with painful medical procedures. In: Bush JP, Harkins SW (Eds). *Children in Pain: Clinical and Research Issues from a Developmental Perspective*. New York: Springer-Verlag, 1991.

Rusy LM, Troshynski TJ, Weisman SJ. Gabapentin in phantom limb pain management in children and young adults: report of seven cases. *J Pain Symptom Manage* 2001; 21:78–82.

Sanders MR, Shepard RW, Cleghorn G, et al. The treatment of recurrent abdominal pain in children: a controlled comparison of cognitive-behavioral family intervention and standard pediatric care. *J Consult Clin Psychol* 1994; 62:306–314.

Schanberg LE, Keefe FJ, Lefebvre JC, Kredich DW, Gil KM. Social context of pain in children with juvenile primary fibromyalgia syndrome: parental pain history and family environment. *Clin J Pain* 1998; 14:107–115.

Scharff L, Leichtner AM, Rappaport LA. Recurrent abdominal pain. In: Schechter N, Berde C, Yaster M (Eds). *Pain in Infants, Children and Adolescents,* 2nd ed. Philadelphia: Lippincott, Williams and Wilkins, 2003, pp 719–731.

Schechter NL. Pain and pain control in children. *Curr Prob Pediatr* 1985; 15(5):1–67.

Schechter NL. Management of common pain problems in the primary care pediatric setting. In: Schechter N, Berde C, Yaster M (Eds). *Pain in Infants, Children and Adolescents,* 2nd ed. Philadelphia: Lippincott, Williams and Wilkins, 2003, pp 693–706.

Schechter NL, Bernstein BA, Beck A, Hart L, Scherzer L. Individual differences in children's response to pain: role of temperament and parental characteristics. *Pediatrics* 1991; 87(2):171–177.

Selbst SM, Zempsky WT. Sedation and analgesia in the emergency department. In: Schechter N, Berde C, Yaster M (Eds). *Pain in Infants, Children and Adolescents,* 2nd ed. Philadelphia: Lippincott, Williams and Wilkins, 2003, pp 651–668.

Siegel LJ, Smith KE. Coping and adaptation in children's pain. In: Bush JP, Harkins SW (Eds). *Children in Pain: Clinical and Research Issues from A Developmental Perspective.* New York: Springer-Verlag, 1991, pp 149–170.

Smith JL, Madsen JR. Neurosurgical procedures for the treatment of pediatric pain. In: Schechter N, Berde C, Yaster M (Eds). *Pain in Infants, Children and Adolescents,* 2nd ed. Philadelphia: Lippincott, Williams and Wilkins, 2003, pp 329–338.

Sourkes BM. The broken heart: anticipatory grief in the child facing death. *J Palliat Care* 1996; 12:56–59.

Spigelblatt L, Laine-Ammara G, Pless IB, Guyver A. The use of alternative medicine by children. *Pediatrics* 1994; 94(6 Pt 1):811–814.

Stallard P, Williams L, Velleman R, et al. The development and evaluation of the pain indicator for communicatively impaired children (PICIC). *Pain* 2002; 98(1–2):145–149.

Stevens B. Acute pain management in infants in the neonatal intensive care unit. In: Finley GA, McGrath PJ (Eds). *Acute and Procedural Pain in Infants and Children,* Progress in Pain Research and Management, Vol. 20. Seattle: IASP Press, 2001.

Stevens B, Johnston C, Gibbins S. Pain assessment in neonates. *Pain in Neonates,* 2nd ed. Amsterdam: Elsevier, 2000, pp 101–134.

Stevens B, Yamada J, Ohlsson A. Sucrose for analgesia in newborn infants undergoing painful procedures. *Cochrane Database Syst Rev* 2004; 3:CD001069.

Stevens MM. Care of the dying child and adolescent: family adjustment and support. In: Doyle D, Hanks GWC, MacDonald N (Eds). *Oxford Textbook of Palliative Medicine,* 2nd ed. Oxford: Oxford University Press, 1998, pp 1045–1056.

Sweet S, McGrath PJ. Physiological measures of pain. In: Finley GA, McGrath PJ (Eds). *Measurement of Pain in Infants and Children,* Progress in Pain Research and Management, Vol. 10. Seattle: IASP Press, 1998, pp 59–82.

Szyfelbein SK, Osgood PF, Carr DB. The assessment of pain and plasma beta-endorphin immunoactivity in burned children. *Pain* 1985; 22:173–182.

Taddio A, Goldbach M, Ipp M, Stevens B, Koren G. Effect of neonatal circumcision on pain responses during vaccination in boys. *Lancet* 1995; 345(8945):291–292.

Terstegen C, Koot HM, de Boer JB, Tibboel D. Measuring pain in children with cognitive impairment: pain response to surgical procedures. *Pain* 2003; 103(1-2):187–198.

Tesler MD, Holzemer WL, Savedra MC. Pain behaviors: postsurgical responses of children and adolescents. *J Pediatr Nurs* 1998; 13:41–47.

Thastum M, Zachariae R. Herlin T. Pain experience and pain coping strategies in children with juvenile idiopathic arthritis. *J Rheumatol* 2001; 28(5):1091–1098.

Tobias JD. Pain management for the critically ill child in the Pediatric Intensive Care Unit. In: Schechter N, Berde C, Yaster M (Eds). *Pain in Infants, Children and Adolescents,* 2nd ed. Philadelphia: Lippincott, Williams and Wilkins, 2003, pp 807–840.

Tobias JD, Rasmussen GE. Pain management and sedation in the pediatric intensive care unit. *Pediatr Clin North Am* 1994; 41(6):1269–1292.

Varni JW, Walco GA, Katz ER. Assessment and management of chronic and recurrent pain in children with chronic diseases. *Pediatrician* 1989; 16(1-2):56–63.

Walco GA, Sterling CM, Conte PM, Engel RG. Empirically supported treatments in pediatric psychology: disease-related pain. *J Pediatr Psychol* 1999; 24(2):155–167; discussion 168–171.

Walco GA, Burns JP, Cassidy RC. The ethics of pain control in infants and children. In: Schechter N, Berde C, Yaster M (Eds). *Pain in Infants, Children and Adolescents,* 2nd ed. Philadelphia: Lippincott, Williams and Wilkins, 2003, pp 157–168.

Walker LS. The evolution of research on recurrent abdominal pain: history, assumptions, and a conceptual model. In: McGrath PJ, Finley GA (Eds). *Chronic and Recurrent Pain in Children and Adolescents,* Progress in Pain Research and Management, Vol. 10. Seattle: IASP Press, 1999, pp 141–172.

Walker LS, Garber J, Greene JW. Somatic complaints in pediatric patients: a prospective study of the role of negative life events, child social and academic competence, and parental somatic symptoms. *J Consult Clin Psychol* 1994; 62:1213–1221.

Wallace MR. Temperament: a variable in children's pain management. *Pediatr Nurs* 1989; 15:118–121.

Weydert JA, Ball TM, Davis MF. Systematic review of treatments for recurrent abdominal pain. *Pediatrics* 2003; 111: e1–11

Wilder RT. Regional anesthetic techniques for chronic pain management in children. In: Schechter N, Berde C, Yaster M (Eds). *Pain in Infants, Children and Adolescents,* 2nd ed. Philadelphia: Lippincott, Williams and Wilkins, 2003, pp 396–416.

Wolf AR. Local and Regional Analgesia. In: Finley GA, McGrath PJ (Eds). *Acute and Procedural Pain in Infants and Children.* Progress in Pain Research and Management, Vol. 20. Seattle: IASP Press, 2001.

Wong CM, McIntosh NM, Menon G, Franck LS. The pain (and stress) in infants in a neonatal intensive care unit. In: Schechter N, Berde C, Yaster M (Eds). *Pain in Infants, Children and Adolescents,* 2nd ed. Philadelphia: Lippincott, Williams and Wilkins, 2003, pp 669–692.

World Health Organization. *Cancer Pain Relief and Palliative Care in Children.* Geneva: World Health Organization, 1998.

Yaster M. Clinical pharmacology. In: Schechter N, Berde C, Yaster M (Eds). *Pain in Infants, Children and Adolescents,* 2nd ed. Philadelphia: Lippincott, Williams and Wilkins, 2003, pp 71–84.

Yaster M, Kost-Byerly S, Maxwell LG. Opioid agonists and antagonists. In: Schechter N, Berde C, Yaster M (Eds). *Pain in Infants, Children and Adolescents,* 2nd ed. Philadelphia: Lippincott, Williams and Wilkins, 2003a, pp 181–224.

Yaster M, Tobin JR, Kost-Byerly S. Local Anesthetics. In: Schechter N, Berde C, Yaster M (Eds). *Pain in Infants, Children and Adolescents,* 2nd ed. Philadelphia: Lippincott, Williams and Wilkins, 2003b, pp 241–264.

Zeltzer L, LeBaron S. Hypnosis and nonhypnotic techniques for re-duction of pain and anxiety during painful procedures in children and adolescents with cancer. *J Pediatr* 1982; 101(6):1032–1035.

Zeltzer LK, LeBaron S. Does ethnicity constitute a risk factor in the psychological distress of adolescents with cancer? *J Adolesc Health Care* 1985; 6(1):8–11.

Zeltzer LK, Fanurik D, LeBaron S. The cold pressor pain paradigm in children: feasibility of an intervention model (Part II). *Pain* 1989; 37(3):305–313.

Zeltzer L, Bursch B, Walco G. Pain responsiveness and chronic pain: a psychobiological perspective. *J Develop Behav Pediatr* 1997; 18:413–422

Zeltzer LK, Tsao JC, Stelling C, et al. A phase I study on the feasibil-ity and acceptability of an acupuncture/hypnosis intervention for chronic pediatric pain. *J Pain Symptom Manage* 2002; 24(4):437–446.

Zwaigenbaum L, Szatmari P, Boyle MH, Offord DR. Highly somatizing young adolescents and the risk of depression. *Pediat-rics* 1999; 103:1203–1209.

Core Curriculum for Professional Education in Pain, edited by J. Edmond Charlton, IASP Press, Seattle, © 2005.

42

Pain in Older Adults

I. Epidemiology

   A. Know that the presence of acute pain remains approximately the same across the adult life span, but there is an age-related increase in the prevalence of chronic pain at least until the seventh decade of life. There is also limited evidence to suggest a plateau or even a slight reduction in the frequency of pain complaints beyond this age (Brattberg et al. 1997; Helme and Gibson 2001).

   B. Recognize that pain is a very common problem for adults of advanced age, with persistent or bothersome (chronic) pain affecting more than 50% of older persons living in a community setting and greater than 80% of nursing home residents (Ferrell et al. 1995; Helme and Gibson 2001).

   C. Understand that while chronic pain is prevalent among older adults, it is not a normal part of aging. Rather, physical pathology and/or psychopathology are always involved (Harkins et al. 1994).

II. Issues related to age differences

   A. Be familiar with age-related changes in the function of nociceptive pathways, including alterations in afferent transmission and descending modulation (Gibson and Farrell 2003).

   B. Be aware of the evidence and current controversy surrounding the notion of altered pain perception in older adults (studies of reduced experimental pain threshold, pain tolerance, and reduced pain symptoms in certain clinical conditions—myocardial pain, abdominal pain, malignancy, and postoperative pain). Also understand that reduced pain sensitivity does not mean that older adults experience less pain when they report it. To the contrary, it may suggest even greater levels of underlying pathology in those older persons who choose to report pain (Harkins et al. 1994; Gagliese and Melzack 1997; Gibson and Helme 2001).

   C. Know of age-related differences in psychological mediators of pain, including altered pain beliefs and attitudes, coping strategy use, misattribution of symptoms, report bias, and stoicism (Yong et al. 2001; Gibson and Chambers 2003).

   D. Be aware of common age-associated psychosocial issues (e.g., loss of family and friends, retirement from the workforce, bereavement, loss of independence/institutionalization) and how such factors may influence the expression, maintenance, and treatment of pain (Roy 2001).

III. Pain assessment

   A. Know of available self-report pain assessment tools that have demonstrated reliability and validity for use in older adults (e.g., verbal descriptor scales, numeric scales, and faces scales) (Herr and Garand 2001; Gagliese 2002). Appreciate that many older persons with dementia can also use such scales in an appropriate fashion (Chibnall and Tait 2001), although one may need to solicit the report of pain.

   B. Understand the role of other important pain-related outcome measures when assessing chronic pain in older adults. For example, depression (including suicide risk), anxiety, sleep disruption, appetite disturbance/weight loss, cognitive impairment, and interference with performance of activities of daily living might be directly related to pain and, therefore, would be expected to improve with effective pain management (Flor et al. 1992; Helme et al. 1996; American Geriatrics Society 2002).

C. Recognize potential indicators of pain (pain behaviors, e.g., bracing, rubbing, guarding, agitation, delirium, altered mobility/activity status, and facial expressions) in those who are unable to report pain (e.g., those having suffered a stroke or those with Alzheimer's disease) and know the most effective way to observe these behaviors (i.e., against an established baseline or during movement) (Weiner et al. 1996; Feldt 2000; Hadjistavropoulos et al. 2000, 2002a,b). While caregivers are often used as surrogates in the assessment of pain, know that the validity of this approach is uncertain (Weiner et al. 1999).

D. Understand the importance of a comprehensive medical history and physical examination when assessing the older pain patient. Know how to perform a comprehensive musculoskeletal examination including that of joints, soft tissues, and the axial skeleton. Also know that chronic pain in older adults is often contributed to by more than one diagnosis, so comprehensive assessment should be performed routinely (Weiner et al. 1999; Herr and Garand 2001).

E. Appreciate the increased likelihood of atypical pain presentations in older people due to diminished physiological reserves and interacting comorbidities (Harkins 1994; Gibson and Helme 2001).

F. Recognize the high prevalence of incidental pathology (e.g., radiographic osteoarthritis in the absence of symptoms) and know that the history and physical examination should guide the acquisition of additional diagnostic studies and tests. Also know that identifiable pathology may be elusive in some older adults with chronic pain, but that pain itself is a treatable disorder and should be recognized as a discrete entity (Weiner et al. 1994).

IV. Pain management

A. Recognize that treatment protocols and treatment goals may need to be adjusted in order to accommodate the special needs of older persons (American Geriatrics Society 2002).

B. Be aware of possible age-related bias against the referral of older adults for pain management as well as bias against prognosis and against the perceived effectiveness of many pharmacological and nonpharmacological treatments when used in older persons. This type of age bias may be found in staff involved in treatment, in the community at large, and in older persons themselves (Kee et al. 1998).

C. Have knowledge and clinical experience in dealing with recurrent and chronic pain conditions that are common in adults of advanced age (e.g., osteoarthritis, postherpetic neuralgia, spinal canal stenosis, malignancy, myofascial pain, fibromyalgia, post-stroke pain syndrome, and diabetic peripheral neuropathy).

D. Be aware that pain is often undertreated in older persons with dementia (Morrison and Siu 2000). Also understand that a proactive, but cautiously aggressive treatment approach should be adopted, due to the higher risk-benefit ratio of pain interventions in this group (American Geriatrics Society 2002).

E. Understand the important influence of concurrent medications and the potential impact of comorbid medical and psychosocial problems when formulating a treatment plan. Also know important drug-drug interactions, relative/absolute contraindications, and side effects related to analgesics that are commonly used in the older adult (American Geriatrics Society 2002).

F. Know pharmacokinetic and pharmacodynamic changes that occur in the action of analgesics (e.g., nonsteroidal anti-inflammatory drugs, opioids) and adjunctive agents (i.e., drugs that are not primarily analgesic, but have analgesic properties, such as tricyclic antidepressants, anticonvulsants, and corticosteroids) for use in older adults. The implications of such changes in terms of dose adjustment and the likelihood of adverse side effects should also be recognized (Weiner and Hanlon 2001; American Geriatrics Society 2002).

G. Be aware of available anesthetic/interventional procedures for the management of pain in older persons (e.g., morphine pumps, spinal stimulators, and surgical ablation) and the demonstrated benefits and limitations of their use in this population (Prager 1996).

H. Recognize that pharmacological therapy for chronic pain is always more effective when combined with nonpharmacological approaches designed to optimize pain management and that pharmacological therapy should be viewed as a means of facilitating compliance with rehabilitation (American Geriatrics Society 2002).

I. Understand the role of psychological therapies in the management of the older adult with chronic pain (e.g., cognitive-behavioral therapy, relaxation, biofeedback, principles of secondary gain and operant conditioning, and hypnosis) (Cook 1998; Kerns et al. 2001).

J. Understand the role of physical therapies in the management of pain in older adults (e.g., exercise programs, assistive devices, TENS, vibration, massage, manipulation, heat and cold, and acupuncture) (Ferrell et al. 1997; Gloth and Matesi 2001).

K. Know the role of the multidisciplinary pain clinic in the management of the older adult with chronic pain, and know when it is appropriate to refer older persons to these clinics (Gibson et al. 1996; Helme et al. 1996).

V. General issues

A. Recognize that all older people are not the same. There is substantial heterogeneity in the extent of physiological, psychological, and functional capacity among individuals of the same chronological age (Busse and Maddox 1985).

REFERENCES

American Geriatrics Society Panel on Persistent Pain in Older Persons. The management of persistent pain in older persons. *J Amer Geriatr Soc* 2002; 50:S205–S224.

Brattberg G, Parker MG, Thorslund M. A longitudinal study of pain: reported pain from middle age to old age. *Clin J Pain* 1997; 13:144–149.

Busse E, Maddox G. *The Duke Longitudinal Studies of Normal Aging: 1955–1980.* New York: Springer, 1985.

Chibnall J, Tait R. Pain assessment in cognitively impaired and unimpaired older adults: a comparison of four scales. *Pain* 2001; 92:173–186.

Cook AJ. Cognitive-behavioral pain management for elderly nursing home residents. *J Gerontol* 1998; 53B:P51–P59.

Feldt K. The checklist of nonverbal pain indicators (CNPI). *Pain Manage Nurs* 2000; 1:13–21.

Ferrell BA. Pain evaluation and management in the nursing home. *Ann Intern Med* 1995; 123:681–695.

Ferrell BA, Josephson KR, Pollan AM, Loy S, Ferrell BR. A randomized trial of walking versus physical methods for chronic pain management. *Aging (Milano)* 1997; 9:99–105.

Flor H, Fydrich T, Turk DC. Efficacy of multidisciplinary pain treatment centers: a meta-analytic review. *Pain* 1992; 49:221–230.

Gagliese L. Assessment of pain in elderly people. Turk DC, Melzack R (Eds). *Handbook of Pain Assessment.* New York: Guilford Press, 2002, pp 119–133.

Gagliese L, Melzack R. Chronic pain in elderly people. *Pain* 1997; 70:3–14.

Gibson SJ, Chambers C. Pain across the life span: a developmental perspective. In: Hadjistavropoulos T, Craig KD (Eds). *Pain: Psychological Perspectives.* Mahwah, NJ: Lawrence Erlbaum, 2003.

Gibson SJ, Farrell MJ. A review of age differences in the neurophysiology of nociception and the perceptual experience of pain. *Clin J Pain* 2004; 20(2):227–239.

Gibson SJ, Helme RD. Age-related differences in pain perception and report. *Clin Geriatr Med* 2001; 17:433–456.

Gibson SJ, Farrell M, Katz B, Helme RD. Multidisciplinary management of chronic non-malignant pain in older adults. In: Ferrell BR, Ferrell BA (Eds). *Pain in the Elderly.* Seattle: IASP Press, 1996, pp 91–99.

Gloth MJ, Matesi AM. Physical therapy and exercise in pain management. *Clin Geriatr Med* 2001; 17:525–535.

Hadjistavropoulos T, LaChapelle DL, MacLeod FK, Snider B, Craig KD. Measuring movement-exacerbated pain in cognitively impaired frail elders. *Clin J Pain* 2000; 16:54–63.

Hadjistavropoulos T, von Baeyer C, Craig KD. Pain assessment in persons with limited ability to communicate. In: Turk D, Melzack R (Eds). *Handbook of Pain Assessment.* New York: Guilford, 2002a, pp 134–149.

Hadjistavropoulos T, LaChapelle DL, Hadjistavropoulos HD, Green S, Asmundson GJ. Using facial expressions to assess musculoskeletal pain in older persons. *Eur J Pain* 2002b; 6(3):179–187.

Harkins SW, Price DD, Bush FM. Geriatric pain. In: Wall PD, Melzack R (Eds). *Textbook of Pain.* New York: Churchill Livingstone, 1994, pp 769–787.

Helme RD, Gibson SJ. The epidemiology of pain in elderly people. *Clin Geriatr Med* 2001; 17:417–431.

Helme RD, Katz B, Gibson SJ, et al. Multidisciplinary pain clinics for older people: do they have a role? *Clin Geriatr Med* 1996; 12:563–582.

Herr K, Garand L. Assessment and measurement of pain in older adults: pain management in the elderly. *Clin Geriatr Med* 2001; 17:457–478.

Kee WG, Middaugh SJ, Redpath S, Hargadon R. Age as a factor in admission to chronic pain rehabilitation. *Clin J Pain* 1998; 14:121–128.

Kerns RD, Otis JD, Marcus KS. Cognitive-behavioral therapy for chronic pain in the elderly. *Clin Geriatr Med* 2001; 17:503–523.

Morrison RS, Siu AL. A comparison of pain and its treatment in advanced dementia and cognitively intact patients with hip fracture. *J Pain Symptom Manage* 2000; 19:240–248.

Prager JP. Invasive modalities for the diagnosis and treatment of pain in the elderly. *Clin Geriatr Med* 1996; 12:549–561.

Roy R. *Social Relations and Chronic Pain.* New York: Academic/Plenum, 2001.

Weiner DK, Hanlon JT. Pain in nursing home residents—management strategies. *Drugs Aging* 2001; 18(1):13–29.

Weiner DK, Distell B, Studenski S, et al. Does radiographic osteoarthritis correlate with flexibility of the lumbar spine? *J Amer Geriatr Soc* 1994; 42:257–263.

Weiner D, Pieper C, McConnell E, Martinez S, Keefe F. Pain measurement in elders with chronic low back pain: traditional and alternative approaches. *Pain* 1996; 67:461–467.

Weiner D, Peterson B, Keefe F. Chronic pain-associated behaviors in the nursing home: resident versus caregiver perceptions. *Pain* 1999; 80:577–588.

Yong H, Gibson SJ, Horne DJ, Helme RD. Development of a pain attitudes questionnaire to assess stoicism and cautiousness for possible age differences. *J Gerontol* 2001; 56:279–284.

Core Curriculum for Professional Education in Pain, edited by J. Edmond Charlton, IASP Press, Seattle, © 2005.

43

Pain Issues in Individuals with Limited Ability to Communicate Due to Cognitive Impairment

I. General

Understand the full range of conditions (e.g., dementia, developmental disabilities, severe head injury, stroke, and autism) that can lead to limitations in ability to communicate due to cognitive impairment (Kolb and Wishaw 1996; Hadjistavropoulos et al. 2001; Breau et al. 2004a; Nader et al. 2004).

Recognize that individuals may have multiple impairments that can affect motor, cognitive, language, and social/emotional capabilities to communicate pain and distress.

Know about the pain conditions and sources of pain that are frequently encountered in individuals with cognitive impairments and limitations in ability to communicate (Miller et al. 1997; Stallard et al. 2001; Breau et al. 2003a; Jansen et al. 2004).

A. Pain sources

  1. Recognize that pain is a frequent complication of motor impairment in certain populations with cognitive and neurological impairments (e.g., cerebral palsy).
  2. Recognize that individuals with cognitive and motor impairments have multiple potential sources of pain.
  3. Be aware that people with cognitive impairments are not immune from the everyday pains suffered by non-impaired individuals, e.g. headaches, menstrual pains, toothache, and earache.
  4. Be aware of the other pains that are commonly reported in patients with cognitive impairments, e.g., musculoskeletal pain, pain from reflux esophagitis, constipation, and spasticity (Gilbert-Macleod et al. 2000).

B. Know the effects that many neurological disorders associated with limited ability to communicate have on the experience of pain (Farrell et al. 1996; Benedetti et al. 1999; Oberlander et al. 1999; Gibson et al. 2001; Hadjistavropoulos et al. 2001).

C. Understand the risk factors that may increase the prevalence of pain in these individuals because of:

  1. Comorbidities that increase risk for pain e.g. central damage, gastroesophageal reflux, contractures (Hennequin et al. 2000; Breau et al. 2004a).
  2. The increased number of medical procedures (especially, but not only, in neonates and children) that these individuals may experience (Stevens et al. 2003).
  3. Increased risk of accidental injury (Leland et al. 1994; Hsieh et al. 2001; Braden et al. 2003) and intentional injury (Homer and Gilleard 1990; Sullivan and Knutson 1998; Goldson 2001).
  4. Likelihood of difficulties in communication.
  5. Devaluing of these individuals by society.
  6. Poor services for these populations (Ziring et al. 1999).
  7. Limited lobbying on behalf of these populations.

D. Know that the level of physical disability does not necessarily reflect the level of intellectual disability. (Smith and Phillips 1992).

E. Know the developmental abilities that children of differing mental ages would display and how these may be affected by their level of physical disability (Smith and Phillips 1992).

221

F.   Know the neurological factors that could affect pain sensation, processing, or expression, and know that this effect could lead to a lesser or greater pain experience.

G.   Know the medical conditions that could affect pain sensation, processing, or expression, and know that this effect could lead to a lesser or greater pain experience.

H.   Know the pharmacological treatments that may be given to people with intellectual or physical disabilities for associated medical conditions; know that these could affect pain sensation, processing, or expression, and know that this effect could lead to a lesser or greater pain experience.

I.   Be aware that pain sensitization (being more sensitive to stimuli) can result from repeated pain and that many people with physical or intellectual disabilities are subjected to repeated painful procedures or have long-term recurrent or chronic painful conditions.

J.   Know the medical conditions that may lead to true pain insensitivity and be aware of the rarity of these conditions (Oberlander et al. 1999, 2000; Oberlander 2001; Shorer et al. 2001).

K.   Know that the presence of self-injury does not necessarily mean that a person is insensitive or indifferent to pain (Breau et al. 2001b).

L.   Know the short- and long term impact of pain on children's and adults' functioning (Houlihan et al. 2004).

II.   Assessment and treatment

A.   General

1.   Recognize that pain is often underestimated and undertreated in these populations.
2.   Be aware of the reasons for underestimation and undertreatment of pain in these populations, i.e., attitudes and misconceptions of health care professionals. Be aware of the legal consequences of the underestimation and undertreatment of pain.

B.   Assessment

1.   Be aware of the assessment procedures suitable for specific populations with cognitive impairments (Hadjistavropoulos et al. 1998, 2000, 2001; McGrath et al. 1998; LaChapelle et al. 1999; Breau et al. 2000, 2001a,b, 2002a; Feldt 2000; Hunt et al. 2003; Abbey et al. 2004; Fuchs-Lacelle and Hadjistavropoulos 2004; Hunt et al. 2004; Stolee et al. 2005) and understand how measures intended for other populations may be modified (Breau et al. 2002a,b; Stallard et al. 2002; Boldingh et al. 2004).
2.   Be familiar with possible applications of certain self-report tools among subsamples of persons with cognitive impairments (Fanurik et al. 1998; Hadjistavropoulos et al. 1998, 2001; Chibnall and Tait 2001; Benini et al. 2004). Be aware that pain assessment/measurement methods that are not specifically designed for this population may lead to underestimation of their pain (Defrin et al. 2004).
3.   Ensure that individuals with limitations in ability to communicate are assessed for pain on a regular basis.
4.   Be familiar with the literature concerning the undertreatment of pain among certain populations with cognitive impairment and the negative implications of undertreatment (Biersdorff 1991; Marzinski 1991; Kaasalainen et al. 1998; Koh et al. 2004).
5.   Be familiar with environmental, situational, and emotional factors that can affect an individual's response to pain.
6.   Be familiar with psychosocial interventions that could be adapted to treat the negative psychological consequences of pain among persons with cognitive impairments (Teri and Gallagher-Thompson 1991).
7.   Be aware of the most frequent causes of pain in this group and the relation of risk for these pain causes to child factors (Hunt and Burne 1995; Breau et al. 2000a,b).

8. Be aware of the characteristics of pain due to specific causes (location, duration, intensity, etc.) (Stallard et al. 2001, Breau et al. 2003a; Hunt et al. 2003).

9. Know behaviors associated with pain in this group, including the importance of facial expression. Learn to attend to and be vigilant for behavioral pain cues. Recognize that behavioral cues of pain can be similar to other populations and/or idiosyncratic (Coffman et al. 1997; Fanurik et al. 1999a; Benini et al. 2004).

10. Be aware that observational procedures for assessing pain that only include a small number of items may be failing to identify important, idiosyncratic pain behaviors that can be characteristic of many persons with severe cognitive and neurological impairments.

11. Know the limitations of self-report by persons with intellectual disabilities (Fanurik et al. 1998).

12. Know about factors that may affect people's expression of pain, such as intellectual functioning, physical disabilities, and autistic features (Fanurik et al. 1999a; Nader et al. 2004).

13. Learn to attend to the reports of caregivers. Be aware of the importance of context in assessing pain in people who are cognitively impaired. Respect the judgements of those who know the individual well.

14. Recognize that many persons with cognitive impairment may have the capacity to self-report pain and may be familiar with pain assessment tools that can facilitate self-report of pain (Closs et al. 2004).

15. Take into account diagnostic and results of medical tests, where possible, when assessing for the presence of pain in persons with cognitive impairment.

16. Be aware of personal and societal beliefs or attitudes that may affect judgments of pain (Breau et al. 2003b, 2004b).

C. Treatment

1. Be familiar with various treatment modalities that either are suitable for persons with cognitive impairments, or could be modified for such individuals (Ferrell 1995).

2. Understand the significant issues regarding pharmacological and other interventions with this population, including difficulties in using cognitive or behavioral methods.

   a. Note that there is limited literature on pharmacological treatment in this population. Koh et al. (2004), on finding that children with cognitive impairment received lower opioid doses in the perioperative (but not postoperative) period than children without cognitive impairment, suggested there may be a belief that children with cognitive impairment are more sensitive to side effects of opioids, but there is no research to substantiate this assertion. Malviya et al. (2001) found that children with cognitive impairment undergoing surgery received smaller opioid doses than children without impairment.

3. Given the wide variety of pain manifestations among people with severe neurological impairments (McGrath et al. 1998), be prepared to match intervention and assessment procedures to the needs and abilities of each patient (Hadjistavropoulos et al. 2000).

4. Ensure that qualified health professionals are responsible for prescribing and administering pain medications.

5. Recognize the importance of multidisciplinary intervention in the pain management of individuals with limitations in ability to communicate.

6. Be knowledgeable about methods of institutionalizing programmes (e.g., CARES 2005) to meet the needs of individuals with limited ability to communicate due to cognitive impairment.

7. Know the most validated pain management techniques available for the painful conditions most likely to affect this group (e.g., gastrointestinal pain, orthopedic pain, and pain due to respiratory infections) (Oberlander 2001).

8. Be aware of common medical conditions that could affect pain management (e.g. seizure disorders, motor disorders) and how to adapt pain control to manage these conditions.

9. Be aware that mental age may differ from chronological age and that pain management should take this factor into account.

10. Be aware of pain management techniques commonly used by caregivers, or in self-management, as appropriate (Breau et al. 2001a, 2003a).

11. Be familiar with the treatments for the most commonly occurring pains, e.g. nonsteroidal anti-inflammatories, muscle relaxants, anticonvulsants, proton pump inhibitors, and treatments for neuropathic pain.

12. Be aware that surgical interventions may be necessary but can have reduced effectiveness in people who are severely neurologically impaired.

13. Be prepared to refer patients to specialists in the management of painful conditions.

III. Caregivers and social context

A. Recognize the importance of the social context and social support when attempting to understand the pain experience of persons with limited ability to communicate.

B. Know about the role of caregivers in assessing pain among persons with limitations in ability to communicate (McGrath et al. 1998; Feldt 2000; Breau et al. 2003b).

C. Be familiar with issues related to stress and burden experienced by caregivers of patients with severe limitations in ability to communicate, because high levels of caregiver burden can lead to difficulties in ability to provide care (Zarit et al. 1985). Accordingly, be familiar with necessary community resources aimed at assisting caregivers to help the patient.

D. Be familiar with family system management approaches suitable for families of individuals with severe neurological impairments and limitations in ability to communicate (Gwyther and Blazer 1984).

E. Be aware of societal attitudes toward children and adults with impairments and understand how these attitudes could influence assessment and treatment of pain (Savage 1998; Fanurik et al. 1999a,b; MacLaren et al. 2001; Malviya et al. 2001; Breau et al. 2002a, 2004b).

F. Be aware of personal beliefs that could affect your assessment or treatment of pain in a child or adult with physical or intellectual disabilities.

REFERENCES

Abbey J, Piller N, De Bellis A, et al. The Abbey pain scale: a 1-minute numerical indicator for people with end-stage dementia. *Int J Palliat Nurs* 2004; 10:6–13.

Benedetti F, Vighetti S, Ricco C, et al. Pain threshold and tolerance in Alzheimer's disease. *Pain* 1999; 80:377–382.

Benini F, Trapanotto M, Gobber D, et al. Evaluating pain induced by venipuncture in pediatric patients with developmental delay. *Clin J Pain* 2004; 20:156–163.

Biersdorff KK. Pain insensitivity and indifference: alternative explanations for some medical catastrophes. *Ment Retard* 1991; 29:259–262.

Boldingh EJ, Jacobs-van der Bruggen MA, Lankhorst GJ, Bouter LM. Assessing pain in patients with severe cerebral palsy: development, reliability, and validity of a pain assessment instrument for cerebral palsy. *Arch Phys Med Rehabil* 2004; 85:758–766.

Braden K, Swanson S, Di Scala C. Injuries to children who had preinjury cognitive impairment: a 10-year retrospective review. *Arch Pediatr Adolesc Med* 2003; 157:336–340.

Breau LM, McGrath PJ, Camfield C, Rosmus C, Finley GA. Preliminary validation of an observational pain checklist for persons with cognitive impairments and inability to communicate verbally. *Dev Med Child Neurol* 2000; 42(9):609–616.

Breau LM, Camfield C, McGrath PJ, Rosmus C, Finley GA. Measuring pain accurately in children with cognitive impairments: refinement of a caregiver scale. *J Pediatr* 2001a; 138(5):721–727.

Breau LM, Boll P, McKay A, et al. Pain and self-injurious behaviour in neurologically impaired children. *Can Psychol* 2001b; 42(2a):13.

Breau LM, Finley GA, McGrath PJ, Camfield CS. Validation of the Non-Communicating Children's Pain Checklist—Postoperative Version. *Anesthesiology* 2002a; 96:528–535.

Breau LM, McGrath PJ, Camfield CS, Finley GA. Psychometric properties of the Non-Communicating Children's Checklist—Revised. *Pain* 2002b; 99(1–1):349–357.

Breau LM, Camfield CS, McGrath PJ, Finley GA. The incidence of pain in children with severe neurological impairments. *Arch Pediatr Adolesc Med* 2003a; 157(12):1219–1226.

Breau LM, MacLaren J, McGrath PJ, Camfield CS, Finley GA. Caregivers' beliefs regarding pain in children with severe neurological impairment: relation between pain sensation and reaction increases with severity of impairment. *Clin J Pain* 2003b; 19(6):335–344.

Breau LM, Camfield CS, McGrath PJ, Finley GA. Risk factors for pain in children with severe neurological impairments. *Dev Med Child Neurol* 2004a; 46(6):364–371.

Breau LM, McGrath PJ, Stevens B. Healthcare professionals' perceptions of pain in infants at risk for neurological impairment. *BMC Pediatr* 2004b; 4:23.

CARES. *CARES Model for Institutionalizing Pain Management.* Medical College of Wisconsin. Available at: www.mcw.edu/display/router.asp?docid=3256. Accessed 31 July, 2005.

Chibnall J, Tait R. Pain assessment in cognitively impaired and unimpaired older adults: a comparison of four scales. *Pain* 2001; 92:173–186.

Closs SJ, Barr B, Briggs M, Cash K, Seers K. A comparison of five pain assessment scales for nursing home residents with varying degrees of cognitive impairment. *J Pain Symptom Manage* 2004; 27(3):196–205.

Coffman S, Alvarez Y, Pyngolil M, et al. Nursing assessment and management of pain in critically ill children. *Heart Lung* 1997; 26:221–228.

Defrin R, Pick CG, Peretz C, Carmeli E. A quantitative somatosensory testing of pain threshold in individuals with mental retardation. *Pain* 2004; 108:58–66.

Fanurik D, Koh JL, Harrison RD, Conrad TM, Tomerlin C. Pain assessment in children with cognitive impairment: an exploration of self-report skills. *Clin Nurs Research* 1998; 7:103–124.

Fanurik D, Koh JL, Schmitz ML, Harrison RD, Conrad TM. Children with cognitive impairment: parent report of pain and coping. *J Dev Behav Pediatr* 1999a; 20:228–234.

Fanurik D, Koh JL, Schmitz ML, et al. Pain assessment and treatment in children with cognitive impairment: a survey of nurses' and physicians' beliefs. *Clin J Pain* 1999b; 15:304–312.

Farrell MJ, Katz B, Helme RD. The impact of dementia on the pain experience. *Pain* 1996; 67:7–15.

Ferrell BA. Pain evaluation and management in the nursing home. *Ann Intern Med* 1995; 123:681–687.

Feldt KS. The Checklist of Nonverbal Pain Indicators (CNPI). *Pain Manage Nurs* 2000; 1:13–21.

Fuchs-Lacelle S, Hadjistavropoulos T. Development and preliminary validation of the pain assessment checklist for seniors with limited ability to communicate (PACSLAC). *Pain Manage Nurs* 2004; 5(1):37–49.

Gibson SJ, Voukelatos X, Ames D, Flicker L, Helme RD. An examination of pain perception and cerebral event-related potentials following carbon dioxide laser stimulation in patients with Alzheimer's disease and age-matched control volunteers. *Pain Res Manage* 2001; 6:126–132.

Gilbert-Macleod CA, Craig KD, Rocha EM, Mathias MD. Everyday pain responses in children with and without developmental delays. *J Pediatr Psychol* 2000; 25(5):301–308.

Goldson E. Maltreatment among children with disabilities. *Infants Young Child* 2001; 13:44–54.

Gwyther L, Blazer D. Family therapy and the dementia patient. *Am Fam Physician* 1984; 29:149–156.

Hadjistavropoulos T, LaChapelle D, MacLeod F, et al. Cognitive functioning and pain reactions in hospitalized elders. *Pain Res Manage* 1998; 3:145–151.

Hadjistavropoulos T, LaChapelle D, MacLeod F, Snider B, Craig KD. Measuring movement exacerbated pain in cognitively impaired frail elders. *Clin J Pain* 2000; 16:54–63.

Hadjistavropoulos T, von Baeyer C, Craig KD. Pain assessment in persons with limited ability to communicate. In Turk D, Melzack R (Eds). *Handbook of Pain Assessment,* 2nd ed. New York: Guilford Press, 2001, pp 134–149.

Hennequin M, Allison PJ, Veyrune JL. Prevalence of oral health problems in a group of individuals with Down syndrome in France. *Dev Med Child Neurol* 2000; 42:691–698.

Homer AC, Gilleard C. Abuse of elderly people by their carers. *BMJ* 1990; 301:1359-1362.

Houlihan, CM, O'Donnell M, Conaway M, Stevenson RD. Bodily pain and health-related quality of life in children with cerebral palsy. *Dev Med Child Neurol* 2004; 46:305–310.

Hsieh K, Heller T, Miller AB. Risk factors for injuries and falls among adults with developmental disabilities. *J Intellect Disabil Res* 2001; 45:76–82.

Hunt AM. Towards an understanding of pain in the child with severe neurological impairment. Development of a behaviour rating scale for assessing pain. PhD Thesis. University of Manchester, 2001.

Hunt A, Burne R. Medical and nursing problems of children with neurodegenerative disease. *Palliat Med* 1995; 9:19–26.

Hunt A, Mastroyannopoulou K, Goldman A, Seers K. Not knowing—the problem of pain in children with severe neurological impairment. *Int J Nurs Stud* 2003; 40(2):171–183.

Hunt A, Goldman A, Seers K, et al. Clinical validation of the paediatric pain profile. *Dev Med Child Neurol* 2004; 46(1):9–18.

Jansen DEMC, Krol B, Groothoff JW, Post D. People with intellectual disability and their health problems: a review of comparative studies. *J Intellect Disabil Res* 2004; 48:93–102.

Kaasalainen S, Middleton J, Knezacek S, et al. Pain and cognitive status in institutionalised elderly: perceptions and interventions. *J Gerontol Nurs* 1998; 24:24–31.

Koh JL, Fanurik D, Harrison RD, Schmitz ML, Norvell D. Analgesia following surgery in children with and without cognitive impairment. *Pain* 2004; 111:239–244.

Kolb B, Whishaw IQ. *Fundamentals of Human Neuropsychology,* 4th ed. New York: W.H. Freeman, 1996.

LaChapelle D, Hadjistavropoulos T, Craig KD. Pain measurement in persons with intellectual disabilities. *Clin J Pain* 1999; 15:13–23.

Leland NL, Garrard J, Smith DK. Comparison of injuries to children with and without disabilities in a day-care center. J Dev Behav Pediatr 1994; 15:402–408.

McGrath PJ, Rosmus C, Canfield C, Campbell MA, Hennigar A. Behaviours caregivers use to determine pain in non-verbal, cognitively impaired individuals. *Dev Med Child Neurol* 1998; 40(5):340–343.

MacLaren J, Breau LM, McGrath PJ, Finley GA, Camfield C. Caregivers beliefs regarding pain in cognitively impaired children. *Canadian Psychol* 2001; 42(2a):11.

Malviya S, Voepel-Lewis T, Tait AR, et al. Pain management in children with and without cognitive impairment following spine fusion surgery. *Paediatr Anaesth* 2001; 11(4):453–458.

Marzinski LR. The tragedy of dementia: clinically assessing pain in the confused, nonverbal elderly. *J Gerontol Nurs* 1991; 17:25–28.

Miller AC, Johann-Murphy M, Cate IM. Pain, anxiety and cooperativeness in children with rhizotomy: changes throughout rehabilitation. *J Pediatr Psychol* 1997; 22(5):689–705.

Nader R, Oberlander TF, Chambers C, Craig KD. Expression of pain in children with autism. *Clin J Pain* 2004; 20(2):88–97.

McGrath PJ, Rosmus C, Camfield C, Campbell MA, Hennigar A. Behaviours caregivers use to determine pain in non-verbal, cognitively impaired people. *Dev Med Child Neurol* 1998; 40:340–343.

Oberlander TF. Pain assessment and management in infants and young children with developmental disabilities. *Infants Young Child* 2001; 14(2):33–47.

Oberlander TF, Gilbert CA, Chambers CT, O'Donnell ME, Craig KD. Biobehavioral responses to acute pain in adolescents with significant neurological impairment. *Clin J Pain* 1999a; 15:201–209.

Oberlander TF, O'Donnell ME, Montgomery CJ. Pain in children with significant neurological impairment. *J Dev Behav Pediatr* 1999b; 20:235–243.

Savage TA. Children with severe and profound disabilities and the issue of social justice. *Adv Pract Nurs Q* 1998; 4:53–58.

Shorer Z, Moses SW, Hershkovitz E, Pinsk V, Levy J. Neurophysiologic studies in congenital insensitivity to pain with anhidrosis. *Pediatr Neurol* 2001; 25:397–400.

Smith B, Phillips CJ. Attainments of severely mentally retarded adolescents by aetiology. *J Child Psychol Psychiatry* 1992; 33:1039–1058.

Stallard P, Williams L, Lenton S, Velleman R. Pain in cognitively impaired, non-communicating children. *Arch Dis Child* 2001; 85:460–462.

Stallard P, Williams L, Velleman R, et al. The development and evaluation of the pain indicator for communicatively impaired children (PICIC). *Pain* 2002; 98:145–149.

Stevens B, McGrath PJ, Gibbins S, et al. Procedural pain in neonates at risk for neurological impairment. *Pain* 2003; 105:27–35.

Stolee P, Hillier LM, Esbaugh J, et al. Instruments for the assessment of pain in older persons with cognitive impairment. *J Am Geriatr Soc* 2005; 53:319–326.

Sullivan PM, Knutson JF. The association between child maltreatment and disabilities in a hospital-based epidemiological study. *Child Abuse Neglect* 1998; 22:271–288.

Teri L, Gallagher-Thompson D. Cognitive-behavioral interventions for treatment of depression in Alzheimer patients. *Gerontologist* 1991; 31:413–416.

Terstegen C, Koot HM, de Boer JB, Tibboel D. Measuring pain in children with cognitive impairment: pain response to surgical procedures. *Pain* 2003; 103(1–2):187–198

Theodorou SD, Klimentopoulou AE, Papalouka E. Congenital insensitivity to pain with anhidrosis. Report of a case and review of the literature. *Acta Orthop Belg* 2000; 66:137–145.

Voepel-Lewis T, Merkel S, Tait AR, Trzcinka A, Malviya S. The reliability and validity of the Face, Legs, Activity, Cry, Consolability Observational Tool as a measure of pain in children with cognitive impairment. *Anesth Analg* 2002; 95(5):1224–1229.

Zarit SH, Orr NK, Zarit JM. *The Hidden Victims of Alzheimer's Disease: Families Under Stress*. New York: New York University Press, 1985.

Ziring PR, Brazdziunas D, Cooley WC, et al. American Academy of Pediatrics Committee on Children with Disabilities. Care coordination: integrating health and related systems of care for children with special health care needs. *Pediatrics* 1999; 104: 978–981.

ADDITIONAL RESOURCE LIST

SPASTICITY

Armstrong RW, Steinbok P, Cochrane DD, et al. Intrathecally administered baclofen for treatment of children with spasticity of cerebral origin. *J Neurosurg* 87(3):409–414.

Barwood S, Baillieu C, Boyd R, et al. Analgesic effects of botulinum toxin A: a randomized, placebo- controlled clinical trial. *Dev Med Child Neurol* 42 (2):116–121.

Grazko MA, Polo KB, Jabbari B. Botulinum toxin A for spasticity, muscle spasms, and rigidity. *Neurology* 1995; 45(4): 712–717.

Kurlemann G, Palm DG. Vigabatrin in metachromatic leucodystrophy; positive influence on spasticity. *Dev Med Child Neurol* 1991; 33(2):182.

REFLUX ESOPHAGITIS

Bohmer CJ, Niezen-de Boer MC, Klinkenberg-Knol EC, Nadorp JH, Meuwissen SG. Gastro-oesophageal reflux disease in institutionalised intellectually disabled individuals. *Neth J Med* 1997; 514:134–139.

Gustafsson PM, Tibbling L. Gastro-oesophageal reflux and oesophageal dysfunction in children and adolescents with brain damage. *Acta Paediatr* 1994; 83:1081–1085.

Kimber C, Kiely EM, Spitz L. The failure rate of surgery for gastro-oesophageal reflux. *J Pediatr Surg* 1998; 33(1):64–66.

Motil KJ, Schultz RJ, Browning K, Trautwein L, Glaze DG. Oropharyngeal dysfunction and gastroesophageal dysmotility are present in girls and women with Rett syndrome. *J Pediatr Gastroenterol Nutr* 1999; 29(1):31–37.

Reyes AL, Cash AJ, Green SH, Booth IW. Gastroesophageal reflux in children with cerebral palsy. *Child Care Health Dev* 1993; 19:109–118.

Spillane AJ, Currie B, Shi E. Fundoplication in children: experience with 106 cases. *Aust N Z J Surg* 1996; 66(11):753–756.

HIP DISLOCATION

Bagg MR, Farber J, Miller F. Long-term follow-up of hip subluxation in cerebral palsy patients. *J Pediatr Orthop* 1993; 13(1):32–36.

Brunner R, Baumann JU. Clinical benefit of reconstruction of dislocated or subluxated hip joints in patients with spastic cerebral palsy. *J Pediatr Orthop* 1994; 14(3):290–294.

McHale KA, Bagg M, Nason SS. Treatment of the chronically dislocated hip in adolescents with cerebral palsy with femoral head resection and subtrochanteric valgus osteotomy. *J Pediatr Orthop* 1990; 10(4):504–509.

Pritchett JW. Treated and untreated unstable hips in severe cerebral palsy. *Dev Med Child Neurol* 1990; 32(1):3–6.

Root L, Laplaza FJ, Brourman SN, Angel DH. The severely unstable hip in cerebral palsy. Treatment with open reduction, pelvic osteotomy, and femoral osteotomy with shortening. *J Bone Joint Surg Am* 1995; 77(5):703–712.

ASSESSMENT AND TREATMENT OF PAIN

Bell ML. Postoperative pain management for the cognitively impaired older adult. *Semin Perioper Nurs* 1997; 6(1):37–41.

Breau LM, Finley GA, McGrath PJ, Camfield CS Validation of the Non-communicating Children's Pain Check Postoperative Version. *Anesthesiology* 2002c; 96(3):528–535

Closs SJ, Cash K, Barr B, Briggs M. Cues for the identification of pain in nursing home residents. *Int J Nurs Stud* 2005; 42(1):3–12.

Collignon P, Giusiano B. Validation of a pain evaluation scale for patients with severe cerebral palsy. *Eur J Pain* 2001; 5(4):433–442.

Cook AKR, Niven CA, Downs MG. Assessing the pain of people with cognitive impairment. *Int J Geriatr Psych* 1999; 14(6):421–425.

Feldt KS, Ryden MB, Miles S. Treatment of pain in cognitively impaired compared with cognitively intact older patients with hip-fracture. *J Am Geriatr Soc* 1998; 46(9):1079–1085.

Ferrell BA, Ferrell BR, Rivera L. Pain in cognitively impaired nursing home patients. *J Pain Symptom Manage* 1995; 10(8):591–598.

Fanurik D, Koh JL, Schmitz ML, et al. Children with cognitive impairment: parent report of pain and coping. *J Dev Behav Pediatr* 1999; 20(4):228–234.

Fuchs-Lacelle S, Hadjistavropoulos T. Development and preliminary validation of the pain assessment checklist for seniors with limited ability to communicate (PACSLAC). *Pain Manage Nurs* 2004; 5(1):37–49.

Galloway S, Turner L. Pain assessment in older adults who are cognitively impaired. *J Gerontol Nurs* 1999; 25(7):34–39.

Giusiano B, Jimeno MT, Collignon P, Chau Y. Utilization of neural network in the elaboration of an evaluation scale for pain in cerebral palsy. *Methods Inf Med* 1995; 34(5):498–502.

Hadden KL, von Baeyer CL. Global and specific behavioural measures of pain in children with cerebral palsy. *Clin J Pain* 2005; 21(2):140–146.

Hadjistavropoulos T, LaChapelle D, Hadjistavropoulos HD, Green S, Asmundson GJG. Using facial expressions to assess musculoskeletal pain in older persons. *Eur J Pain* 2002; 6(3):179–187.

Hurley AC, Volicer BJ, Hanrahan PA, Houde S, Volicer L. Assessment of discomfort in advanced Alzheimer patients. *Res Nurs Health* 1992; 15(5):369–377.

Jancar J, Speller CJ. Fatal intestinal obstruction in the mentally handicapped. *J Intellect Disabil Res* 1994; 38(Pt 4):413–422.

Kaasalainen S, Middleton J, Knezacek S, et al. Pain and cognitive status in the institutionalized elderly: perceptions and interventions. *J Gerontol Nurs* 1998; 24(8)24–31, quiz 50–21.

Koh JL, Fanurik D, Harrison RD, Schmitz ML, Norvell D. Analgesia following surgery in children with and without cognitive impairment. *Pain* 2004; 111(3):239–244.

Lefebvre-Chapiro S, the Doloplus Group. The Doloplus® 2 scale—evaluating pain in the elderly. *Eur J Palliat Care* 2001; 8:191–194.

McDonald M. Assessment and management of cancer pain in the cognitively impaired elderly. *Geriatr Nurs* 1999; 20(5):249–254.

Miller J, Neelon V, Dalton J, et al. The assessment of discomfort in elderly confused patients: a preliminary study. *J Neurosci Nurs* 1996; 28 (3):175–182.

Morrison RS, Siu AL. A comparison of pain and its treatment in advanced dementia and cognitively intact patients with hip fracture. *J Pain Symptom Manage* 2000; 19(4):240–248.

Parmelee PA. Pain in cognitively impaired older persons. *Clin Geriatr Med* 1996; 12(3):473–487.

Sengstaken EA, King SA. The problems of pain and its detection among geriatric nursing home residents. *J Am Geriatr Soc* 1993; 41(5):541–544.

Snow AL, Weber JB, O'Malley KJ, et al. NOPPAIN: a nursing assistant-administered pain assessment instrument for use in dementia. *Dement Geriatr Cogn Disord* 2004; 17:240–246.

Stallard P, Williams L, Lenton S, Velleman R. Pain in cognitively impaired, non-communicating children. *Arch Dis Child* 2001; 85(6):460–462.

Twycross A, Mayfield C, Savory J. Pain management for children with special needs: a neglected area. *Paediatr Nurs* 1999; 11(6):43–45.

Zwakhalen SM, van Dongen KA, Hamers JP, Abu-Saad HH. Pain assessment in intellectually disabled people: non-verbal indicators. *J Adv Nurs* 2004; 45(3):236–245.

OTHER

Baker A, Bowring L, Brignell A, Kafford D. Chronic pain management in cognitively impaired patients: a preliminary research project. *Perspectives* 1996; 20(2):4–8.

Blackman JA. Crying in the child with a disability: the special challenge of crying as a signal. In: Barr RD, Hopkins B, Green JA (Eds). *Crying as a Sign, a Symptom and a Signal: Clinical, Emotional and Developmental Aspects of Infant and Toddler Crying.* Cambridge, MA: McKeith Press, Cambridge University Press, 2000, pp 106–120.

Bosch J, Van Dyke C, Smith SM, et al. Role of medical conditions in the exacerbation of self-injurious behavior: an exploratory study. *Ment Retard* 1997; 35(2):124–130.

Brady M. Treatment of common symptoms in paediatric palliative care. *Palliat Med* 1999; 1(3):63–68.

Donovan J. Learning disability nurses' experiences of being with clients who may be in pain. *J Adv Nurs* 2002; 38(5):458–466.

Feldt KS, Warne MA, Ryden MB. Examining pain in aggressive cognitively impaired older adults. *J Gerontol Nurs* 1998; 24(11):14–22.

Pickering G, Eschalier A, Dubray C. Pain and Alzheimer's disease. *Gerontology* 2000; 46(5):235–241.

Regnard C, Mathews D, Gibson L, Clarke C. Difficulties in identifying distress and its causes in people with severe communication problems. *Int J Palliat Nurs* 2003; 9(4):173–176.

Scherder E, Oosterman J, Swaab D, et al. Recent developments in pain in dementia. *BMJ* 2005; 330:461–464.

Symons F, Oberlander TF (Eds). Pain in individuals with developmental disabilities. Baltimore: Paul H. Brookes Publishing, 2005.

Core Curriculum for Professional Education in Pain, edited by J. Edmond Charlton, IASP Press, Seattle, © 2005.

44

Pain Relief in Substance Abusers

I.   Understand the disease of addiction and know its basis in the biopharmacology and neurophysiology of the central nervous system.

    A.   Be aware of the joint statement of the American Academy of Pain Medicine (AAPM), the American Pain Society (APS), and the American Society of Addiction Medicine (ASAM) defining addiction: "Addiction is a primary, chronic, neurobiologic disease, with genetic, psychosocial, and environmental factors influencing its development and manifestations. It is characterized by behaviors that include one or more of the following: impaired control over drug use, compulsive use, continued use despite harm, and craving" (Savage et al. 2002).

    B.   Know that the behavioral, emotional, and cognitive changes of addiction in large part reflect alterations in brain biopharmacology caused by drugs of abuse, and that the risk of addiction is partially influenced by genetic predisposition (Leshner 1999; Lichterman et al. 2000; Koob and Moal 2001; Nestler 2001).

    C.   Know that all drugs of abuse share the ability to activate specific dopaminergic pathways in the brain known as the "reward center" and share the ability to drive motivational systems and behaviors; there is genetically determined variability in the intracellular and physiological response to the drugs (Compton and Gebhart 2003; Wise 2003).

    D.   Know that alcohol is an important drug of abuse or addiction; in this outline the term "drug" includes alcohol.

II.   Understand the interactions between addiction and pain (Compton et al. 2003; Savage 2003a).

    A.   Know that nociception and the physiological and behavioral responses to pain can be altered by the acute and chronic neurobiological and systemic physiological changes caused by drugs of abuse and by the physiological states consistent with drug addiction.

    B.   Know that many abused drugs have analgesic properties, including central nervous system (CNS) depressants; CNS stimulants; NMDA antagonists; alcohol in high doses; and cannabinoids, for which the clinical role is not yet established (Cichewicz 2004).

    C.   Know that drugs of abuse may induce psychological sequelae, including sleep disorders, anxiety, depression, cognitive impairment, and other psychiatric symptoms or illnesses, and that such sequelae can increase the experience of pain and decrease the response to treatment of pain (Bair et al. 2003; Goldsmith and Reis 2003; Savage 2003a).

    D.   Know that addiction commonly occurs concurrently with anxiety and affective disorders, including post-traumatic stress disorder and the sequelae of childhood sexual abuse (Breslau et al. 1997; Kendler 2000), and that such disorders may be associated with an increased experience of pain.

    E.   Know that the sequelae of active addiction and those of untreated pain are often similar, including sleep disturbance, alterations in mood, cognitive abnormalities, increased stress, aberrant drug use patterns, and problems with work and recreation. Adequate pain treatment will be difficult or may fail without concurrent treatment of addiction.

F. Be aware that fear, anxiety, stress, undertreatment of pain, and/or exposure to mind- and mood-altering drugs used to treat pain may trigger craving and influence the risk of relapse to active addiction in a patient in recovery from addiction (Halikas 1997).

III. Know how to screen for drug abuse or addiction problems in patients with pain.

A. Be knowledgeable regarding, and comfortable asking, questions that may indicate abuse or addiction issues, including use of standard, culturally appropriate screening tests (Conigliaro et al. 2003; Gastfriend et al. 2003; Graham 2003).

B. Be aware that patients may not disclose a history of addiction, or may under- or over-report drug use, for fear that pain will not be treated or will be inadequately treated (Savage 2003a).

C. Know the biochemical and physical markers for alcoholism and for intravenous drug abuse (Warner 2003).

D. Understand the therapeutic use and limitations of urine drug tests, and be aware of false-positives, false-negatives, the sensitivity and specificity of tests, and the time course for detecting drugs in different body fluids (Heit 2003b; Heit and Gourlay 2004).

E. Be familiar with, and inquire about, medical conditions that occur more frequently in the presence of substance use/addiction disorders, for example trauma, alcoholic or viral hepatitis, esophagitis/gastritis, HIV, or skin abscesses (Jaffe 1997; Selwyn and Merino 1997; Blondell 2003; Saitz 2003).

F. Understand that tolerance, physical dependency/abstinence syndrome, and concern (preoccupation) with securing medications to control pain meet the American Psychiatric Association criteria for dependency (DSM-IV-TR), but are insufficient for the diagnosis of addiction in patients maintained on psychoactive medication for control of pain, especially opioids (Portenoy and Payne 1997; American Psychiatric Association 2000).

G. Recognize behaviors that raise concern about abuse, diversion, or addiction, including apparent loss of control over medication use, adverse consequences due to the prescribed medications or other drug use, preoccupation with medications due to craving, noncompliance with other recommended treatment approaches, and failure to improve function. Also be aware that diversion of drugs may occur in patients without addiction (Heit 2003a; Ling et al. 2003; Savage 2003a; Passik and Kirsh 2004).

H. Understand that patients with a poor response to certain opioids or to low doses of opioids may appear opioid seeking, and may be falsely labeled as addicted and be undertreated for pain when opioids are indicated; such drug-seeking behavior, called "pseudoaddiction," is corrected by adequate pain relief, including adequate prescribing of opioids (Weissman and Haddox 1989; Compton et al. 2003).

IV. Understand the general principles for the comprehensive approach to pain management in patients with addictive disease, whether with active disease or in recovery (Portenoy and Payne 1997; Covington and Kotz 2003; Curie et al. 2003; Ireck 2003; Savage 2003a; Portenoy et al. 2005).

A. Know the stages of addiction (active/currently using, in treatment or recently abstinent, or long-term abstinent with or without recovery support) and the significance of each stage to pain management.

B. Understand the multidimensional approach to pain management, including cognitive-behavioral techniques, physical conditioning, pharmacological management, and rehabilitation strategies; such comprehensive treatment enhances pain management, may decrease the need for medications that may be abused or trigger a relapse, and may be effective in addressing addiction as well.

C. Know how to prescribe, and when to refer, patients for adjunctive pain therapies including physical approaches, psychological interventions, and invasive therapies.

D. Know the principles of establishing a supportive environment and therapeutic relationship that improve the outcome of pain treatment; hyperadrenergic states, such as fear and anxiety, may mimic or increase the abstinence syndrome and thus influence pain management.

E. Be aware that cancer patients, and other patients with progressive painful conditions, may experience fear, grief, depression, anger, and spiritual conflict; such symptoms may affect management of both pain and addiction.

F. Be aware that patients may be more receptive to referral for addiction assessment and/or treatment after experiencing adverse consequences of drug or alcohol use, such as trauma or medical complications (Gentilello et al. 1995; Blondell 2003).

G. Identify resources and assist patients to initiate or continue participation in 12-step recovery groups and/or addiction treatment, concurrent with pain management.

H. Know that therapeutic urine drug testing may provide a deterrence for use of nonprescribed or illicit drugs and may detect relapses, allowing for earlier interventions.

V. Understand the use of pharmacological agents in patients with addiction (Savage 1999, 2003a).

A. Be aware of environmental strategies and medication management that may reduce the risk of active addiction if opioids or other abusable drugs are needed for pain management. Strategies include: close monitoring of the patient; prescribing manageable quantities of medication including smaller, more frequently dispensed prescriptions; having a trusted person hold and dispense medication if needed; and use of a formal treatment agreement when indicated (Joranson et al. 2002).

B. When prescribing controlled medications, recognize behaviors that raise concern about abuse, diversion, or addiction (see section IIIG).

C. In general, long-acting opioids and medications taken on schedule are preferable except in titrating for acute pain, although the efficacy of short- versus long-acting opioids in patients with addiction has not been demonstrated.

D. In patients who are physically dependent on opioids, whether used for pain management or for agonist (maintenance) treatment of addiction, avoid the use of opioid agonist/antagonist or full antagonist medications (See section IXD).

E. Know that, in some patients, use of sedative hypnotics such as benzodiazepines may be intoxicating and may be a risk factor for relapse. Anxiety and insomnia can usually be managed with drugs that will not produce euphoria, such as sedating antidepressants or antihistamines for insomnia and buspirone for anxiety; however, buspirone may be ineffective for patients on methadone agonist (maintenance) therapy (McRae et al. 2004).

F. Know how to taper opioids and sedative-hypnotics, providing substitution therapy when appropriate, and how to modulate abstinence effects from these drugs and from alcohol with adjuvant medications. Patients with prior addiction may require intensive structure and medical supervision (Dickinson et al. 2003; Mayo-Smith 2003; O'Connor et al. 2003).

G. Avoid oral medications containing alcohol (elixirs) in general, and especially for patients in recovery. Know that patients on disulfiram should not take alcohol-based medications (elixirs, tinctures), nor should alcohol-based skin preparations be used.

VI. Know the principles of acute pain management, including perioperative management, for patients with active addiction or in recovery (Alford 2003; Compton and Athanasos 2003; Saitz 2003).

A. Recognize the characteristic symptoms of intoxication, overdose, and withdrawal for each class of drugs of abuse, including alcohol. Understand that a patient may be intoxicated with one drug while withdrawing from a different drug. Recognition of all active drug responses will improve management of intoxication and withdrawal, which will facilitate pain management and minimize disruptive behaviors (Myrick et al. 2003).

B. Treat to prevent the development of perioperative abstinence syndromes, especially from alcohol, opioids, and sedative hypnotics. Loading doses of a long-acting opioid or sedative hypnotic will help to prevent withdrawal (see section IVE; Compton et al. 2003).

C. Know that patients dependent on opioids or sedative hypnotics, whether from prescriptions for pain, from opioid maintenance therapy for addiction, or from illicit use, should not be purposefully withdrawn from these classes of drugs during acute medical or surgical interventions.

D. Know that parenteral and/or oral opioid analgesics should not be withheld if needed for acute pain control. Be aware that patients with tolerance to opioids require higher than usual doses, often for a longer time, for management of acute pain and that ineffective doses of opioid analgesics for pain will result in "drug-seeking" behaviors (Scimeca et al. 2000; Payte et al. 2003; Savage 2003b).

VII. Understand how the analgesic response to opioids is complicated in patients with addiction (Harden 2002; Joranson et al. 2002; Ling et al. 2003, 2005; Savage 2003b).

A. Know that multiple factors can influence the opioid dose required for effective analgesia, including a high tolerance for opioids (South and Smith 2001), variations in receptor binding to specific opioids (Pasternak 2001), and alterations in drug metabolism (Lawford et al. 2000; Lichtermann et al. 2000; Pasternak 2001; Compton and Ling 2002; Andersen et al. 2003).

B. Be aware that some patients on chronic opioid therapy for addiction, i.e., agonist or "maintenance" treatment, may have a lowered threshold for, and decreased tolerance to, some types of experimental acute pain, and be aware that chronic opioid therapy may increase the sensitivity to some types of pain, thus complicating the response to pain management in patients with prior exposure and a high tolerance to opioids (Chavkin et al. 2001; Doverty et al. 2001).

VIII. Understand the potential risks and benefits concerning the use of opioids in the treatment of chronic pain and cancer pain in patients with abuse or addiction (Adams et al. 2001; Harden 2002; Joranson et al. 2002; Nedeljkovic et al. 2002; Andersen et al. 2003; Savage 2003b; Zacny et al. 2003).

A. Know that approaches to the treatment of cancer pain and of chronic pain in patients with addiction follow the treatment of cancer pain and chronic pain in general: physical modalities, cognitive-behavioral interventions, invasive treatments, and non-opioid and opioid medications (Covington and Kotz 2003; Otis 2003; Savage 2003a).

B. Be aware that undertreatment of pain may trigger craving and increase the risk of relapse to active addiction.

C. Know that cancer may occur somewhat more frequently in persons with addictive disorders, probably because of the pathological effects of alcohol and tobacco, which are used with higher frequency. In such patients, be comfortable using the World Health Organization therapeutic ladder, while addressing the addiction disorder and offering appropriate treatment and psychospiritual intervention and support.

D. In the treatment of cancer-related pain, opioids should never be withheld when needed for effective pain relief because of concerns regarding the development or diagnosis of addiction; however, increased patient monitoring and attention to prescriptions are indicated.

E. Be aware of the lack of controlled studies concerning the use of opioids for chronic pain in patients with abuse and/or addiction. Reports of clinical observations include cases with improved function and decreased pain, without concomitant observation of aberrant behaviors, when opioids are carefully prescribed.

F.   When opioids are indicated for chronic noncancer pain, good prescribing practices should be followed (see section VA). Know how to use opioids with other pharmacological and adjuvant approaches (Ireck 2003). Detailed medical records are important and should include the rationale for use of opioids, goals of treatment, and response to treatment.

G.   When pain persists beyond apparent healing, the patient should be thoroughly assessed for nociceptive and neurogenic causes. If no physical origin of the pain is detected, pain in some patients may resolve or may improve following discontinuation of opioid medications and with treatment of addiction.

IX.   Understand the needs of special populations or treatment groups of patients with addiction.

A.   Know that pregnant women with addiction have special needs regarding management of non-obstetric pain, obstetric pain, and pain during lactation (Jarvis et al. 1999; Rathmell et al. 2002; Weaver 2003; Finnegan and Kandall 2004).

B.   Know that patients with HIV infections often have a variety of painful conditions and that the World Health Organization recommends that HIV-related pain be treated aggressively using a cancer pain model of treatment. In patients with HIV, opioids should never be withheld when needed for effective pain relief (see VIIIB) (Swica and Breitbart 2002; Pohl 2003).

C.   Know that the pain of sickle cell crisis requires a prompt and effective response, because the physical sequelae of unrelieved pain can worsen the crisis (Pohl 2003).

D.   Know how to manage acute and chronic pain in patients on opioid agonist (maintenance) therapy, for example methadone or levo-alpha methadyl acetate (LAAM) maintenance (Rosenblum et al. 2003). Important points include:

   1.   Maintenance doses do not provide analgesia for acute pain, but should be maintained as a baseline during pain management with opioids.
   2.   Tolerance to opioids is increased; higher than usual doses, in addition to baseline opioid maintenance, are needed for analgesia.
   3.   Antagonist or agonist-antagonist drugs will produce an immediate and painful abstinence syndrome and should not be used.
   4.   When methadone is used for analgesia, dosing is usually every 6 to 8 hours, not once daily as used for agonist maintenance (Scimeca et al. 2000; Payte et al. 2003).

E.   Know that sublingual buprenorphine, a long-acting partial mu agonist that is used for opioid maintenance therapy, may significantly decrease the effectiveness of usual doses of mu-opioid analgesics, and that patients maintained on buprenorphine have special needs for acute pain management (Johnson 2003).

F.   Know that naltrexone, a long acting mu-opioid antagonist, is used in the treatment of patients with alcoholism to decrease craving and in opioid addiction to assist in relapse prevention. Naloxone has an extended half-life; therefore, patients presenting in acute pain require management that may include discontinuing naltrexone, adjunctive treatment, regional blockade, and closely monitored high opioid dosing. Potential receptor hypersensitivity to mu opioids may follow cessation of naltrexone, but clinical problems have not been observed (Leavitt 2002; Miotto et al. 2002).

G.   Be aware that many incarcerated persons have addiction problems. Opioid maintenance therapy and opioids for pain management are frequently abruptly discontinued at the time of incarceration, thus pain from any pre-existing condition will be exacerbated.

X.   Be aware of legal, regulatory, and reimbursement issues that limit access to care for patients with pain and addiction (Joranson and Gilson 2003; Stimmel 2003).

A.   Be familiar with the laws, rules, and regulations that govern the use of opioids for treatment of pain and for the treatment of addiction, at local, regional, and national levels.

B. Know that fear of sanction and misunderstanding of regulations limit physicians' use of opioids for the treatment of pain, especially in patients with addictive disorders.

C. Know the national and regional regulations that apply to confidentiality of medical records for treatment of addictive disease and for treatment of mental health. Understand and respect the patient's concern about confidentiality and the potential negative consequences for the patient if confidentiality regarding addiction diagnosis or treatment is breached.

REFERENCES

Adams NJ, Plane MB, Fleming MF, Mundt MP, Saunders LA. Opioids and the treatment of chronic pain in a primary case sample. *J Pain Symptom Manage* 2001; 22(3)791–796.

Alford DP. Surgical interventions in the alcohol- or drug-using patient. In: Graham AW, Schultz TK, May-Smith MF, Ries RR, Wilford BB (Eds). *Principles of Addiction Medicine,* 3rd ed. Chevy Chase, MD: American Society of Addiction Medicine, 2003, pp 1205–1216.

American Psychiatric Association. *Diagnostic and Statistical Manual of Mental Disorders,* 4th ed. Washington, DC: American Psychiatric Association, 2000.

Andersen G, Christup L, Sjorgren P. Relationships among morphine metabolism, pain and side effects during long-term treatment: an update. *J Pain Symptom Manage* 2003; 25(1):74–91.

Bair MJ, Robinson RL, Katon W, Kroenke K. Depression and pain comorbidity. *Arch Intern Med* 2003; 163:2433–2445.

Blondell RD. Trauma case finding. In: Graham AW, Schultz TK, May-Smith MF, Ries RR, Wilford BB (Eds). *Principles of Addiction Medicine,* 3rd ed. Chevy Chase, MD: American Society of Addiction Medicine, 2003, pp 349–359.

Breslau N, Davis G, Peterson E, Schultz L. Psychiatric sequelae of posttraumatic stress disorder in women. *Arch Gen Psychiatry* 1997; 54:81–87.

Chavkin C, McLaughlin JP, Celver JP. Regulation of opioid receptor function by chronic agonist exposure: constitutive activity and desensitization. *Mol Pharmacol* 2001; 60(1):20–25.

Cichewicz DL. Synergistic interactions between cannabinoid and opioid analgesics. *Life Sci* 2004; 73(11):1317–1324.

Compton P, Athanasos P. Chronic pain, substance abuse and addiction. *Nurs Clin North Am* 2003; 38(3):525–537.

Compton P, Gebhart GF. The neurophysiology of pain and interfaces with addiction. In: Graham AW, Schultz TK, May-Smith MF, Ries RR, Wilford BB (Eds). *Principles of Addiction Medicine,* 3rd ed. Chevy Chase, MD: American Society of Addiction Medicine, 2003, pp 1385–1404.

Compton PA, Ling W. Pain tolerance and analgesic response in methadone-maintained individuals. *J Addict Dis* 2002; 18(2):109.

Compton P, Athanasos P, Elashoff D. Withdrawal hyperalgesia after acute opioid physical dependence in nonaddicted humans: a preliminary study. *J Pain* 2003; 4(9)511–519.

Conigliaro J, Reyes CD, Parran TV, Schulz JE. Principles of screening and early intervention. In: Graham AW, Schultz TK, May-Smith MF, Ries RR, Wilford BB (Eds). *Principles of Addiction Medicine,* 3rd ed. Chevy Chase, MD: American Society of Addiction Medicine, 2003, pp 325–335.

Covington EC, Kotz MK. Psychological approaches to the management of pain. In: Graham AW, Schultz TK, May-Smith MF, Ries RR, Wilford BB (Eds). *Principles of Addiction Medicine,* 3rd ed. Chevy Chase, MD: American Society of Addiction Medicine, 2003, pp 1385–1404.

Curie SR, Hodgins DC, Crabtree A, Jacobi J, Armstrong S. Outcome from integrated pain management treatment for recovering substance abusers. *J Pain* 2003; 4(2):91–100.

Doverty MJ, White JM, Somogy I AA, et al. Hyperalgesic responses in methadone maintenance patients. *Pain* 2001; 90:91–96.

Dickinson WF, Mayo-Smith MF, Eickelberg SJ. Management of sedative-hypnotic intoxication and withdrawal. In: Graham AW, Schultz TK, May-Smith MF, Ries RR, Wilford BB (Eds). *Principles of Addiction Medicine,* 3rd ed. Chevy Chase, MD: American Society of Addiction Medicine, 2003, pp 621–632.

Finnegan LP, Kandall SR. Maternal and Neonatal effects of alcohol and drugs. In: Lowinson J, Ruiz P, Millman R, Langrod J (Eds). *Substance Abuse: A Comprehensive Textbook,* 4th ed. Baltimore: Lippincott, Williams and Wilkins, 2004.

Gastfriend DR, Reif S, Baker SS, Najavits LM. Assessment. In: Graham AW, Schultz TK, May-Smith MF, Ries RR, Wilford BB (Eds). *Principles of Addiction Medicine,* 3rd ed. Chevy Chase, MD: American Society of Addiction Medicine, 2003, pp 373–382.

Gentilello LM, Donovan DM, Dunn CW, Rivara FP. Alcohol intervention in trauma centers: current practice and future directions. *JAMA* 1995; 274:1043–1048.

Goldsmith RJ, Ries RK. Substance-induced mental disorders. In: Graham AW, Schultz TK, May-Smith MF, Ries RR, Wilford BB (Eds). *Principles of Addiction Medicine,* 3rd ed. Chevy Chase, MD: American Society of Addiction Medicine, 2003; 1263–1276.

Graham AW. Appendix 4: Screening and assessment instruments. In: Graham AW, Schultz TK, May-Smith MF, Ries RR, Wilford BB (Eds). *Principles of Addiction Medicine,* 3rd ed. Chevy Chase, MD: American Society of Addiction Medicine, 2003, pp 1607–1610.

Halikas JA, Cravings. In: Lowinson J, Ruiz P, Millman R, Langrod J (Eds). *Substance Abuse, A Comprehensive Textbook,* 3rd ed. Baltimore: Lippincott, Williams and Wilkins, 1997, pp 85–90.

Harden RN. Chronic opioid therapy: another reappraisal. *APS Bull* 2002; 12(1)8–12.

Heit HA. Addiction, physical dependence and tolerance: precise definitions to help clinicians evaluate and treat chronic pain patients. *J Pain Palliat Care Pharmacother* 2003a; 17(1):15–29.

Heit HA. Use of urine toxicology tests in a chronic pain practice. In: Graham AW, Schultz TK, May-Smith MF, Ries RR, Wilford BB (Eds). *Principles of Addiction Medicine,* 3rd ed. Chevy Chase, MD: American Society of Addiction Medicine, 2003b, pp 1455–1456.

Heit HA, Gourlay DL. Urine drug testing in pain medicine. *J Pain Symptom Manage* 2004; 27:260–267.

Ireck N. Practical issues in the management of pain. In: Graham AW, Schultz TK, May-Smith MF, Ries RR, Wilford BB (Eds). *Principles of Addiction Medicine,* 3rd ed. Chevy Chase, MD: American Society of Addiction Medicine, 2003, pp 1475–1478.

Jaffe JH. Opiates: clinical aspects. In: Lowinson J, Ruiz P, Millman R, Langrod J (Eds). *Substance Abuse: A Comprehensive Textbook,* 3rd ed. Baltimore: Lippincott, Williams and Wilkins, 1997, pp 158–166.

Jarvis MA, Wu-Pong S, Kniseley JS, Schnoll SH. Alterations in methadone metabolism during late pregnancy. *J Addict Dis* 1999; 18(4):51–61.

Johnson RE, Strain EC, Amass L. Buprenorphine: how to use it right. *Drug Alcohol Depend* 2003; 70:S59–S77.

Joranson DE, Gilson AM. Legal and regulatory issues in the management of pain. In: Graham AW, Schultz TK, May-Smith MF, Ries RR, Wilford BB (Eds). *Principles of Addiction Medicine,* 3rd ed. Chevy Chase, MD: American Society of Addiction Medicine, 2003, pp 1465–1473

Joranson DE, Carrow GM, Ryan KM, et al. Pain management and prescription monitoring. *J Pain Symptom Manage* 2002; 23:231–238.

Kendler KS. Childhood sexual abuse and adult psychiatric and substance use disorders in women: an epidemiological and co-twin control analysis. *Arch Gen Psychiatry* 2000; 57(10):953–959.

Koob GF, Moal ML. Drug addiction, dysregulation of reward and allostasis. *Neuropsychopharmacology* 2001; 24(2)97–129.

Lawford BR, Young RM, Noble EP, et al. The D(2) dopamine receptor A(1) allele and opioid dependence: association with heroin use and response to methadone treatment. *Am J Med Genet* 2000; 96(5):592–598.

Leavitt SB. Naltrexone in the prevention of opioid relapse. *Addiction Treatment Forum* 2002; August. Available at: www.atforum.com.

Leshner AI. Science-based views of drug addiction and its treatment. *JAMA* 1999; 284(14):1314–1316.

Lichtermann D, Franke P, Maier W, Rao ML. Pharmacogenomics and addiction to opiates. *Eur J Pharmacol* 2000; 410(2–3):269–279.

Ling W, Wesson DR, Smith DE. Abuse of prescription opioids. In: Graham AW, Schultz TK, May-Smith MF, Ries RR, Wilford BB (Eds). *Principles of Addiction Medicine,* 3rd ed. Chevy Chase, MD: American Society of Addiction Medicine, 2003, pp 1483–1492.

Ling W, Wessin D, Smith D. Prescription opiate abuse. In: Lowinson J, Ruiz P, Millman R, Langrod J (Eds). *Substance Abuse: A Comprehensive Textbook,* 4th ed. Philadelphia: Lippincott, Williams and Wilkins, 2005, pp 459–468.

Mayo-Smith MF. Management of alcohol intoxication and withdrawal. In: Graham AW, Schultz TK, May-Smith MF, Ries RR, Wilford BB (Eds). *Principles of Addiction Medicine,* 3rd ed. Chevy Chase, MD: American Society of Addiction Medicine, 2003, pp 621–620.

McRae AL, Sonne SC, Brady KT, Durkalski V, Palesch Y. A randomized, placebo-controlled trial of buspirone for the treatment of anxiety in opioid-dependent individuals. *Am J Addict* 2004; 13(1):53–63.

Miotto K, McCann M, Basch J, Rawson R, Ling W. Naltrexone and dysphoria: fact or myth? *Am J Addict* 2002; 11:151–160.

Myrick H, Anton R, Kasser CL. Management of intoxication and withdrawal: general principles. In: Graham AW, Schultz TK, May-Smith MF, Ries RR, Wilford BB (Eds). *Principles of Addiction Medicine,* 3rd ed. Chevy Chase, MD: American Society of Addiction Medicine, 2003, pp 611–618.

Nedeljkovic SS, Wasan A, Jamison RN. Assessment of efficacy of longterm opioid therapy in patients with substance abuse potential. *Clin J Pain* 2002; 18:S39–S51.

Nestler EJ. Molecular basis of long-term plasticity underlying addiction. *Nat Rev Neurosci* 2001; 2:34–43.

O'Connor PG, Kosten TR, Stine SM. Management of opioid intoxication and withdrawal. In: Graham AW, Schultz TK, May-Smith MF, Ries RR, Wilford BB (Eds). *Principles of Addiction Medicine,* 3rd ed. Chevy Chase, MD: American Society of Addiction Medicine, 2003, pp 651–669.

Otis JAD. Non-opioid medications in the management of pain. In: Graham AW, Schultz TK, May-Smith MF, Ries RR, Wilford BB (Eds). *Principles of Addiction Medicine,* 3rd ed. Chevy Chase, MD: American Society of Addiction Medicine, 2003, pp 1439–1449.

Passik SD, Kirsh KL. Opioid therapy in patients with a history of substance abuse. *CNS Drugs* 2004; 18(1):13–25.

Pasternak GW. The pharmacology of mu analgesics: from patients to genes. *Neuroscientist* 2001; 7(3):220–231.

Payte JR, Zweben JE, Martin J. Opioid maintenance treatment. In: Graham AW, Schultz TK, May-Smith MF, Ries RR, Wilford BB (Eds). *Principles of Addiction Medicine,* 3rd ed. Chevy Chase, MD: American Society of Addiction Medicine, 2003, pp 751–766.

Pohl MI. Pain in special populations. In: Graham AW, Schultz TK, May-Smith MF, Ries RR, Wilford BB (Eds). *Principles of Addiction Medicine,* 3rd ed. Chevy Chase, MD: American Society of Addiction Medicine, 2003, pp 1417–1419.

Portenoy R, Payne R. Acute and chronic pain. In: Lowinson J, Ruiz P, Millman R, Langrod J (Eds). *Substance Abuse: A Comprehensive Textbook,* 3rd ed. Baltimore: Lippincott, Williams and Wilkins, 1997, pp 563–598.

Portenoy R, Payne R, Passik D. Acute and chronic pain. In: Lowinson J, Ruiz P, Millman R, Langrod J (Eds). *Substance Abuse: A Comprehensive Textbook,* 4th ed. Philadelphia: Lippincott, Williams and Wilkins, 2005, pp 863–904.

Rathmell JP, Viscomi CM, Ashburm MA. Management of nonobstetric pain during pregnancy and lactation. *Anesth Analg* 2002; 85(5):1074–1084.

Rosenblum A, Joseph H, Fong C, et al. Prevalence and characteristics of chronic pain among chemically dependent patients in methadone maintenance and residential treatment facilities. *JAMA* 2003; 289(18):2370–2378.

Saitz R. Medical and surgical complications of addiction. In: Graham AW, Schultz TK, May-Smith MF, Ries RR, Wilford BB (Eds). *Principles of Addiction Medicine,* 3rd ed. Chevy Chase, MD: American Society of Addiction Medicine, 2003, pp 1027–1052.

Savage SR. Opioid use in the management of chronic pain. *Med Clin North Am* 1999; 83:761–768

Savage SR. Principles of pain management in the addicted patient. In: Graham AW, Schultz TK, May-Smith MF, Ries RR, Wilford BB (Eds). *Principles of Addiction Medicine,* 3rd ed. Chevy Chase, MD: American Society of Addiction Medicine, 2003a, pp 1405–1416.

Savage SR. Opioid medications in the management of pain. In: Graham AW, Schultz TK, May-Smith MF, Ries RR, Wilford BB (Eds). *Principles of Addiction Medicine,* 3rd ed. Chevy Chase, MD: American Society of Addiction Medicine, 2003b, pp 1451–1463.

Savage SR, Covington EC, Heit HA, et al. Consensus document. Definitions related to the use of opioids for the treatment of pain. The American Academy of Pain Medicine, The American Pain Society, and the American Society of Addiction Medicine, 2002. Available at: www.asam.org/pain/definitions2.pdf.

Selwyn PA, Merino FS. Medical Complications and Treatment. In: In: Lowinson J, Ruiz P, Millman R, Langrod J (Eds). *Substance Abuse: A Comprehensive Textbook,* 3rd ed. Baltimore: Lippincott, Williams and Wilkins, 1997, pp 597–628.

Scimeca MM, Savage SR, Portenoy R, Lowinson J. Treatment of pain in methadone-maintained patients. *Mt Sinai J Med* 2000; 67(5–6):412–422.

South S, Smith M. Analgesic tolerance to opioids. *Pain Clin Updates* 2001; IX(5).

Stimmel B. Constraints on prescribing and the relief of pain. In: Graham AW, Schultz TK, May-Smith MF, Ries RR, Wilford BB (Eds). *Principles of Addiction Medicine,* 3rd ed. Chevy Chase, MD: American Society of Addiction Medicine, 2003, pp 1479–1481.

Swica Y, Breitbart W. Treating pain in patients with AIDS and a history of substance abuse. *West J Med* 2002; 176:33–39.

Warner EA. Laboratory diagnosis. In: Graham AW, Schultz TK, May-Smith MF, Ries RR, Wilford BB (Eds). *Principles of Addiction Medicine,* 3rd ed. Chevy Chase, MD: American Society of Addiction Medicine, 2003, pp 337–348.

Weaver JMF. Perinatal addiction. In: Graham AW, Schultz TK, May-Smith MF, Ries RR, Wilford BB (Eds). *Principles of Addiction Medicine,* 3rd ed. Chevy Chase, MD: American Society of Addiction Medicine, 2003, pp 1231–1246.

Weissman DE, Haddox JD. Opioid pseudoaddiction—an iatrogenic syndrome. *Pain* 1989; 36:363–366.

Wise RA. Brain reward circuitry: insights from unsensed incentives. In: Graham AW, Schultz TK, May-Smith MF, Ries RR, Wilford BB (Eds). *Principles of Addiction Medicine,* 3rd ed. Chevy Chase, MD: American Society of Addiction Medicine, 2003, pp 57–71.

Zacny J, Bigelow G, Compton P, et al. College on Problems of Drug Dependence taskforce on prescription opioid non-medical use and abuse: position statement. *Drug Alcohol Depend* 2003; 69:215–232.

Core Curriculum for Professional Education in Pain, edited by J. Edmond Charlton, IASP Press, Seattle, © 2005.

45

Pain Relief in Areas of Deprivation and Conflict

I. Introduction

A. Be aware that some countries have fewer resources and lower life expectancies than others (World Health Organization 2003).

B. Be aware that most of the conflicts in the world occur in poorer countries. Countries with fragile economies and health care systems may be further damaged by war or by a natural disaster. These may be made worse by overcrowding, malnutrition, and preexisting disease.

C. Know that there are insufficient health care workers in many countries (Lertakyamanee et al. 1999).

D. Some diseases are endemic in poorer countries and lead to a cycle of deprivation (Commission on Macroeconomics and Health 2001).

E. Know that there are large numbers of displaced and traumatized people due to conflict in the world and that continuity of contact with medical services is impaired and thus treatment is difficult (Norwegian Refugee Council Web site, www.idpproject.org; de Jong et al. 2001).

F. There is a significant burden of pain and disability in developing countries (Gureje et al. 1998, 2001; Mwafongo and Zubin 2001; Chopra et al. 2002; Omokhodion 2004).

G. Know that same general approaches to measuring and treating pain are probably applicable worldwide (McIvor and Turner 1995; Rajagopal et al. 2001; Lacoux and Ford 2002; Lacoux et al. 2002).

II. Disease

A. The disease pattern in the developing world is different and influences the pain syndromes seen. In many developing countries people do not live long enough to have cancer; however, this is changing. For example, the increase in smoking is one cause of cancer (World Health Organization 2003).

B. Know that HIV infection and AIDS are a greater problem in poorer countries and that the problem of HIV/AIDS pain is similar to that of cancer and is undertreated (Glare 2001; Breitbart and Dibiase 2002; Coughlan 2003).

C. Trauma, including road traffic accidents, is increasing and is often poorly managed resulting in increased acute and chronic pain (World Health Organization 2003; Ghaffar et al. 2004).

D. Know that there is a major problem with landmine injuries and pain (de Smet et al. 1998; Husum et al. 2002, 2003).

E. Know that the management of torture requires careful assessment and treatment by a multidisciplinary team (McIvor and Turner 1995; Thomsen et al. 2000).

F. Know that that some torture aims not to leave signs, so that pain is often denied by health workers who seek confirmation in signs. Know that the decision to document or not document pain from torture has psychological implications for the tortured individual and political implications for those who practice or condone torture (Thomsen et al. 2000; Williams et al. 2003).

III. Providers

    A. Understand that there is a wide spectrum of different providers that may be international, governmental, and nongovernmental; all have different remits (Griekspoor and Collins 2001; Robertson et al. 2002; World Health Organization 2003).

IV. Education and awareness

    A. Understand that training, knowledge, and education may be limited (Maltby et al. 1987; World Health Organization Web site, Statistical Information System, www3.who.int/whosis) and that many countries have few anesthetists per capita (Lertakyamanee et al. 1999).

    B. Know that cooperative ventures might increase knowledge and care (Williams et al. 2001).

    C. Understand that beliefs about pain around the world are not well understood or communicated. The need for translation may contribute to poor understanding (Edwards et al. 2001; Morris 2001; Aboud et al. 2003).

    D. Know that local social networks may be among the best ways to support those with pain (Dominguez and Olvera 2003).

V. Ethics and research

    A. Know that research is important and, as stated by the World Health Organization Constitution, "the extension to all peoples of the benefits of medical, psychological and related knowledge is essential to the fullest attainment of health" (Sadana and Pang 2003; World Health Organization 2005).

    B. Ethical and political issues exist in research, especially where ethical committees do not exist or have less stature, resulting in possible exploitation (Bhutta 2002; Robertson et al. 2002; Hyder et al. 2004).

    C. Know that there is a lack of knowledge about pain in many of the common diseases present in deprived settings (Kumar 2004).

    D. Consider the following dilemmas:

        1. Should we be promoting pain management when general health care is poor?
        2. Inducing a short-term change in medical behavior is easier than creating a sustainable change.
        3. Payment by poor communities for health care (which is advocated by some international donors) results in a fall in attendance at medical facilities by the population.

VI. Treatment

    A. Understand the problems with worldwide opioid access (Joranson et al. 2000). Morphine is a cheap drug. Diversion from medical sources seems uncommon (Rajagopal et al. 2001). Understand that opioids are underused around the world due to excessive legal control (Joranson et al. 2000) but use is inhibited also by the myths about addiction, rapidly developing tolerance and shortening of life. Global opioid use is lower in poorer countries (Joranson 1993, 1994; University of Wisconsin Comprehensive Cancer Center Pain and Policy Studies Group Web site, www.medsch.wisc.edu/painpolicy/index.htm).

    B. Know that palliative care is inadequate in many countries (Joranson et al. 2000; Williams et al. 2001; Bruera et al. 2002; Sepulveda et al. 2002).

    C. Pain scoring is desirable and has been shown to work in various settings (Jelsma et al. 1997; Soyannwo et al. 2000; Lacoux and Ford 2002; Aboud et al. 2003; Clark et al. 2003).

    D. Simple measures such as having relatives present, good quality translation, explanation, and listening are important.

    E. Understand the value of just being there. In a conflict any place of medical care can represent safety and hope, resulting in the wider benefits that also assist analgesia (Robertson et al. 2002).

F. Many factors result in a lack of drugs: lack of money, poor infrastructure, accessibility and transport, and lack of education of health care workers. Understand that there are concerns about the quality of drugs in many countries.

G. Complex medical procedures and equipment are unlikely to be available or appropriate.

REFERENCES

Aboud FE, Hiwot MG, Arega A, et al. The McGill Pain Questionnaire in Amharic: Zwai Health Center patients' reports on the experience of pain. *Ethiop Med J* 2003; 41:45–61.

Bhutta ZA. Ethics in international health research: a perspective from the developing world. *Bull World Health Organ* 2002; 80:114–120.

Breitbart W, Dibiase L. Current perspectives on pain in AIDS. *Oncology (Huntington)* 2002; 16:964–968.

Bruera E, De Lima L, Woodruff R. The International Association for Hospice and Palliative Care: international activities and initiatives. *J Pain Symptom Manage* 2002; 24:102–105.

Chopra A, Saluja M, Patil J, Tandale HS. Pain and disability, perceptions and beliefs of a rural Indian population: a WHO-ILAR COPCORD study. WHO-International League of Associations for Rheumatology. Community Oriented Program for Control of Rheumatic Diseases. *J Rheumatol* 2002; 29:614–621.

Clark P, Lavielle P, Martinez H. Learning from pain scales: patient perspective. *J Rheumatol* 2003; 30:1584–1588.

Commission on Macroeconomics and Health. *Macroeconomics and Health: Investing in Health for Economic Development.* Geneva: World Health Organization, 2001.

Coughlan M. Pain and palliative care for people living with HIV/AIDS in Asia. *J Pain Palliat Care Pharmacother* 2003; 17:91–104.

de Jong JT, Komproe IH, Van Ommeren M, et al. Lifetime events and posttraumatic stress disorder in 4 postconflict settings. *JAMA* 2001; 286:555–562.

de Smet J, Charlton JE, Meynadier J. Pain and rehabilitation from landmine injury. *Pain Clin Updates* 1998; VI(2).

Dominguez B, Olvera Y. Termografía y control psicologico del dolor cronico. In: Bistre S, Araujo M (Eds). *Dolor, Síndrome, y Padecimiento.* Mexico: Azerta Comunicación Creativa, 2003, pp 41–48.

Edwards CL, Fillingim RB, Keefe F. Race, ethnicity and pain. *Pain* 2001; 94:133–137.

Ghaffar A, Hyder AA, Masud TI. The burden of road traffic injuries in developing countries: the 1st national injury survey of Pakistan. *Public Health* 2004; 118:211–217.

Glare PA. Pain in patients with HIV infection: issues for the new millennium. *Eur J Pain* 2001; 5(Suppl A):43–48.

Griekspoor A, Collins S. Raising standards in emergency relief: how useful are Sphere minimum standards for humanitarian assistance? *BMJ* 2001; 323:740–742.

Gureje O, Von Korff M, Simon GE, Gater R. Persistent pain and well-being: a World Health Organization study in primary care. *JAMA* 1998: 280:147–151.

Gureje O, Simon GE, Von Korff M. A cross-national study of the course of persistent pain in primary care. *Pain* 2001; 92:195–200.

Husum H, Resell K, Vorren G, et al. Chronic pain in land mine accident survivors in Cambodia and Kurdistan. *Soc Sci Med* 2002; 55:1813–1816.

Husum H, Gilbert M, Wisborg T, Van Heng Y, Murad M. Land mine injuries: a study of 708 victims in North Iraq and Cambodia. *Mil Med* 2003; 168:934–940.

Hyder AA, Wali SA, Khan AN, et al. Ethical review of health research: a perspective from developing country researchers. *J Med Ethics* 2004; 30:68–72.

Jelsma JM, Machiri G, Madzivire DM. The use of pain measurement scales in the Zimbabwean context. *Cent Afr J Med* 1997; 43:256–259.

Joranson D. Availability of opioids for cancer pain: recent trends, assessment of system barriers. New WHO guidelines and the risk of diversion. *J Pain Symptom Manage* 1993; 8:353–360.

Joranson D. Global opioid consumption: trends, barriers, diversion. *IASP Newsletter* 1994; Sept–Oct.

Joranson DE, Ryan KM, Gilson AM, Dahl JL. Trends in medical use and abuse of opioid analgesics. *JAMA* 2000; 283:1710–1714.

Kumar A. Organization and development of pain clinics and palliative care in developing countries. *Eur J Anaesthesiol* 2004; 21:169–172.

Lacoux P, Ford N. Treatment of neuropathic pain in Sierra Leone. *Lancet Neurol* 2002; 1:190–195.

Lacoux PA, Crombie IK, Macrae WA. Pain in traumatic upper limb amputees in Sierra Leone. *Pain* 2002; 99:309–312.

Lertakyamanee JTT. Anaesthesia manpower shortage in Asia. *World Anaesth Reports* 1999; 3:Article 8.

Maltby JR, Rana NB, Amatya R, Shrestha BM. Anaesthesia training in Nepal. *Can J Anaesth* 1987; 34:51–55.

McIvor RJ, Turner SW. Assessment and treatment approaches for survivors of torture. *Br J Psychiatry* 1995; 166:705–711.

Morris D. Ethnicity and pain. *Pain: Clin Updates* 2001; IX(4).

Mwafongo V, Zubin M. The pattern of pain as seen among Dar es Salaam residents. *Trop Doct* 2001; 31:227–228.

Omokhodion FO. Low back pain in an urban population in Southwest Nigeria. *Trop Doct* 2004; 34:17–20.

Rajagopal MR, Joranson DE, Gilson AM. Medical use, misuse, and diversion of opioids in India. *Lancet* 2001; 358:139–143.

Robertson DW, Bedell R, Lavery JV, Upshur R. What kind of evidence do we need to justify humanitarian medical aid? *Lancet* 2002; 360:330–333.

Sadana R, Pang T. Health research systems: a framework for the future. *Bull World Health Organ* 2003; 81:159.

Sepulveda C, Marlin A, Yoshida T, Ullrich A. Palliative care: the World Health Organization's global perspective. *J Pain Symptom Manage* 2002; 24:91–96.

Soyannwo OA, Amanor–Boadu SD, Sanya AO, Gureje O. Pain assessment in Nigerians—Visual Analogue Scale and Verbal Rating Scale compared. *West Afr J Med* 2000; 19:242–245.

Thomsen AB, Eriksen J, Smidt-Nielsen K. Chronic pain in torture survivors. *Forensic Sci Int* 2000; 108:155–63.

Williams AC de C, Amris K, Van der Merwe J. Pain in survivors of torture and organized violence. In: Dostrovsky JO, Carr DB, Koltzenburg M (Eds). *Proceedings of the 10th World Congress on Pain,* Progress in Pain Research and Management, Vol. 24. Seattle: IASP Press, 2003, pp. 791–802.

Williams JE, Chandler A, Ranwala R, DeSilva BS, Amarasinghe I. Establishing a cancer pain clinic in a developing country: effect of a collaborative link project with a UK cancer pain center. *J Pain Symptom Manage* 2001; 22:872–878.

World Health Organization. *WHO Health Report 2003—Shaping the Future.* Geneva: World Health Organization, 2003.

World Health Organization. *Constitution of the World Health Organization, July 22, 1946.* Available at: www.yale.edu/lawweb/avalon/decade/decad051.htm. Accessed August 10, 2005.